BASIC STEPS
IN PLANNING
NURSING RESEARCH

From Question to Proposal

SEVENTH EDITION

MARILYNN J. WOOD, DrPH, BSN
Faculty of Nursing
University of Alberta
Edmonton, Alberta
Canada

JANET C. ROSS-KERR, PhD, BScN
Faculty of Nursing
University of Alberta
Edmonton, Alberta
Canada

JONES AND BARTLETT PUBLISHERS
Sudbury, Massachusetts
BOSTON   TORONTO   LONDON   SINGAPORE

World Headquarters
Jones and Bartlett Publishers
40 Tall Pine Drive
Sudbury, MA 01776
978-443-5000
info@jbpub.com
www.jbpub.com

Jones and Bartlett Publishers
Canada
6339 Ormindale Way
Mississauga, Ontario L5V 1J2
Canada

Jones and Bartlett Publishers
International
Barb House, Barb Mews
London W6 7PA
United Kingdom

Jones and Bartlett's books and products are available through most bookstores and online booksellers. To contact Jones and Bartlett Publishers directly, call 800-832-0034, fax 978-443-8000, or visit our website, www.jbpub.com.

Substantial discounts on bulk quantities of Jones and Bartlett's publications are available to corporations, professional associations, and other qualified organizations. For details and specific discount information, contact the special sales department at Jones and Bartlett via the above contact information or send an email to specialsales@jbpub.com.

The authors, editor, and publisher have made every effort to provide accurate information. However, they are not responsible for errors, omissions, or for any outcomes related to the use of the contents of this book and take no responsibility for the use of the products and procedures described. Treatments and side effects described in this book may not be applicable to all people; likewise, some people may require a dose or experience a side effect that is not described herein. Drugs and medical devices are discussed that may have limited availability controlled by the Food and Drug Administration (FDA) for use only in a research study or clinical trial. Research, clinical practice, and government regulations often change the accepted standard in this field. When consideration is being given to use of any drug in the clinical setting, the health care provider or reader is responsible for determining FDA status of the drug, reading the package insert, and reviewing prescribing information for the most up-to-date recommendations on dose, precautions, and contraindications, and determining the appropriate usage for the product. This is especially important in the case of drugs that are new or seldom used.

Production Credits
Publisher: Kevin Sullivan
Acquisitions Editor: Amy Sibley
Associate Editor: Patricia Donnelly
Editorial Assistant: Rachel Shuster
Associate Production Editor: Lisa Cerrone
Marketing Manager: Rebecca Wasley
V.P., Manufacturing and Inventory Control: Therese Connell

Composition: Arlene Apone
Cover and Title Page Design: Kristin E. Parker
Cover and Title Page Image: © Yuri Ivanov/ShutterStock, Inc.
Printing and Binding: Malloy, Inc.
Cover Printing: Malloy, Inc.

Library of Congress Cataloging-in-Publication Data
Wood, Marilynn J.
  Basic steps in planning nursing research : from question to proposal / Marilynn J. Wood, Janet C. Ross-Kerr. — 7th ed.
    p. ; cm.
  Includes bibliographical references and index.
  ISBN 978-0-7637-7179-9 (pbk.)
  1. Nursing—Research—Planning. I. Kerr, Janet C., 1940- II. Title.
  [DNLM: 1. Nursing Research—methods. 2. Research Design. WY 20.5 W877b 2011]
  RT81.5.W647 2011
  610.73072—dc22
                                                                    2010001536

6048
Printed in the United States of America
14 13 12 11 10   10 9 8 7 6 5 4 3 2 1

Contents

Preface

Research is a critical process in the ongoing development of any discipline. We believe that all members of that discipline have important roles to play in research that range from user to investigator. Because it is helpful to have a basic knowledge of research to enhance understanding, we have written this book for beginners as an introduction to the research process. We focus mainly on developing a workable research plan, beginning with finding a research topic and ending with a written research proposal. We do not intend that this book should cover all aspects of research. Rather it treats the planning process as an art in and of itself. Thus, it is an excellent tool for beginners and is also relevant to people at all levels of expertise who need to focus on developing a good research plan.

The basic thesis of this book is that research is only as good as the plan and that a well-conceived plan will see the research through to completion. However, planning takes thought, organization, and hard work; researchers must learn where to find information, how to organize their thinking, and how to clearly communicate their questions, ideas, and plans. We have found this approach to be a sound introduction for beginners and an excellent review for experienced researchers.

The essence of this book is found in the idea that the way you ask a question will irrevocably determine the way you will answer that question. This is the unique feature of our approach to research and distinguishes this book from others that offer different views of research and the research process. The focus on the clarification and exemplification of the question before proceeding to plan the study has helped many individuals organize their thinking and come up with outstanding research proposals.

In our approach, the question remains at the forefront throughout the planning process, providing a touchstone for assessment of decisions made every step of the way. Without this touchstone, research planning can wander off in many directions and can end up far removed from the original idea. The planning process is presented as a series of steps, each one based on the previous stage.

Although based on previous stages, each phase requires different skills, levels of information, and solutions to the problems that inevitably arise. This book attempts to take the student of research through these steps in a logical manner and demonstrates how decisions at each stage affect what can be done at the next step. The focus always remains on finding the answer to the research question.

Deciding what to study and considering all the options is a serious and sometimes frustrating task. Although this decision is ultimately the responsibility of the researcher, it requires discussion with others and reading what others have written about the subject. Perhaps the hardest task of all is deciding on one well-defined study on one well-defined topic. There is so much to do that it is hard to not want to do it all at once. We have found that the refocusing and redirecting process of deciding on the topic is assisted by learning a few simple rules about how to ask a researchable question.

Although research questions can lead to all kinds of research approaches, this book is limited to those within the scientific paradigm. The major thrust in this approach is on finding and clarifying cause-and-effect relationships to build theory in the scientific mode. We have chosen this approach to simplify the process for beginners, not because we do not believe other research approaches are effective. On the contrary, we have great appreciation for other philosophic approaches. We believe, however, that research stemming from each different philosophic base deserves a book of its own because it is difficult, if not impossible, to address all approaches adequately in a beginning text such as this.

This book, then, offers what we believe are the basic steps in planning nursing research based on the first and primary step: asking a researchable question. We hope you enjoy it and would welcome your feedback on what you have read and whether or not it has been helpful to you.

Acknowledgments

The authors and the publisher would like to acknowledge the following individuals who contributed the sample research proposals found in the appendices at the end of the book: Leanne Fontanie, Jocelyn M. Jubinville, Susan M. Neufeld, Safina Hassan McIntyre, Colleen M. Astle, and Karina Black.

CHAPTER ONE

How to Write a Researchable Question

➤ **TOPICS**

Research Topics
What Is a Researchable Question?
Asking Research Questions
Examining Components of a Research Question
Be Interested in Your Idea
Bibliography

➤ **LEARNING OBJECTIVES**

- Define a researchable question.
- Describe the components of a research question.
- Write a research question at all three levels.

Ever since the first person said there must be a better way, people have been asking questions and trying to improve the quality of life. The invention of the wheel, the electric light, and the automobile all resulted from painstaking thought, trial and error, problem solving, and research to find that better way. The same is true of new surgical techniques and new drugs—both are products of a need to improve the human environment.

The human mind is always questioning. As children we asked, Why is the grass green? What makes the sun go down? Why does my dog bark? What causes lightning? Most adults would answer the questions with an explanation "because . . ." which satisfies us as a statement of fact. But if we found a different opinion in every answer, or if we heard "I don't know," we kept asking questions because, as human beings, we had to know.

The purpose of research is to answer questions, whether they arise from a practical need or simple curiosity. But not all questions can or need to be answered by research. Some questions already have answers. Others, by their very nature, can only elicit an opinion—for example, How many angels can dance on the head of a pin? Other questions can be satisfied with an immediate answer: What's the fastest way of getting to your house? Questions asking What should I do? or Where should I go? require opinions and, therefore, are not suitable for research.

What, then, is a research question?

A research question is an explicit query about a problem or issue that can be challenged, examined, and analyzed, and that will yield useful new information.

Answers to research questions add to our general knowledge. They can be used by other people in other places because the answers are valid no matter who asked the question or where the answer was found. This is the critical feature of research findings—they must be facts, not opinions.

Identical duplication of research questions, although possible, is rare. Similar questions occur over and over again and give rise to replication studies that can be useful in themselves, but identical questions that are significant and usable are extremely unusual. If you have thought of a specific, clear research question, in all probability no one else has asked exactly that same question. Whether your question explores an entirely new avenue of thought or examines an area that has been explored before, the exact question is yours.

If you can support your position and document your procedure, you have done something unique: no one else has thought of your exact question.

The research question is a reflection of the opinions, past experience, and ideas of the researcher. The questions and the problems chosen for study are as varied as the people who choose them. Some people are interested in minute detail, others in the overall picture. Some are interested in people, others in mechanical objects. Some are interested in ideas, others in actions. All such topics are amenable to research, and they can all be the subject of a research question.

To do research, the first step is to find a topic to research. Where can topics be found, and how do you know they are researchable?

Research Topics

Finding a research topic isn't as hard as it first seems. When you develop the ability to look for researchable topics, they appear everywhere. Experienced researchers become so good at spotting research problems that they usually have at least a dozen ideas waiting to be investigated. But finding topics can be intimidating at first.

Where do you look for research topics? The most fruitful area for research topics is your own thoughts, observations, and experiences. What have you been reading lately? Who have you been talking to, and what did you talk about? Where have you been? When you read a book, you may find yourself disagreeing with the author, or you may think that the author didn't prove the point to your satisfaction. You may think of several arguments to refute the author's position. You may find yourself annoyed with the author's bias. Whenever you disagree with something you have read, you have the beginning of a research topic. If you have experienced a similar reaction to a conversation or someone's behavior, you also have a potential research topic.

That research topics arise out of these areas is natural. You know something about the subject. You have some facts or opinions that contrast with another's point of view. You read something that contradicted the position you just heard. You were taught a slightly different approach. Your personal experiences did not agree with the generalizations being made. Or you found a flaw in the logical development of the argument. Whatever the source of your disagreement, you found yourself frustrated by the fact that you could not positively prove that the other person was wrong. This is the basis for the research question.

The second aspect of topic selection is that irritation or frustration indicates interest in the subject being discussed. Just how interested you are depends on how long your reactions linger. If you immediately forget your irritation, you aren't that interested. If it keeps nagging at you, you probably have an interest that will sustain you throughout the research. Because you need a subject that will interest you long enough to complete the research process, use this rule to gauge your interest level. Knowing enough about your topic and being interested in it are basic requirements for selection.

How do you know if your knowledge is extensive enough? Take stock of what you do know. Where did you learn it? If your entire stock of information is based on accidental, personal experience, you may find that this amount of knowledge is not enough to sustain you. If, on the other hand, you have talked to many people about this subject and have been reading in the area, and if your personal observations have reinforced what you have read and heard, you certainly know enough to begin.

If you want to do research on nursing managers and their leadership strategies, but your entire stock of information is based on being a staff nurse, you may not know enough to do a study of managers. What you do know about is being a staff nurse who is subjected to different administrative strategies. If you have talked to other nurses about different managers and have read about management and how it is best accomplished, you are well on your way to doing research on nurses' responses to various administrative strategies. But you would have some difficulty with managers' perceptions and decisions on management strategies because that's not where your real interest lies. You might, in fact, bias your research against the manager simply because your interest is in the staff nurses. Knowing enough about your topic means that you know what you are specifically interested in and why. Then you can identify your point of view, which will help you to keep your study unbiased.

Judging the extent of your knowledge about a particular subject depends on how specific the problem is. The more general the problem, the more people share facts and opinions about the problem. Suppose your research problem was nursing and your research question was, What is nursing? You wouldn't be providing anything new one way or another because a general description of nursing already exists. On the other hand, a question such as, What interventions by cardiac rehabilitation nurses are most effective in preventing another heart attack? requires more specific information about cardiac rehabilitation nursing. You would have to read about the subject, determine the types of interventions carried out by nurses with patients who have suffered heart attacks, find out how successful these have been, and use this information to formulate your opinion, which must be susceptible to testing with new facts.

Nursing research topics include studies of patient populations and potential patient populations, or studies of people's responses to health problems or potential health problems. A student once said about her research question, "I only chose this topic for my research because it is a nursing topic." When questioned further, she revealed that she was very interested in middle-aged women and their self-perceptions; in fact she had read everything published on the subject but had hesitated to write her proposal on that topic because she did not think it was a nursing subject. She was quickly disabused of that notion, and she happily wrote an excellent proposal on her topic. If you are particularly interested in a topic, as this woman was, and have read exhaustively in the area on your own, try to find something about the topic that you can research. You will be much happier if you do.

Fortunately, you have been studying nursing and command a wealth of information that you may not realize you have. This knowledge can provide rich sources for research problems. In the area of patient care, you know about a variety of nursing diagnoses and interventions. You also know that there are different nursing care strategies based on which health agency the patient comes to and for what health problem. Have you formed any opinion on how to improve patient care in any of these areas? Do you think you would be able to document it? If so, how? You may have noticed that certain patients within the same agency and with the same health problems receive different care. You wonder if this is because of something about the individual patient. You have been reading about stereotyping and wonder if patients are being stereotyped and treated according to the label.

Theoretical issues provide an entire area of research topics. Role theory offers innumerable ideas, whether relating to singular roles, such as the sick role, or studies of roles in interaction, such as the patient role versus the nurse role. Concepts concerning the patient's psychological and social reactions, such as grief, loss, denial, anger, alienation, and uncertainty, can be applied to almost any patient situation for testing.

Testing assessment and intervention strategies is another field for exploration. How these strategies are used and developed, and who uses them and for what, are areas open to divergent opinion and fact building. Behavior modification, crisis intervention, and providing comfort are interventions that need to be tested on a variety of patients in a variety of settings.

No single theory, hunch, opinion, or even fact is ever totally researched. There is always room for further challenges and explorations. The less that is known about a particular subject, the more work needs to be done. The more work that has been done, the more refinement is necessary.

Now that you have a general idea about research topics and where to find them, the next step is to ask a question about the topic.

What Is a Researchable Question?

A researchable question is one that yields facts to help solve a problem, produce new knowledge, add to theory, and/or improve nursing practice. A question that yields opinion rather than facts can lead to an interesting article or essay but is not researchable. Research deals with facts—that is, with observable phenomena in the real world. A question that will provide answers that explain, describe, identify, substantiate, predict, or qualify is a researchable question.

For this reason nursing research must be usable. Because research deals with the real world, the findings should add to knowledge that can be used by other researchers, theorists, or practitioners. Whether the question deals with improving patient care, administration, services, or educational strategies, the answer should actually help to improve those areas. Whoever reads the published report with the intention of using the findings relies on the researcher having been ethical in writing the report—that the facts as presented are true and based on a valid and reliable study. If findings are to be used, the study must be honest and reliable.

To be of use, nursing research questions should be now questions that have relevance in the present. No matter how good the research is, if the society does not need or want the research findings, they will be ignored. Therefore, questions should be relevant to the issues of the day. In nursing, clinical questions, in particular, are now questions. Nursing desperately needs answers to clinical questions that are practical and immediately usable.

Research questions need to be clear. Fuzzy questions yield fuzzy answers. A fuzzy answer is neither usable nor ethical. Therefore, the clearer the question, the clearer the answer and the more usable in clinical settings.

Finally, a researchable question lends direction to the rest of the research process. If the research question were about an event, directive questions would ask, What happened? When did it happen? In what way did it happen? To whom did it happen? What difference did it make, now that it has happened? These questions demand more of an answer than a simple yes, no, or maybe. Without some movement in it, the question is just a "sitter," without impetus or direction. Sitters are questions that elicit answers such as Yes, that's interesting, or And then what? or even worse for the researcher, Well, now, what are you going to do about it?

Now is the time to examine the research question in more detail, to show how it is written, what the parts are, and what each part of the question does. Because people often find research a difficult process and feel overwhelmed before they are through, they may stop before they have any sense of completion or accomplishment. This might be either because they did not have a clearly stated question to work with or because they chose an overly complex question as their first effort. Both are guaranteed to produce a sense of hopelessness before the plan is completed. As a research novice, starting with a simple, clearly stated question practically assures you of seeing the research plan through to the finished proposal. A simple question is less likely to lead to a complicated research design than a complex question, which assuredly will. The simpler the question, the greater the chance of satisfaction from this, your first effort.

Everything in your research plan depends on the question. It represents the point you want to make, to explore, to describe, or to know, stripped clean of any superfluous verbiage. It is your research purpose stated in one simple, comprehensive sentence. To arrive at this point, you will have to eliminate all interesting but irrelevant distractions, seek out the essence of what you want to know, and move from a very broad subject to one specific point you want to make. Now let's build research questions and see how the process works.

Asking Research Questions

Although there are no hard-and-fast rules for asking research questions, there are guidelines that you can follow that will simplify the process. The way research questions are worded can have a profound effect on the research process that follows, so the more you know about asking questions, the closer you become to being a skillful researcher.

There are two basic components to every question: the stem and the topic. Who stole the cookies? In this question, the stem is who and the topic is stolen cookies. The question could as easily have been, What nurses wear uniforms? in which case the stem is what and the topic is nurses wear uniforms. A simple question has one stem and one topic. You may recall in the last section we recommended that beginning researchers start with a simple question (our first rule of thumb) to keep from feeling overwhelmed by the research process. That means a question with one stem and one topic.

After simplicity, the next most important thing about research questions is that they be action oriented, demanding some activity on your part to provide the answer (our second rule of thumb).

How to Write a Researchable Question

The type of question you ask about your topic becomes the basis for the design of your research plan. Whether you go to the library or out into the community, whether you observe a group of children playing or you work in a laboratory to find the answer, your particular activity is inherent in the question you have asked. For this reason, the next rule is to ask an active question.

You may have noticed in published reports of research that the author presented a statement or a hypothesis rather than a question. This is appropriate for a finished report or a published study, as you will see later, but at the beginning of the research plan you need something that will provide direction. Because you are concerned with the planning phase of the research project, you are dealing in future tense—what you will and won't do when you start to collect your data. A question, rather than a statement, is called for in this instance. Notice the difference in the following sentences:

Mastectomy has an effect on women.

What are the reactions of women to mastectomy?

In the first sentence, the statement is a declaration of fact requiring no action on anyone's part. The question, on the other hand, demands an answer. The following series of statements and questions illustrates the differences between a question and a statement:

Age has an effect on convalescence.

What is the relationship between age and convalescence?

Italian women have smaller (or bigger) babies than Chinese women.

What is the relationship between ethnicity and birth size of infants?

Ice water increases heart rate.

What is the relationship between temperature of ingested drinking water and heart rate?

As you can see, a statement of fact demands no action, whereas a question does.

You will find as you start to write questions that some do not require action. Any question that can be answered by a yes or no is not action oriented. These questions are not researchable. The question has been answered, obviating the need to do any research. Questions that begin with should or could are also not researchable; they elicit opinions, not facts. For example:

Should nurses wear white uniforms?

Should nurses allow patients to participate in care planning?

What should patients do about noisy roommates?

Could patients bathe in the morning?

Everyone has an opinion on each of these questions. If your question can be answered by a simple yes, no, or I don't know, then you don't need to do research to find the answer. Try rewriting each of your should questions into action questions that require some investigation to find the answer. You will notice a great difference between action and opinion questions.

As you write your initial questions, try to write questions that begin with what, what is the relationship, and why. Avoid using inactive verbs such as do at the beginning of your question. Questions that begin with do, like questions that begin with should, can be answered by yes, no, maybe, or I don't know, and they are considered to be stoppers. They elicit an opinion rather than some activity directed toward research. Notice how questions that begin with do look.

Do nurses neglect patients?

Do all patients respond to pain in the same way?

Do patients with coronary heart disease tend to keep their clinic appointments more regularly than other types of patients?

Look at each of these questions in relation to its basic components, the topic, and the question. In the first example the topic is nurses neglect patients, and the question is do. Do doesn't imply much action, does it? Change do to what, and the question becomes, What nurses neglect patients? If what were substituted for do in the second question, the same change would take place: What patients respond to pain in the same way? The answers can no longer be simple yes or no opinions; some form of action is needed to find an answer.

As you are trying to write your questions as simply as possible, don't be discouraged if you find yourself writing yes or no questions—even the most advanced researchers have to think carefully about the best way to word a question. Your first task is to try to write your question as simply as possible, which may entail writing a complex question first and breaking it down into its simple component questions. After you have done that, you can look at the type of question you have asked.

Active questions require some form of observation or measurement for an answer. Active questions imply that the researcher will have to observe something, participate in something, or question someone to arrive at an answer. The way the question is worded determines how the researcher intends to measure the quantity or quality of the topic. Measurement, in the research sense, means examining an abstract idea to derive a concrete answer. Whether the answer is in numeric form or a description, it is observable and concrete. An active question, then, provides some direction for the researcher to answer the question in a measurable (concrete) form.

As you begin working with your research questions, keep a record of your initial questions and your final, perfected questions. In addition, write working definitions of the major terms or ideas in your question. A working definition is your statement of what the term or word means to you in the context of your question; in other words, a working definition is a definition that is specific to your study. Working definitions, at the beginning of your study, are not dictionary definitions; they are your personal descriptions of the terms. Right or wrong, they are what you mean, not what Webster says.

Keep your initial research questions and working definitions together so that you can refer to them as you develop your project. As you progress, you may change your mind on your project. Sometimes you change your mind because someone else has done the study, sometimes because someone talked you out of what you wanted to do, and sometimes because you hadn't clearly formulated what you wanted to do initially. In any case, keep the research questions and definitions close by so you can refer to them as necessary.

Examining Components of a Research Question

Now that you have a general understanding of research questions, you can look at each component of your question in more detail. The two basic components, the stem and the topic, need to be examined separately to see what they do and how they will affect the rest of your plan.

Because all research requires some plan for collecting information to answer a question, the way you ask the question determines how you will answer it. A Chinese philosopher once said, "The answer is in the question." This statement is just as true in research as it is in philosophy.

The first step in phrasing a research question is to use an active stem. In the section on writing questions, changing the question from an opinion question to an active question required replacing words such as should or do with words such as what or why. By altering the stem, we have changed the question from passive to active voice.

The second half of the research question, the topic, is simply what the question is about. The topic can be simple, embodying a single concept or idea; it can be complex, with multiple concepts; or it can be global theory. Asking research questions involves some narrowing of focus into a topic that can be attached to a stem to form a simple question. Let's look at some examples:

Stem	Topic
What	are the concerns of clients in fertility clinics?
What	are the characteristics of successful dieters?
What	are the health beliefs of the Amish?

In these examples, the topic is a fairly simple, specific concept. In the first question, the topic is concerns of a specific group of people. The second topic examines characteristics, and the third topic examines health beliefs. Simple topics such as these are concerned with only one idea. As topics become more complex, they deal with two or more ideas in relationship to one another, and they require a different stem.

Stem	Topic
What	is the relationship between mothers' dietary intake and infant birth weight?
What	is the relationship between preoperative teaching and postoperative pain?
What	is the relationship between obesity and locus of control?

These topics contain two ideas or concepts. The stem asks if there is a relationship between them. These are still simple questions with one stem and one topic, even though the topic has become more complex. The stem is adjusted to fit the topic and vice versa. You can ask what is dietary intake or what is birth weight, but if you want to put them together in one question, you must change your stem to what is the relationship to fit the change in your topic from a single idea to two such ideas or concepts.

The topic is even more complex when you ask a question beginning with a why stem. Why questions start with a set of relationships that have already been established through research, and the theoretical explanation for the relationship is being questioned. For example:

Stem	Topic
Why	do North American aboriginals have a higher incidence of tuberculosis than other ethnic groups?
Why	does preoperative teaching decrease postoperative anxiety?
Why	does increased assertiveness in nurses lead to lower nosocomial infection rates?

These questions are still simple from the standpoint that they have one stem and one topic; however, a topic developed for a why stem becomes quite complex because it shows that a cause-and-effect relationship has been established between the two concepts.

Levels of Questions

All research falls into one of three major levels; each level is based on the amount of knowledge or theory about the topic under study. At the first level, there is little to no literature available on either the topic or the population, and the purpose is to describe what is found as it exists naturally. At the second level, there is knowledge about the topic and about the population, but the intent of the researcher is to do a statistical description of the relationship among the variables. At the third level, there is a great deal of knowledge and theory about the topic, and the intent of the study is to test the theory through direct manipulation of the variables. Each level of knowledge limits the type of study that can be done.

Questions at Level I are designed to elicit descriptions of a single topic or a single population that has previously been ignored in the literature. There may be literature about the topic but not in relation to a specific population, or there may be no literature at all that you can find anywhere on the topic. On the other hand, the topic may have been studied before, but you want to take a fresh look at it, perhaps from an entirely different viewpoint. Other Level I questions are based on some piece of missing data that other studies have overlooked. Level I studies are exploratory by their very nature (their intent is to explore all facets of a topic or a population), and their intent is to describe what is found. Level I studies take place in natural settings to describe what exists, as it exists. Answers to these questions provide complete descriptions of the topics.

If your topic has already been fully described and you have found a description in research literature, then you know too much for a Level I question and you must move to the second level. Level II questions focus on the relationships between two or more variables previously described but never before studied together. (A variable, in research, is defined as anything that varies or changes, that has two or more properties, or that has two or more qualities. Age, gender, height, and weight are all examples of variables.) At this level, you have considerably more knowledge about the topic than you did at the first level, but you don't yet know enough to predict the relationship between your variables. You can, however, develop a good rationale for why they should be related. If, when you read about your topic, you find that you have enough information to predict that one variable influences the other in a certain way, then you know too much for a Level II question and you should move on to the third level.

Questions at Level III require considerable knowledge of the topic. These studies test predictive hypotheses about the variables. The knowledge required for the development of hypotheses is based on the results of Level II studies, which allow you to predict the action of your variables.

Finding the appropriate level for your question determines your subsequent course of action. Because this is such a critical step, we will give you detailed guidelines to follow. These guidelines will save time and energy and, at the same time, will help you focus on what you want to study. Now let's look at each level in detail.

Level I Questions

At this level there is little or no prior knowledge of the topic. The stem question is always what is or what are, and the topic is a single entity or concept. Level I questions are asked in such a way that they lead to exploration (by the researcher) and result in a complete description of the topic. Here are some examples:

Stem	Topic
What	are the eating problems of handicapped children?
What	are the characteristics of suicidal patients?
What	are the spiritual needs of transplant patients?

All these questions have the same stem and address a single topic: eating problems, characteristics, and spiritual needs. Each contains a reference to the population that the researcher wants to study: handicapped children, suicidal patients, and transplant patients. Most research questions refer to the study population in some way so that they focus on the researcher's interest. When the topic is broad, such as problems, needs, or characteristics, it will need further clarification so that the question clearly asks what you want to know. Thus, you specify eating problems, spiritual needs, and characteristics of suicidal patients so that there is no doubt about your meaning. Each question spells out both the concept to be studied and the population in which it will be studied. These are the components of a good Level I question. In addition, these questions require that some type of activity, such as observing, questioning, or listening, be undertaken by the researcher to describe the topic completely.

The most important characteristic about Level I questions is that they are based on topics that either have not been studied before or have not been studied in that particular population. If you look at the previous examples, you can see the idea. In the first question the topic is eating problems, and the subjects are handicapped children. There may be a great deal of literature on eating problems but little or no literature on eating problems that are specific to handicapped children. The second question refers to population characteristics. In sociology, an entire field of demography is devoted exclusively to studying population characteristics, but at the time this question was asked no study had described characteristics of suicidal patients. The third question deals with the needs of patients. There may be many studies in nursing literature on patient needs, but at the time this question was asked there was little information on the specific topic of spiritual needs. There may be studies on spiritual needs of other populations, such as soldiers, the dying, or children, but little literature specific to the spiritual needs of patients. These questions ask about one concept only. No reference to relationships, causes, or effects should be included in a Level I question.

Whenever you write a question at the first level, go back over that question and read it critically to see if it has the following characteristics: one variable, concept, or topic; and a reference to the population in which that variable, concept, or topic will be found.

A question such as What causes nurses to avoid suicidal patients? has two variables. One is nurses' avoidance, and the other is the cause, which is unspecified but implied. Even if you don't know the cause, you have assumed that there is one and that the nurses' behavior is the effect. When you review your question and find that you have assumed a cause-and-effect relationship, try the second level. The same is true of questions that include words such as influences or effects or results from. These are red flags. Whenever you see these words in a Level I question you know you will need to rethink and rewrite the question. All of these words assume a second variable, and at Level I there can be only one variable.

Level II Questions

Second-level research questions build on the results of studies at the first level. When a topic has been thoroughly described, it is possible to identify measurable variables. The next step is to look for relationships among these variables. At Level II, the stem question asks, What is the relationship? and the topic contains two or more variables. The answer to the question at the second level is determined by the statistical significance of the relationship between the variables.

Because Level II questions are built on existing knowledge, some research literature must always be available on all of the variables in the question. You know something about the variables even though they have not been examined together before. When you study variables together, you need to have a rationale to explain their proposed relationship. You need to discuss the concepts behind the variables and propose that a relationship may exist between (or among) them. The answer to the question will verify whether such a relationship exists.

Here are some Level II questions:

Stem	Topic
What	is the relationship between relaxation and severity of pain in postoperative patients?
What	is the relationship between severity of pain and length of convalescence from hysterectomy?
What	is the relationship between the educational level of nurses and their attitudes toward professional organizations?
What	is the relationship between preoperative teaching and post-operative anxiety?
What	is the relationship among prenatal nutrition, birth weight of infants, and age of the mothers?

Each of these questions begins with the stem What is the relationship? and has a topic with at least two variables. For each question, a rationale must be developed to explain why the variables could be related. Be sure that you can identify a minimum of two separate variables in your question.

When we say that each variable must vary, it is because there is no sense in doing research on something that does not change or has only one characteristic. It (whatever it is) simply exists, and we don't have to do research on it. We do research on phenomena that have more than one property so that we can describe or measure that property and look at its relationship to other properties. When we are studying an attribute of a person, such as an attitude, there must be at least two categories of that attribute to say that it varies. Attitudes, for example, may be measured as positive, negative, and neutral. The minimum measurement of an attribute is to say that it is present or absent—two categories of measurement. If we specify that the variable is always present, it is no longer a variable and becomes a fixed entity. For example, look at the question What is the relationship between the Leboyer method of childbirth and the weight gain of infants during the first month? The way this question is written, the Leboyer method is the only method that will be looked at in relation to weight gain so there is no variation, that is, no other method to compare to Leboyer in terms of weight gain. Each variable must be written so that it can have at least two categories. In this example, the first variable should have been method of childbirth, allowing for more than one method to occur. The second variable, weight gain during the first month, is written properly because it does not restrict itself to any one amount of weight gain but rather allows for variable weight gains to be measured. This is an easy mistake to make, especially when you have something in mind that you are hoping to prove, such as that the Leboyer method is better than any other method of childbirth. Remember that you must measure the others, too, or you have nothing to relate to the amount of weight gain in your sample. Later on in the planning of your study, you will discover that you will be collecting data only on the variables in your question and, if something is not in your question, it won't be measured. This may help you to see the importance of writing the variables so they can vary.

When writing questions at Level II, examine them critically. Each question must have a minimum of two variables written in such a way that they both vary.

A question that asks What is the relationship between nurses' positive and negative attitudes toward alcoholics? has only one variable, nurses' attitudes. Positive and negative are merely two categories of attitude. When a Level II question is written properly, it will ask about the relationship between _____ and _____. If you look carefully, it is easy to spot a missing variable. This question needs another variable that will be examined in relation to nurses' attitudes, such as patient satisfaction with treatment.

The process of writing research questions involves deciding the appropriate level of your question. After this has been done, the rest of the research process follows easily in a series of steps, all of which depend on the level of the question. So, when you are analyzing your Level II question, there are a couple of red flags to watch for that will help you decide if you are at the right level. If you find that you can predict the exact relationship between your variables (that is, you know which one influences the other and what direction the influence will take), this is a red flag. Try a Level III question. Also, if you cannot study your variables without testing a cause-and-effect relationship between them, you have run into another red flag. These questions may belong at Level III.

Although you may know one variable occurs first in time (for example, pain), at Level II you really don't know if pain, in fact, is related to convalescence. If there were to be a relationship, you would not be able to predict the direction of the relationship. In other words, you do not know whether the intensity of pain was associated with a shorter or longer convalescence. If you do know this from your literature search, your study can be moved from Level II to Level III.

Level III Questions

The third level of research builds on the results of previous research. Research at this level begins with a significant relationship between variables. At Level III, the question asks why this relationship exists, and you must provide the answer, which always begins with because and ends with an explanation. Assume that at Level II you had asked the question, What is the relationship between sensory stimulation and weight gain in depressed nursing home residents? You found that, of the four types of sensory stimuli examined, two of them were more effective in increasing weight gain than the other two. You are now in a position to ask the Level III question, Why are these two more effective than the other two? You will have to check the research and theory literature on sensory stimulation, breaking it down into its component parts regarding weight gain until you find something that provides an explanation. You can then safely design a study that begins, If I manipulate this variable, then that particular result will occur. Now you have the basis for a predictive hypothesis and an experimental design. All Level III questions lead to experimental designs. The questions look like this:

Stem	Topic
Why	does patient satisfaction increase with positive attitudes toward self-care?
Why	does increased vitamin C in the diet decrease skin fragility in elderly people?
Why	does isolation from other patients increase signs of sensory deprivation in hospitalized patients?

Each of these why questions has two variables, and each question specifies that one variable either causes or influences the action of the other variable in a certain way. The why question is answered by you, the researcher, who searches the literature for the theory necessary to explain the relationship. The study resulting from a Level III question will test the theory. The process of asking a Level III question is more complex than either of the other levels because much more information is needed to begin. You must answer the initial why question before you can propose to test the exact relationship between your variables. Here is an example:

Stem	Topic
Why	is urinary tract infection lower among spinal cord injury patients who drink cranberry juice? (Kinney & Blount, 1979)

The information used in this study to explain the relationship between urinary tract infection and cranberry juice was developed from other research findings and began with:

Because the metabolism of cranberry juice results in acidic urine. This lowered urinary pH may provide a bacteriostatic medium within the urinary tract.

This question is based on both actual observations in a clinical setting and research findings. Patients who drink cranberry juice were noted to have fewer urinary tract infections than those who don't drink cranberry juice. The researcher wondered why. The answer came from physiological literature as well as through research and theory. The researcher, after reviewing the literature, proceeds with any one of several new why questions: Why does cranberry juice metabolism result in acidic urine? Why does a bacteriostatic medium result in decreased urinary tract infections? Why does lowered urinary pH provide a bacteriostatic medium? If each of these questions can be answered through the literature, then the researcher can test the assumptions in the original question and set up an experimental design to show, beyond question, that increased cranberry juice ingestion decreases the incidence of urinary tract infections. Level III questions require thinking through the answer as well as reviewing the literature to support the researcher's educated guess as being on the right track. Here is another example:

Stem	Topic
Why	does a focused educational and counseling intervention reduce delay in older adults seeking help for symptoms of acute myocardial infarction (AMI)?

Theoretical explanation: The self-regulatory model (SRM) proposes that both internal and environmental stimuli influence the adaptive behavior of an individual toward a health threat. Three stages are proposed to occur that would regulate adaptive behavior during a crisis such as AMI. Each stage has a cognitive and emotional level. During these three stages, the person's response is influenced by his or her perceived control over the health threat and how much anxiety is produced by the threat. An educational and counseling intervention that makes use of what is known from the SRM about producing adaptive behavior will promote help-seeking behavior at the time of AMI symptoms. This will result in the person seeking help sooner than would otherwise be the case (Tullmann, Haugh, Dracup, & Bourguignon, 2007).

At Level III you can predict what will happen and provide a theory based on previous research findings to explain it. At Level II you propose that two variables might be related, based on what you know about each one individually, but you cannot predict how or even if they are related. If you find a significant relationship at Level II, you move on to Level III because you will want to explain the why and document the precise nature of the relationship.

Remember that at Level III you must be able to design an experiment to test the action of your variables. Some questions, however, simply are not amenable to Level III studies. These are the why questions that require studies of variables that we have no ethical right to manipulate on human subjects or that are impossible to manipulate. Look at these examples:

Stem	Topic
Why	does age increase convalescence time for postsurgical patients?
Why	does gender influence the number of postoperative medications a patient takes?
Why	does smoking increase the probability of lung cancer?

In the first two examples, the causes, or influencing variables, are age and gender. Neither of these can be altered or manipulated by the researcher. You can, however, study them as they occur naturally in a Level II study. In the third question, the causal variable is smoking. A study manipulating smoking with human subjects to see if lung cancer could be increased would be unethical. With questions such as these, rewrite them at Level II and see how they fit:

Stem	Topic
What	is the relationship between age and length of convalescence?
What	is the relationship between gender and amount of postoperative medication?
What	is the relationship between the amount of cigarette smoking and incidence of lung cancer?

In each case, the study can be done quite easily at Level II by finding a sample where these conditions occur naturally—that is, patients who have lung cancer already and whose smoking habits can be documented, or patients who are convalescing from surgery and whose age can be related to the length of time they take to convalesce.

At Level III, you can (and must) specify the direction of each variable in relation to the other, and the causative variable must be amenable to manipulation by you. Many studies can be done on the same two variables but at different levels. For example, you might ask the Level II question, What is the relationship between preoperative teaching and patients' postoperative anxiety levels? To answer this question at Level II, you would need to find comparable groups of patients in areas where some nurses did preoperative teaching and others did not so that you could compare the patients' anxiety levels. The same two variables could be studied based on a why question asking, Why does structured preoperative teaching significantly decrease the patients' postoperative level of anxiety? In this study, you would design an experiment to test different kinds of structured preoperative teaching strategies and determine which one was more effective in reducing the anxiety. To do this study, however, you would first develop a theoretical explanation for why the particular teaching strategy is likely to be more successful at decreasing anxiety.

Rewriting Your Question

Many people who begin research think that their written questions are perfectly clear, yet not everyone will be able to understand what they mean. We have found that practicing the writing of research questions greatly improves their clarity. Table 1-1 presents examples of questions that were written by nurses of various backgrounds and, following group discussion, were rewritten more clearly. You may find these examples useful.

As you read these questions and their revisions, several common problems become apparent: Level I questions can have only one variable. Words like effect, cause, factors, and reasons for all refer to an assumed variable that the author failed to include. If you don't know enough to specify what those variables are, rewrite the question at Level I. If you know what the variables are, rewrite the question at Level II. If you know what the variables are but cannot specify the cause and effect (or if it would be unethical to manipulate the causal variable), rewrite the question at Level II. If you know the cause and effect and want to test the relationship experimentally, write a why question at Level III. Many of the examples in Table 1-1 were written by people who knew too much about their topics but still tried to use Level I questions. When rewritten at Level II or III, the questions suddenly made sense.

When two or more variables exist in the topic, write the question at Level II before trying to write it at Level III to be sure you have the answer before proceeding. Remember, Level III questions are based on the answers to Level II questions.

In attempting to write a Level II question, you may be writing about one variable with two extremes (such as the high and low incidence of medication errors) rather than writing about two variables. Questions such as this one need to be rewritten at Level I.

The following simple rules summarize the problems you may encounter and will help you write more effective research questions.

- At Level I, have only one variable and one population in the topic.
- If you have a cause or effect in your question, write the question at Level II or III.
- If the words cause, effect, or any of their synonyms appear in your question, either eliminate those words or specify what they are and how they vary.
- At Level II you need a minimum of two variables.
- All variables must be written so that they vary.
- At Level III there must be two variables that specify a cause and an effect.
- If you have written a Level III why question, make sure it is both ethical and possible to manipulate the causal variable. If not, rewrite the question at Level II.

Be Interested in Your Idea

A solid research topic is always worth doing and doing well, but research is only as good as the time and effort put into it. Don't choose a research topic because it looks easy. All research requires painstaking thought, writing, and reading before the proposal is finished, not to mention carrying out the research. You might get by with a minimal effort, but you will have lost an opportunity to explore something meaningful to you. On the other hand, don't choose a topic that is so grandiose or complex that it can't possibly be done effectively. Instead, choose a question that interests you, yet is clear and simple.

Choose a topic that truly interests you and will keep you going back again and again to search the literature, your notes, or your own thoughts. You need not necessarily retain the first thoughts you had when you began to

TABLE 1-1
Examples of Rewritten Questions

Original Question	Rewritten Question	
What are the effects of a child's admission to a psychiatric unit on the siblings?	Level I:	What are the feelings of children who have had a sibling admitted to a psychiatric unit?
What is the clinical significance of oliguria in the postoperative patient?	Level I:	What are the characteristics of patients who have oliguria postoperatively?
What is the level of pain relief in pediatric postoperative patients having received TENS (transcutaneous electric nerve stimulation) instruction?	Level I:	What methods of pain relief are available to pediatric surgery patients?
	Level II:	What is the relationship between level of pain and type of pain relief instruction (including TENS) among pediatric postoperative patients?
	Level III:	Why does preoperative TENS instruction significantly decrease postoperative pain levels in pediatric patients?
What is the relationship between medication nurses with low error incidence and high error incidence?	Level I:	What are the characteristics of nurses with high medication error incidence?
	Level II:	What is the relationship between error incidence and years of experience among medication nurses?
What is the relationship between administrative and staff nurses?	Level I:	What are the administrative characteristics of nurses?
	Level II:	What is the relationship between interpersonal skills of nursing staff and their job titles?
What happens to quality of nursing care with nursing registries?	Level II:	What is the relationship between quality of nursing care and type of nursing personnel (registry vs. hospital-based)?
What is the reason for hip fractures being more prevalent in women than men?	Level I:	What are the characteristics of patients with hip fractures?
	Level II:	What is the relationship between gender and hip fractures in elderly people?
What effect does discharge planning have on post-MI patient?	Level II:	What is the relationship between discharge planning and course of recovery at home for the post-MI patient?
What are the effects of relaxation/imagery techniques on asthmatic patients?	Level III:	Why do relaxation/imagery techniques decrease the number of asthmatic attacks in chronic asthmatic patients?

write your question. On the contrary, you may focus on one small aspect of the larger problem that you had never thought of before. But this will not occur without your being intimately involved in the larger topic to begin with. This involvement is necessary if your research project is to be successful.

Bibliography

Diers, D. (1979). *Research in nursing practice*. New York: Lippincott.

Fawcett, J., & Downs, F. S. (1999). *The relationship of theory and research* (3rd ed.). Philadelphia: F. A. Davis.

Hale, E. D., Trehame, G. J., & Kitas, G. D. (2007). Qualitative methodologies: Asking research questions with reflexive insight. *Musculoskeletal Care, 5*(3), 139–147.

Hek, G. (1995). Asking research questions. *Journal of Community Nursing, 9*(1), 19–20.

Johnson, B. K. (1991). How to ask research questions in clinical practice. *American Journal of Nursing, 91*(3), 64–65.

Kinney A.B., & Blount, M. (1979). Effect of cranberry juice on urinary pH. *Nursing Research, 28*(3), 287-290.

Krouse, H. J. (1999). Congress preview: Research forum. Inquisitive minds want to know: Asking research questions. *ORL-Head & Neck Nursing, 17*(3), 22.

Meadows, K. A. (2003). So you want to do research? 1: An overview of the research process. *British Journal of Community Nursing, 8*(8), 369–375.

Meadows, K. A. (2003). So you want to do research? 2: Developing the research question. *British Journal of Community Nursing, 8*(9), 397–398, 400–403.

Rempusheski, V. F. (1990). Ask an expert . . . Formulating research questions. *Applied Nursing Research, 3*(1), 44–46.

Rempusheski, V. F. (1990). From where do nursing research questions emerge? *Applied Nursing Research, 3*(1), 44–46.

Smith, M., Buckhalter, K. C., Kang, H., Shultz, S. K., & Ellingrod, V. (2008). Tales from the field: What the nursing research textbooks will not tell you. *Applied Nursing Research, 21*(4), 232–236.

Tullmann, D. F., Haugh, K. H., Dracup, K., & Bourguignon, C. (2007). A randomized controlled trial to reduce delay in older adults seeking help for symptoms of acute myocardial infarction. *Research in Nursing and Health, 20*, 485–497.

Wright, D. J. (1999). Developing an effective research question. *Professional Nurse, 14*(11), 786–789.

From Question to Problem

➤ LEARNING OBJECTIVES

- Understand how to find the level of knowledge on a given topic.
- Relate the level of theory to the level of question.
- Describe how the research problem evolves from the literature review.
- Discuss how to start a literature review from your question.

Whether you need to find the best treatment of decubiti for a patient whose skin is beginning to break down or whether you want to design a study to test one or more treatments for decubiti, the initial process is the same. You want to find the current level of knowledge on this topic. What research has been done, and what was the outcome?

Throughout the first chapter, the words research topic, research problem, and research subject were used interchangeably. This was done quite deliberately. In research, the research problem stands by itself as the moving force behind the research plan. It is developed from the research question and is the final and complete synthesis of everything you have thought, read, argued over, and written. It substantiates what you propose to do and why. Before this point, however, you have been talking about problems that occur in real life, situations that need solutions, topics or ideas that interest you, and subject areas that you want to explore. As they were used in the first chapter, the terms subjects, topics, and problems referred to a less sophisticated order of thinking than the research problem for your proposal.

The research problem is the full exposition of the idea that you want to study. The problem statement or the problem definition—however you prefer to think of it—is a logical progression of ideas and arguments about your research idea. The problem introduces your topic, explains its importance, condenses facts and theories about the topic, and then in a final, decisive section justifies conclusively your choice of topic. The full statement of the problem answers all of the possible who, what, where, when, and why questions that anyone not involved in your project would ever dream of asking. And those answers are firm, so definitive that there are no loose ends, no gaps, and no fuzziness in the reader's mind.

In essence, the research problem is an essay about your research topic. An essay is a statement of opinion, substantiated by facts, that supports the position taken on a subject. A good essay offers an orderly progression of ideas that carries the reader through to the logical conclusion. Research problems should be written in the same way as good essays.

Because many research reports begin with the research problem, you may wonder why this book began by asking a question. The question serves the same purpose in research as the thesis serves for an essay. In an essay, the thesis is the author's opinion boiled down to one arguable statement. The research question does the same thing—it is the entire research design boiled down to one measurable question. Just as the entire essay is built on the thesis statement, the entire research proposal is built from the research question. Explaining how to build a research plan from your research question is the major subject of this book.

In the previous chapter, you were introduced to some of the functions of the research question and how to pin down your subject. In this section, you will refine your question into its clearest, most concise form and move into the development of the research problem.

Finding the Level of Knowledge About a Topic

Now that you have written your question, your next step is critical analysis of your question with the ultimate aim of using it to search the literature on your topic. In Chapter 1 you were introduced to the idea of three levels of research based on three levels of knowledge and theory development. Take a moment right now, if you have not already done so, to write out your topic at all three levels. Remember that:

Level I questions have one variable in one population.

Level II questions have two or more variables in one population.

Level III questions have cause and effect.

Suppose you find that you have one variable in two populations, or two or more variables in two or more populations, and cause and effect that cannot be manipulated by the researcher. What do you do?

When you have one variable in two populations, write two simple Level I questions, each with one variable in one population. In this case (for example, What are the characteristics of patients in a typical nursing home in Scotland versus the United States?) you will do two Level I studies, one in each population, and then compare the results of each complete study. You still have a Level I study—you simply have two of them to compare. This type of study is the basis for the Human Relations Area Files at Harvard University. These files are collections of anthropological field studies or single case studies of cultural groups that have been collected into one vast resource for secondary analysis. For the most part they are all Level I studies of single variables in single populations or descriptions of population characteristics. Anyone wishing to use the files can take two or more cultural groups to compare and contrast, but the initial studies were all at Level I.

Suppose you had written a question such as, What is the relationship between ethnicity and response to chemotherapy? How would you know whether this was a Level II question or two Level I questions? The difference lies in (1) the amount of knowledge about the variables and (2) the intent of the investigation. In the case of the single variable in two populations, the purpose would be to do a thorough verbal description of a single variable within the context of its population. The intent of the second-level question is to take selected portions of a previously studied variable (response to chemotherapy) and selected ethnic groups (Anglo and Latino) and see if they relate to one another in a statistically significant way. In the first type of question, the answer is a simple description of a variable in two different groups. In the second, the answer is a statistical relationship in which two or more ethnic groups are considered to be different categories of one variable.

Suppose you know enough about your variables to write a cause-and-effect statement, based on fact rather than hunch, but you know that there is no ethical way you as the researcher can change the independent variable as required for a third-level study. What do you do? Rewrite the question at Level II, but use the theory as the base for your study. Or, if you have access to a laboratory setting, you may leave the question at Level III and use the theory base to answer the question and test the theory on animals, cells, cultures, or other appropriate subjects.

The way you write your question is the way you will answer it, so be perfectly clear at the very beginning about your level of knowledge about the topic. It is your level of knowledge that takes you to the library to discover the level of knowledge available there. Based on your literature review, you may change your question to a different level.

One way of finding out your level of knowledge about the topic you have chosen to study is to try to write questions at all three levels. You will immediately recognize your level of knowledge about the topic. If you cannot write a Level III question, it may be because you don't know the answer to the Level II question. This is what happened to Ginnette Miles, a graduate student at the University of Iowa. Here are her questions and her working definitions of terms:

Level I question: What are the craniofacial features of preterm infants with postnatal cranial molding?

> Craniofacial features: The physical traits of the upper skull and forehead, including head shape and curvature, measurements and anterior-posterior diameter, biparietal diameter, and forehead length and width.

> Preterm infants: Infants who were born before or during the 37th week of gestation.

> Postnatal cranial molding: Symmetrical flattening of the lateral aspects of the cranium and forehead that develops in preterm infants as the head is repositioned from one side to the other on a mattress.

Level II question: What is the relationship between the craniofacial features of preterm infants and their physical attractiveness as perceived by adults?

The answer to this Level II question might have led to a question at Level III, but not knowing that answer means that the Level II study must be done first.

On the other hand, you may know a great deal about your topic right away and will have no difficulty in writing your topic at all three levels. In this case, you need to decide which question you prefer as well as which question has already been answered before you proceed with your research proposal.

The following questions were written by Deborah Sholz when she was a graduate student at the University of Iowa. Notice the amount of knowledge needed to write these questions.

Level I: What are the body positions into which nurses place low-birthweight intubated infants?

> Body position: A configuration of the body that describes whether prone, supine, side-lying toward right or left; whether head is turned 90°, 60°, 45°, 30°, or 0° from midline either to the right or left; whether chest is rotated right or left; whether hips are rotated right or left; whether extremities are extended, flexed, medially or laterally rotated, including hips, knees, ankles, shoulder, elbows, wrists; whether head is in alignment or tilted backward or forward.

> Intubated low-birthweight infants: Infants with an ET tube in trachea weighing less than 1500 grams.

Level II: What is the relationship between body positions and heart rate in the intubated low-birthweight infant?

> Heart rate: Beats per minute as detected by cardiac monitor.

Level III: Why does supine body positioning decrease heart rate in the intubated low-birthweight infant?

> Supine body position: Infant's scapulae and buttocks are flat against bed mattress.

Although there are any number of ideas that you could have chosen to research, most research topics can be grouped into a few primary categories: theory, concepts, observed situations, prior research, and tool development. Each category has different requirements for solutions and different end products. Each has its practical aspects, drawbacks, literature, and logic. Each has its supporters and its detractors. But all are valid. No one is better than another; it's simply a matter of what interests you the most. Some people always start with questioning a theory, some always start by questioning an observed situation. It's really a matter of goodness of fit between the researcher and the topic. If you want to question a clinical situation that has been bothering you, don't drop the idea because it's not a theory question. On the other hand, don't just attach any old theory to your question; your question will direct you to the appropriate one. Conversely, if you are a theorist at heart, your question will direct you to the appropriate situation to study; not every situation will suit your theory. The point is, your question will tell you where you are going and what you are going to do. Remember that it's your question and no one else's; how you develop it is your responsibility.

Now let's take some research topics and divide them into groupings:

Observations:

Some patients refuse medications.

Some patients are called demanding.

Some call lights aren't answered.

Mastectomy seems to affect some women more than others.

Detoxification programs don't always work on addicts.

Behaviors:	**Theories:**
Listening	Loss theory
Eating	Role theory
Touching	Alienation theory
Distancing	Theories of aggression
Avoiding	Psychopathological theories
Talking	Theories of change
Concepts	Learning theory
Addiction	Germ theory
Dependency	Biorhythmical theory
Hopelessness	Ethological theory
Independence	Systems theory
Nausea	
Privacy	

Each category of topic classifies a different order of phenomena. Observations arise from real-life situations that can be seen, smelled, touched, tasted, or heard by any individual. Often an observation is stated as a generalization about a repeating occurrence. It is the generalization that is usually tested in the research project.

Behaviors are specific types of observations that can be seen and thought about. In nursing, research frequently is based on observed behaviors of patients or nurses. Because behavior is frequently seen as purposive or goal directed, however, analysis of behavioral intent is more abstract and more removed from reality than a direct personal observation. Therefore, research on behavior is more abstract than research on observations and should be treated as a different level of abstraction.

Kim defines a concept as "[a procedure for labeling or naming] a symbolic statement for describing a phenomena or class of phenomena" (Kim, 1983, p. 6). Concepts are single abstract ideas, often expressed in a single word, that represent two or more interrelated ideas. A concept can represent a single group of observations or facts that are closely linked to one another in a distinguishable pattern. Research can be done on one concept and its component parts, but the interconnections between the ideas, which form the basis for the study, must be discussed.

You have been exposed to concepts all your life, so when you see one, you will recognize it immediately. Concepts are simply terms that trigger a set of ideas. Isolation is a concept; so are privacy, assertiveness, burnout, patient care, ethnicity, and pain. Each word, as you think about it, stimulates ideas about your past experiences with the concept. Perhaps you have experienced burnout yourself or have known someone who did. Can you describe the experience, what triggered the phenomenon, what helped to alleviate the feelings, what were the behaviors that contributed to the feeling of burnout? Think about pain. What does pain mean to you? Have you had patients who reacted differently to a similar type of pain? Is there a difference between pain threshold and pain tolerance? Is pain physiological or psychological?

When you look at a concept for your study, you will want to answer all of the questions that need answering about the concept as you plan to use it in your study. You will want to determine just what it is you want to know about the concept and write it down before you begin your study.

Theories are explanations for why things are as they are. "A theory may be a description of a particular phenomenon, an explanation of the relationship among phenomena, or the prediction of the effects of one phenomenon on another" (Fawcett, 1995, p. 20). Theories are explanations of two or more interrelated concepts; as such, they are the farthest removed from reality or direct observations. Theories are abstractions of processes, interactions, and observations.

As you can see, each successive category moves farther and farther away from the requirements of being observable and measurable because the level of abstraction increases. Because research deals with observable phenomena that can be described, classified, or explained, the closer the research topic is to observable fact, the easier it will be to pin down the elements in the research question. Not only are observations easier to pin down, but you also are more familiar with them because you have made one or more of these observations for yourself.

At the opposite extreme, theories are the most difficult to pin down because they are the farthest removed from observable facts. You may be familiar with the general idea of the theory and some of the work that has been done on it, but you are not as familiar or knowledgeable about theory as you are with observations. If you can refine a theory into measurable, observable terms, you should be able to pin down concepts and behaviors even more easily.

Because research requires explanation as well as observation, it will always involve some level of abstraction or theory. Whether you build your problem essay from an observation to a theory or begin with a theory and reduce it to measurable terms, you must relate theory to facts.

How to Search the Literature on Your Topic

One of the most troublesome aspects of good research is a thorough review of the literature. You need to be as exhaustive as possible on your topic. Whether you are a staff nurse, student, or faculty member, the library search of the literature will only be as good as the library resources available to you. However, through use of the Internet, your ability to search the literature is unlimited. Begin your search on your topic by the easiest method. After isolating the key ideas from your topic, write synonymous concepts from *Roget's Thesaurus* or from your dictionary. With these synonyms in hand, access the books in your library online or pay a visit to the book catalog in your library and see if there are any books listed under the themes you have listed. Ask your reference librarian for assistance as needed. If there are a great number of books, this is an indication that your question may need to be narrowed down because the answer to your original question is quite likely available in the literature.

Next, begin a search of the research databases available through your university or college library. This will give you access to the periodicals that publish nursing research. You can do this at the library, on the library computer, from a computer terminal in your school, or at home using your computer, provided you have Internet access. If you have not done a search before, it helps to be in the library where you can ask for assistance from a librarian if you run into any problems accessing the databases. By entering keywords related to your topic, you will be able to access all articles that meet your criteria during whatever period of time you specify in the database you have chosen. Here again, if you find thousands of articles that meet your criteria, you may want to narrow down your concept until you find the number of citations to be reasonable. (Two or three hundred citations will not be too many for you to review.) You will be able to print out a list of these articles and their abstracts. You can then review the abstracts and choose which of the articles you wish to read in full. Most articles are now available in full text through the library's database, but others must be obtained by accessing the journal itself in the library. It is likely that your library has arrangements with other libraries that increase your access to the resources you need. If the particular journal or book you need is not available in your library, you may wish to go beyond your own library resources and ask your librarian to assist you in obtaining a copy of the article or to borrow the book on interlibrary loan. Each of these methods of consulting the experts or reviewing the literature can and should be used when appropriate. For your initial review you want to know if anyone has done your particular study before. As you go further, you need to find out what has been done that is central to, as well as peripheral to, your topic. Finally, you need to know just what data-collection techniques have been developed that will be useful to you in your study.

The actual mechanics of a literature review require legwork on your part. Go to the library and look in the journals and books. Talk to the librarian and state precisely what you have read and examined. Direct the computer search of the literature based on what you have done. Because many computer searches are based on recent literature, you may need an additional search for your topic in earlier sources. Remember that there are many other sources. Computer searches are convenient, but they certainly are not exhaustive. You will find that some journals are missing from computer searches, and you will have to search those journals yourself. When you find particularly good studies that are relevant to your topic, check the references at the end of the articles to see if there are some studies listed that you have not found in your search. These might be important for you to read.

Take your time at this stage of your proposal development. Read everything you can on your topic. Learn who the major authors are on your work. Get to know everything they wrote. Whether your question is at Level I, II, or III, you need to be as exhaustive in your search as possible. The more you know about your topic, the better your final project will be. It is certainly worth that effort at the beginning.

You should become familiar with your library's periodical holding list to find out which journals are on file in your library. Make a list of the nursing journals your library has on hand so that as you find a reference, you can check your list to see if you have that journal easily available to you. From the serials list turn to the major nursing indexes, Cumulative Index to Nursing and Allied Health Literature (CINAHL), and the International Nursing Index. Other indexes will also be of use, such as the Hospital Literature Index and Index Medicus. When you have located these sources, look up their major headings and subheadings for your topic and its synonyms. Start with the most recent year and go back a minimum of five years on your topic. At Level I, search broadly; at Level III, search narrowly.

When we get busy or pressured, we tend to forget the resources available to us in our research. Use your reference librarian as much as you need to—that's what a librarian is for. Don't hesitate simply because you aren't sure you know what to look for—ask for help.

Level of Theory and Level of Question

As you saw in Chapter 1, there are three basic levels of research questions. The first level of question deals with a single topic or a population about which you know very little. Your knowledge was limited either about the topic of the question or about the people you wanted to study. Sometimes Level I questions are derived from observations of human or animal behavior that have never been questioned before. If you were interested in how children respond to pain after a burn, you might want to do a Level I study. You may find a great deal of literature on pain, but most of it may relate to adults rather than children. If there is no published literature describing how children respond to pain, then the study will have to be done at Level I.

At Level II, studies have usually been done on the two or three variables that are being correlated. However, you will not find studies that have previously correlated the variables (unless you have found one study you wish to replicate and the purpose of your study is to replicate this particular study).

At Level II, you will usually find some previous research on which to base your rationale for attempting to study these variables together. At this level of research, you will also find concepts derived from Level I studies that are worth exploring or testing further. Sometimes you develop Level II studies from the findings of a Level I study. If, for example, you had read a study about privacy and the hospitalized patient (Schuster, 1975) and you enjoyed the concept that was developed from that study, you may wish to develop your study from that concept. There are many concepts at Level II that need to be developed further than the original paper. Bereavement, pain, privacy, burnout, and helplessness are all concepts that deserve further study. Some of the studies will never go beyond Level II. If you are looking at psychosocial or behavioral variables, you are more likely to stop at Level II studies. If, however, you are looking at physiological variables, you are more likely to go directly to Level III studies because these variables can often be precisely measured and make good outcome variables.

At Level III, you will be dealing with theories or developing your own theoretical framework. Your study will begin with theory, so you go through the process of outlining a theory to make it operational, as described in this chapter. Without the theoretical base, you simply don't have a third-level study. At Level III, however, you trace the linkages among each aspect of the theory. The linkages trace the logical steps from one point of an argument to another. When you ask a *why* question you answer that question with a *because* explanation. The explanation has a series of statements that are linked to one another logically and sequentially. This series of explanations can be diagrammed in a conceptual map of the problem, which will outline how each explanation leads to the next.

At Level III you are testing theory—that is the whole purpose of Level III studies. Your problem will be to find a theoretical framework for your study. You have asked a why question based on a good deal of knowledge. You asked, Why does this particular variable change this other variable in this specific way? You answer your own question by building an explanation for the relationships among those specific variables based on other people's research findings. You would not have been able to ask the question first if you did not know a lot about the way the variables impact one another. The step-by-step explanation of the linkages among these variables, the impact of other variables on them, and how those other variables influence their actions all form the basis for this theoretical framework. How to form those linkages is exemplified in Chapter 5 on how to write hypotheses.

You begin with your theory and you substantiate each point in the theory with the research that has been done by others. If you are right, and you hope you are, your explanation of how and why these variables interact in a particular way can be demonstrated through your project. Your literature review, therefore, is on those two variables and how they have been studied before. You will look for the flaws in design that you will rectify in your proposal, you will look for proven tests that everyone uses because they work, you will look for all possible exceptions to the rule, and you will take notes on each study because you do not want to duplicate mistakes (but you do want to be sure to include all the correct maneuvers). To keep track of all the concepts in your theory, use $5 \times 8''$ cards, make photocopies of the critical articles, and read extensively.

Physiological studies have the greatest literature base; support for your argument will be found in that literature easily. Behavioral studies are the most limited because the conditions under which behaviors will differ are the least known and understood. Studies of human behavior are often culture specific, and to find behaviors that are cross-culturally valid for given circumstances is rare.

The level of theory is dictated by the level of question, but not all questions lead directly to theory because there may not be enough research data on which to build theory. Much basic research needs to be done to advance nursing theory, and, for this reason, we advocate the use of all levels of research design to advance nursing knowledge rapidly. The level of question is based on the level of knowledge about a topic, and the level of knowledge dictates the level of theory. If, after having thoroughly reviewed the literature on your question, you have found little or no data on either the topic or the sample, you remain at a Level I study. If you have found previous research on your variables but no linkage of the two together, you provide that explanation and test your conceptual framework at Level II. If your study shows a significant relationship, then you may proceed to ask why and test your theory at Level III. (A more detailed explanation of how to develop a conceptual or theoretical framework can be found in Chapter 3.)

Developing the Research Problem from the Literature Review ___

The process of putting theory into an observable, measurable research question involves a thorough inventory of your knowledge about the theory—deciding which concepts within the theory most interest you; asking yourself which behaviors best exemplify the concept you have chosen; and, finally, choosing those observations that best represent those behaviors. Because you are narrowing down from abstraction to observation, you are moving from a generalization to a specific. Pinning down theory is a process of identifying what you want to know and filtering out all unnecessary material until you have narrowed your subject to its purest, most refined point. Let's see how it works.

Find Out What You Know

Let's say that your research question involves the concept of the patient role. You know that the term "role" stands for major concepts and theories, and you must decide which aspect of the word interests you. At the same time, you need to find out just how much you know about role to have a starting point for your literature search; you don't want to waste time going over familiar ground.

So you begin with your working definitions of your terms. Simply defined, working definitions refer to what you mean by the terms you are using in context of the research question. A working definition is not the definition of the term found in a dictionary. A working definition refers to the meaning that you, the researcher, have in your head when you are talking about your research topic and its attendant variables. These are the definitions that get you to the literature, but they are probably not going to be the final definitions you will use in your proposal.

You define role as that group of behaviors commonly found among ill persons in a hospital setting. Suddenly you are uncomfortably aware of how far away you are from an observable, measurable definition of the term. As you look at your definition, you can see you need to define just what you mean by that group of behaviors because that phrase is very vague. You also see that you need to define ill person more specifically, and hospital setting isn't exactly the clearest term, either.

Role represents a series of concepts tied together into one word. And you should have a working (measurable) definition of each concept. Each concept must be divided into its component parts, each of which must also be defined in relation to some observable, measurable behavior. So you turn to the dictionary for help. You find that the dictionary defines role in terms of acting a part in a drama. This is not helpful as you attempt to clarify your idea.

Return to your original definition. You are interested in three major interrelated concepts in role theory: ill persons, hospital settings, and grouped behaviors. You have three areas in which to search the literature, look up definitions, plan a computer search, or seek out the reference librarian. On the other hand, you wrote working definitions of each area to narrow down, still further, just which aspects of the theories interest you and how much you know about each.

Ask Questions About the Theory

According to your question, you are most interested in how patients learn their role. Therefore, you ask:

Who teaches the role and how is it taught?

Are there different types of patient roles to be learned?

Is the patient role easy or difficult to learn?

Are patients satisfied or dissatisfied with their roles?

What kind of a role is the patient role?

What other roles interact with the patient role?

Is terminal illness a role situation?

Does the diagnosis of cancer change the patient role?

How does type of hospital affect the patient role?

All of these questions, as well as others you may think of, will need to be answered by some aspect of role theory. As you ask your questions and read what other people have thought or observed, take notes on the answers and opinions that you encounter. You can use index cards for your notes, or you can develop a document file into which you paste various items you find online, making sure that you accurately attach the references to avoid having to look them up again.

Head each entry with a question and, as you read, write notes in answer to the question, citing the author, title, publication date, and page number. When you are finished, group your entries under the appropriate questions. Examine each set of answers and decide which answers you agree with—or feel most comfortable with—and separate them from the other entries. You now have a beginning outline of those aspects of role theory in relation to ill patients that most interest you.

Look Up Interrelated Ideas

Because a concept is made up of at least two ideas, and a theory is made up of at least two concepts, there is always the possibility that at least one of the ideas will lead to an entirely different concept or even a different theory. Therefore, as you search the literature, look up all relevant, related concepts and ideas. You may find a fruitful new line of thought that leads you away from your original idea or reinforces your approach to your question. Look carefully at these ideas. Accept or reject them on the basis of knowledge, not hunch.

This search will also tell you whether you have eliminated too many ideas in the initial development of your question. Use this aspect of the literature review to clarify your topic, making sure you have left out nothing important and are not including anything irrelevant or superfluous.

Outline

Starting with the major heading, break down your theory into the component parts that address your question. (Remember that each major heading has at least two distinct subheadings.) This outlining process helps you become more specific about what aspect of the theory interests you and helps you identify relationships.

As you outline, include only those aspects of the theory that you agree with, and exclude those areas that you consider to be irrelevant or unimportant. From this will emerge your specific point of view. Don't throw away the other arguments; keep them handy where you can refer to them when you are developing your full and final problem.

Role
  I. Role types
      A. Patient roles
          1. Inpatient
          2. Outpatient
          3. Convalescent
          4. Terminal
              a. Patient doesn't know diagnosis
              b. Patient knows diagnosis
                  (1) Recently told
                  (2) Has known for some time
          5. Short term
          6. Long term
          7. Emergency
      B. Staff roles
      C. Family roles
      D. Sick roles
 II. Role learning
III. Achieved versus ascribed roles
 IV. Role distance
  V. Role behaviors
 VI. Role sets
VII. Roles in interaction

Convert Your Topic Outline to a Sentence Outline

For each heading in your outline, write one sentence or one definition that expresses your point of view. As you write your definitions, you may have to revise your outline because you may be moving farther away rather than closer to your original topic. As a handy reminder of your original thinking, you may include an example with your definition. If the definition does not follow from your example, try to rephrase it so that it does.

Role is the set of behaviors attached to a particular social position or status within a society.

   I. Role types are the specific roles attached to a particular position within a social position.

      A. Patient role is the set of behaviors expected of individuals who are receiving healthcare services.

         1. Terminal patient roles are those behaviors expected of patients who are dying.

            a. Those behaviors expected of patients who are dying but don't know it.

            b. Those behaviors associated with patients who do know they are dying.

               (1) Terminal patients who have just been told may react with anger, crying, withdrawal, or a request to see their spiritual advisor.

               (2) Terminal patients who have known about their diagnosis for some time may be used to the idea, may refuse to talk about it, may talk about their death freely, may be clearing up their personal affairs, or may want to be with their families as much as possible.

            c. Those behaviors associated with patients who know they are dying but pretend not to know.

Relate the Theory to the Question

By outlining your theory and writing definitions about each relevant aspect, you now have some new working definitions for each term in your question. Not only do you have your terms defined, you have also added some new qualifying words to your research question. After your thorough review of role theory, your topic may have changed. In fact, you may have a whole new series of topics based on your review of theory. But remember, one topic is all you need for your research; more than one makes an overly complicated study.

    Now that you have asked questions of your theory, defined each term in your question, outlined the relevant aspects of the theory, clarified exactly what you want to observe about each aspect and why, and, finally, substantiated each part of your outline with literature, you have the basic framework of your ideas and your literature review. This outline alone, when written in the form of an essay, constitutes your theoretical framework for the study. (If you had done the same work on one or more concepts, you would have the underpinnings for a conceptual framework.) If you are dealing with more than one theory or concept, your framework must show their relationship to one another as well as to your question.

Beginning with an Observation

Remember that we began this discussion with the comment that starting with a theory and reducing it to specific, observable phenomena is more difficult than starting with an observation and relating it to specific situations. The latter instance requires proceeding from your personal experience and your familiarity with the subject.

You discover how much you know about your topic when you try to write questions at all three levels. If you find you haven't the vaguest idea how to write a cause-and-effect question on your topic, but you can write questions at both Level I and Level II, you are already aware of how much you know about your topic. Begin your literature review with your question. For example:

What are the characteristics of successful dieters?

This is a Level I question about the variable characteristics on a population of successful dieters. You can assume that there have been a number of studies of characteristics of various populations, but have there been any studies on successful dieters? First write working definitions of both characteristics and successful dieters. For example:

Characteristics: The qualities or traits that distinguish individuals or groups of individuals from one another. These qualities or traits may be demographic, such as age, gender, and socioeconomic status; or specific to my population, such as prior dieting history, family history of obesity, onset of obesity, amount of body fat at the time of last diet, and so on.

Successful dieters: Individuals who have deliberately lost at least 15% of their overall body weight and have kept it off for at least one year without gaining back more than five pounds.

With these two definitions in hand, the literature can be searched very carefully to see if there is any study at all that fits this description. Let us say that one or two studies were identified that looked similar to this one or were at least in the same general area of interest. Find those studies and read them. Do they answer the specific question you asked? Do they answer the entire question or do they leave things out?

Start by looking up the terms in your working definitions: successful dieters, diet history, family obesity, and so on. Let us say you found a study on successful dieters, but successful was defined differently. Successful was an individual who had kept the weight off for more than two years.[1] Or not all parts of your definition of characteristics were included. You can still proceed to a Level I study. The population in your study may have different characteristics from the other study's. You may find another study on successful dieters in which the authors defined successful as having been overweight as an adult but not now overweight. In this case, the definition of successful is far more vague than yours, so the findings of the study do not prevent you from pursuing a Level I study. You will take notes on these studies and write up the findings in your literature review. These two studies will help you isolate some other characteristics you did not think of, or they may provide you with useful measures. They provide ideas for your study so you need to refer to them.

Suppose you found only studies of the characteristics of unsuccessful dieters. Look at these studies to see what kinds of characteristics they examined and which ones look promising to you for your study. Be sure to take notes on these studies and refer to them in your proposal, particularly when you develop your method of data collection. (Other studies can provide you with ideas on how to collect data.)

For a Level I study on successful dieters you will probably find studies on the relationship between obesity and many diseases, studies on different dieting programs, and studies on different explanations for the causes of obesity. None of these are directly relevant to your study but are essential reading to give you a general review of your topic. In your final literature review you will probably group many of these studies into summary statements or paragraphs.

Let's take another example. Suppose you had started with an observation that certain patients reacted differently when they learned they had terminal cancer. Some reacted with anger, shouting, crying, and moroseness; others didn't react at all. Your original question might have been, What are the reactions of oncology patients when they are told they are terminally ill?

---

[1] All materials on successful dieters paraphrased from the grant proposal entitled *Characteristics of Successful Dieters* submitted to the Division of Nursing by Pamela Brink in 1986.

This question is already observable and measurable. It relates a particular situation to an abstract explanation. You may end up explaining the differences by using role theory, or you may find an entirely different theory, such as stimulus–response or loss theory. This type of question is easier to write about simply because, as a nurse, you are familiar with the subject. You have experienced these behaviors for yourself. You know what you are looking for and why. And, as a nurse, you can probably use the answer in your practice.

Just because you are familiar with your subject and begin with readily observable terms does not mean that you are free from the responsibility of reviewing the literature on your question. On the contrary, because your question is so specific, it may have already been answered by someone else. Your first task, then, is not to look up the theory but to examine the research literature.

Where Do You Start Your Literature Search?

Just as with the theory question, you begin with each specific idea in your question. In this instance, you may decide to begin with the words oncology patients. Card catalogs and the nursing, medicine, and health databases may turn up citations on oncology but may not have anything specific for oncology patients. Just as in the theory question, you must then look up patients in the literature. But you are interested in specific patients, those with terminal illnesses. To adequately review the literature on this subject, each aspect of your question needs to be investigated for research that relates specifically or remotely.

Certain researchers discuss their findings in relation to new ideas and theories. As you read, take note of these interrelated ideas. One or more of them will strike you as being the one concept or theory that truly fits your question.

Just as with the theory question, keep your references organized and properly annotated. Start a file for research articles, with subheadings for each aspect of your topic. When you search the library databases, you get abstracts of the articles that meet your search criteria. Those abstracts that appear to provide information that helps your understanding of your topic can be pasted into the file under the appropriate heading. Later, you can decide which of the articles you want to read in full. You will probably want headings for each aspect of the question referred to, such as oncology patients. From these headings, an outline will emerge.

Your outline practically writes itself. Your question is the major heading; your minor headings come from the individual words or specific ideas within the question. This outline takes the reverse of the theory outline format. You will move from your specific definitions to an idea or a concept. For example:

I. Oncology patients are inpatients of an oncology unit who were admitted with a tentative diagnosis of a carcinogenic process.

    A. Diagnostic studies have been completed, the diagnosis has been confirmed, and the patient has been informed of the diagnosis of lung cancer. According to the chart, the patient reacted with:

        1. Anger: Explosive and abusive language to the staff and family.

           a. Anger can be a defense mechanism to protect an individual from an intolerable fact.

           b. Anger can be a normal expression for any disagreeable fact or opinion. Cultural behavior?

           c. Anger can be a usual response for some people. Stimulus–response?

        2. No response: After the patient received the diagnosis, the chart states that the patient began to make pleasant conversation with the physician, changed the subject, or otherwise gave no indication of having heard or cared about the diagnosis.

           a. Heard partially. Higher levels of anxiety cause fragmented (spotty) perceptions.

           b. Denied the meaning of what was heard.

           c. May not wish to discuss the issue until given time to think about it. Motivation?

           d. May have the behavioral patterns of not discussing intimate details with strangers. Cultural beliefs?

           e. Explanation given may be so vague and technical that the patient did not understand.

    B. Diagnostic studies have been completed as in A. Patient has been informed of diagnosis of leukemia.

    C. Diagnostics as in A and B. Patient informed of diagnosis of metastatic cancer from prior surgery.

You established your outline through ideas and reading, but because you began with a behavioral observation, your initial definitions are more specific and observable. Your review of research and theory is easier because you knew what you were looking for at the beginning.

When you are developing the literature review for a Level II question, you proceed in exactly the same way. You write working definitions for each of the major variables in your study and begin your outline with your definitions. The following outline was developed by Karen Goebel, a graduate student at the University of Iowa during a beginning research course.

Question: What is the relationship between burnout in the NICU and the types of coping mechanisms used among nurses?

Coping is the cognitive and behavioral efforts used to manage specific internal–external demands that are appraised as taxing or exceeding the resources of the person.

I. Coping mechanisms are specific methods used to decrease stress.
   A. The types of coping mechanisms utilized in the ICU and NICU vary with each individual.
      1. Personal (reactive) strategies are informal methods of communication.
         a. Talking to people outside the unit.
         b. Talking with fellow nurses.
         c. Withdrawing self from the unit.
      2. Management strategies are professionally mediated therapy sessions.
         (1) Attending psychotherapy sessions for discussion.
         (2) Participating in neonatologist-attended meetings.
         a. Personal (proactive) strategies are behaviors initiated by the person.
         (1) Knowledge about the stress-producing situation.
         (2) The amount of control the individual perceives to have over the stressor.
         (3) The ability to laugh.
         (4) Confrontation of the situation.

II. Various stresses within the NICU produce a need for coping mechanisms.
   A. Interpersonal communication problems exist between staff and physicians, nursing office, other departments in the hospital, and other staff members.

B. The nurse's need for an extensive knowledge base in patient teaching, cardiac arrest, pathophysiology of a neonate, and making many rapid decisions.

C. Environmental stressors include numerous pieces of equipment and failure, physical injury to nurse, physical setup, and noise level of the unit.

D. The components of patient care include work load and amount of physical work required, meeting the psychological needs of the patient, meeting the needs of the family, and death of the patient.

III. Coping mechanisms are effective when there is a release of stressful emotions.

IV. Burnout is the loss of motivation for creative involvement resulting from stresses of the NICU.

A. Characteristics of burnout manifest themselves in various ways.

1. Physical manifestations are described.

a. Feelings of chronic fatigue and exhaustion after adequate sleep and rest.

b. Minor ailments, such as colds, headaches, and stomach upsets, occur frequently.

(1) Emotions are altered by burnout. Symptoms of depression.

(2) Hostility and negativism directed toward fellow workers, the unit, or patients and their families.

(3) Guilt for having negative feelings.

2. Burnout affects behavior.

a. Detachment is expressed by avoidance and the use of diagnosis rather than name to identify patient.

b. Overinvolvement is demonstrated by declining to take vacations and the inability to delegate responsibility.

B. The causes of burnout are multivariate.

1. The constant threat of imminent death with resulting guilt.

2. Ethical dilemma about life and death issues.

3. The demands of dealing with and supporting families of NICU patients.

4. New and changing technology that must be learned.

5. Understaffing, which leads to exhaustion and frustration.

6. Interdisciplinary conflicts due to roles not being clearly defined.

7. Intradisciplinary conflicts where strong leadership is required to maintain cohesiveness.

8. Chronic patients who become a source of frustration and strain.

Starting with a problem close to home gives you the advantage of having more information about your question to start with, which, in turn, enables you to direct your reading and outline more specifically and to form working definitions.

The second aspect of starting with a problem close to home is that you are usually involved with the question you select. You either are working with the question on a daily basis or have had a recent experience with it that is likely to occur again. For this reason, the work you do on your problem—your thinking, your reading, and your attempts at clarification—is immediately applicable in your daily life and is not just an isolated incident. The more removed your research question is from you personally, the more removed you will be in the rest of your project. The more intimately involved you are with your question, the more interest you will generate, the more likely you are to sustain your interest, and the more practical your work will be.

On the other hand, if working with theory excites you, don't select a problem just because it's practical. Remember, this is your research project and no one else's—so whatever you want to know is the question you need to ask.

Bibliography

Chinn, P. L. (2008). *Integrated theory and knowledge development in nursing* (7th ed.). St. Louis, MO: Mosby Elsevier.

Cooper, H. M. (1982). Scientific guidelines for conducting integrative research reviews. *Review of Educational Research, 52,* 291–302.

Cooper, H. M. (1984). *The integrative research review.* Newbury Park, CA: Sage.

Cooper, H. M. (1989). *Integrating research: A guide for literature reviews* (2nd ed.). Newbury Park, CA: Sage.

de Chesnay, M., & Anderson, B. A. (2008). *Caring for the vulnerable: Perspectives in nursing theory, practice and research.* Sudbury, MA: Jones and Bartlett.

Fawcett, J. (1995). *Analysis and evaluation of conceptual models of nursing* (3rd ed.). Philadelphia: F. A. Davis.

Harvard, L. (2007). How to conduct an effective and valid literature search. *Nursing Times, 103*(45), 32–33.

Kim, H. S. (1983). *The nature of theoretical thinking in nursing.* Norwalk, CT: Appleton-Century-Crofts.

Lefort, S. M. (1993). The statistical clinical significance debate. *IMAGE: Journal of Nursing Scholarship, 25*(1), 57–62.

McEwan, M., & Mills, E. M. (2007). *Theoretical basis for nursing* (2nd ed.). Philadelphia: Lippincott Williams & Wilkins.

Meleis, A. I. (1997). *Theoretical nursing: Development and progress* (3rd ed.). Philadelphia: J. B. Lippincott.

Oxman, A. D., & Guyatt, G. H. (1988). Guidelines for reading literature reviews. *Canadian Medical Association Journal, 138,* 697–703.

Playle, J. (2000). Developing research questions and searching the literature. *Journal of Community Nursing, 14*(2), 20, 22, 24.

Powers, B. A., & Knapp, T. R. (1990). *A dictionary of nursing theory and research.* Newbury Park, CA: Sage.

Robson, C. (2002). *Real world research* (2nd ed.). London: Blackwell.

Schuster, B. A. (1975). Privacy and the hospitalization experience. In M. V. Batey (Ed.) *Communicating nursing research.* Boulder, CO: Western Council for Higher Education.

Wolf, Z. R., & Heirner, M. M. (1999). Substruction: Illustrating the connections from research question to analysis. *Journal of Professional Nursing, 15*(1), 33–37.

Wright, D. J. (1999). Developing an effective research question. *Professional Nurse, 14*(1), 786–789.

CHAPTER THREE

The Full and Final Research Problem

➤ TOPICS

Elements of a Research Problem
The Psychology of Argument
Strongest Argument Last
Substantiate What You Say
Bibliography

➤ LEARNING OBJECTIVES

- Describe the elements of a research problem.
- Review how to develop a strong argument to support your ideas.
- Understand the importance of substantiating what you say.

In learning how to arrive at your full research problem, you developed all the necessary elements for the entire research plan—your question, your theories, your terms defined, and the type of measurement that you intend to use. Your next step is to put all these components together into a complete package, the research problem. This is very much like putting together a bicycle that you ordered from a catalog. If any of the parts were missing, or if you attached the pedals where the wheels belong, you wouldn't have a workable bicycle. Like the bicycle, the full problem should have a sense of completeness about it; all the parts should operate together, and the problem as a whole should work properly and be aesthetically pleasing. A poorly designed research plan is as useless as a box of parts and bolts.

To extend the analogy, putting a bicycle together is much easier, less time consuming, and less frustrating if you know the relationship among the parts and the whole. If you know the what and why of the parts of a bicycle, then you know if you are putting things together properly and if you have achieved the full and final bicycle. A well-constructed bicycle is achieved because you know how it works, why it works, and what it needs to work.

A well-constructed research problem is achieved in the same way because you know how and why it works and what it needs to work. But before you can build your research problem, you need to understand the basic elements of the problem.

Elements of a Research Problem

Although some research texts and published research papers include all of the introductory matter (problem, rationale, purpose, literature review, and terms) under the heading Problem, it's best to know the elements of the problem itself and how it is developed as a separate and distinct section of the research plan. The elements are:

- Review of the literature
- The rationale for developing the question
- The theoretical or conceptual framework

Each element, for its fullest development, requires a lot of thinking, reorganizing of ideas, and a logical progression of concepts and facts that leads the reader to your statement of purpose. Although research problems can be written in a variety of ways (see the research proposals in the Appendix), the same basic elements are present in all problems.

The problem is your frame of reference for the entire research project, your rationale for choice of literature, your point of view on your subject—all of which are substantiated by facts, theories, and arguments gleaned from your reading. The problem is your statement of what you are doing and why. If you are hesitant about your idea, your problem will be hesitant. If you are uninterested in your study, your problem will be dull. If you haven't done your reading, your problem will be merely a bucket of bolts. Whether you know it or not, your problem is an expression of your personality.

Review of the Literature

The rationale for the development of your question came from some-where—ideas do not develop in a vacuum. Ideas often come from an out-side source, either in written form or in an interview. Your review of the literature simply documents the source of your idea and substantiates the rationale behind your question.

The rationale for incorporating the review of literature in the problem essay is that when you substantiate what you say, you usually substanti-ate it through the literature you have read or through direct personal quotes. Therefore, because you must document your source for your rationale and your theoretical–conceptual framework, why separate your review of literature from the two other elements in the problem defini-tion? You simply waste paper by repeating your sources in a different way.

The literature review is a series of references. It is not a bibliography. Only the literature that you have used to substantiate the background of your problem is included in your literature review and in your subsequent list of references. Not everything that you have read about your problem is relevant to your research, and therefore not everything should be included in the review. Only relevant literature is required in the literature review.

The Rationale for Developing the Question

The amount of space devoted to the rationale will vary, depending on the type of question you have chosen to ask. When a question is at the exploratory level it means there is little or no literature to support a study beyond the exploratory level. In this case, more attention should be given to developing the rationale.

The rationale for asking the question is your statement of why you believe it is an important question to study, why you want the answer, and of what use the answer will be to nursing. What made you think of the question in the first place? You certainly had a series of ideas or questions that led you to ask this final research question. This is your rationale for the development of the question, and if not explicitly stated, it must be clear by the time the reader has finished reading the problem argument. This is your logic, your reasoning, your point of view—and the reader has the right to know what it is.

The Theoretical or Conceptual Framework

Although these words are frightening to the new researcher, they are not as formidable as they sound. The framework for your study is simply an explanation, based on the literature you have read, of how the variables in your study are expected to relate to one another and why. In this book, we put the framework in the form of an essay, and the structure of a good essay is in the form of an argument. The essay supports your rationale for developing the question; it is your explanation of how the theories you have found relate to your study; it provides the justification for your study; and it will give the reader a feeling for the value of the proposed research to nursing, not only in its contribution to the development of theory but also in its relationship to other research on the topic.

The framework is called a conceptual framework when your explanation is based on literature and research about the variables, or when the literature does not contain a particular theory that explains the relationship among your variables. The explanation, therefore, will be your expectation, based on the literature, about the action of your variables. You will evaluate this explanation after you have done the study and, depending on your results, you may or may not find that it actually provides a useful explanation for the action of the variables. Regardless, it will provide the central theme for the discussion of your results.

The framework is called a theoretical framework when the variables have been studied before and have been found to be related to one another. You have available to you either a theory that provides an explanation for the action of your variables or a proposed explanation given by another author to explain the findings of a study of the same variables. In either case, the result would be a theoretical framework for your study. This framework will then be tested by you and will either be supported or not supported by your results. You, therefore, will add to the literature on the theory you are using.

After you have read the literature and have established the existing level of knowledge about your topic, you are ready to develop the framework for your study. We already know that each level of research has its appropriate level of knowledge reflected in the literature. Thus it makes sense that the framework also will be based on the level of knowledge about the topic and will differ for each level of research.

At Level I there may be no framework based on existing literature because there may be no prior research on the topic you have chosen. In this case, a rationale for the study customarily is developed to support the need for exploratory research on the topic and to discuss the potential usefulness of the findings. Sometimes, however, Level I studies are based on theories or concepts that have been studied in other populations. For example, you might decide to explore the sick role in another culture.

Because the theory of sick role was based on research done with a white, middle-class American population, its applicability to other cultures is not known. Your study, therefore, could explore the concept of sick role in another culture, using the existing theory as a starting point for the study. Keeping in mind that it may not fit, you will need flexibility in the design of the study. In this case, the framework for the study would include a discussion of sick-role theory as it would be used for your study and would provide a summary of the previous research on sick-role theory from the standpoint of the cultural or ethnic background of the subjects. In the discussion of your findings, you would be able to contrast your subjects with those of previous studies and might come up with some tentative ideas about the reasons for any differences that you found. These ideas could then provide the basis for further research on sick role.

At Level II, you must provide a conceptual framework for the study in your proposal. From the literature on the variables you plan to study, you will develop a probable explanation for the action that might occur among the variables. For example, in a study of the relationship among grandmother caregiving, family stress and strain, and depressive symptoms, Musil et al. used the resiliency model of family stress, adjustment, and adaptation as the framework to examine the effects of social support and resourcefulness in the relationship between family life stresses and strain and depressive symptoms in grandmothers who were raising grandchildren. Previous research had identified grandmothers raising grandchildren as having significantly more depressive symptoms than other grandmothers. The authors explain that the resiliency model of family stress, adjustment, and adaptation can be used to conceptualize how the demands placed upon the family system might affect the mental health of grandmother caregivers. They propose that family demands, if not moderated by resources and problem solving–coping, may increase the possibility of depression or other emotional problems (Musil, Warner, Zauszniewski, Wykle, & Sanding, 2009). Because not enough was known about these variables in relation to one another (they had not been previously studied together), this framework is conceptual rather than theoretical and represents the authors' best guess about what the findings might mean. Clearly, at Level II, the study is not exploratory but is looking for relationships among specific, predetermined variables to answer questions about these variables. The findings might lead to the development of a theory that could then be tested in further research.

Level III studies always have theoretical frameworks to explain what the researcher expects to find. Because these studies are always based on the results of Level II studies, you always know the relationship among the variables in advance and can predict its direction. Your prediction can be supported by a theoretical framework that explains why the variables affect one another. For example, in an experimental design, McDonald et al. carried out a clinical trial testing the affect of personal relevance on learning. In this case, the theory was that the more personally relevant the information is to the learner, the more likely it is to be learned. This theory comes from the Elaboration Likelihood Model (ELM) (Petty, Barden, & Wheeler, 2002) of persuasion, which identifies two modes of learning: central and peripheral. When people use the central route, they are more likely to think actively and retain the information. This study provided a further test of the theory by utilizing a personally relevant motivational statement, learn about stroke to save someone you love, in a double-blind study using experimental and control groups (McDonald, et al., 2009). As you can see, testing of theory at Level III is done in small increments, all of which eventually contribute to the overall understanding of the topic.

When you develop your problem essay, be sure that you are consistent with the level of your question, and use this as an opportunity to cross-check all the parts of the problem for consistency.

When you write your problem essay, you will be incorporating your rationale for the development of the question, your theoretical or conceptual framework, and your literature review into one (not three) definitive statement of what you are studying and why and its relevance to you and your reader.

Remember, at this point you are the expert on your research. Now all you have to do is demonstrate your expertise in an essay.

When you are looking up your topic initially, don't hesitate to look in theory, history, or even fictional literature for material on your idea. Sometimes there is not much available in the research literature but a great deal in other sources. Use any source available on your topic and check it for accuracy.

Be sure to check sources both in and out of the nursing field. Sometimes, the literature in the area is found only in history books or books on sociology. Check the various professional indexes for sources, look up synonyms and antonyms and check those out, and talk to people and ask them to help you think of sources for your search. Don't hesitate to use any source you can find that substantiates your topic. Nursing is a broad and eclectic field and it is important to understand an amalgam of ideas outside its major areas of interest. The breadth of reading that is possible for any topic is enormous.

Remember that good research is ethical research. If you say that there is no prior research in an area, then you will be believed. Your statements are accepted at face value. If you say you have done your literature review, you will be believed. Think of your statements as your word of honor to your reader.

A major problem that crops up over and over again is losing references. Be sure to keep a record of everything you have read about your topic and keep it secure until well after you have finished the research project in its entirety. Don't throw away your annotated references—you never know when you will need them. It is easy to keep them in a file on your computer, just make sure your work is backed up in case of a glitch in your computer. You can be absolutely sure that if you lose, misplace, or throw away one annotated reference, that is the one you will desperately need when you write your proposal.

The Psychology of Argument

Each element in your research problem is absolutely necessary to persuade the reader that your research project is sound, well thought out, and well documented from observations or reading. This is the essence of argument—to persuade another person that your logic is correct and that your position is well thought through.

To argue your point successfully, you will need to know the opposing position as well as you know your position. For many of us, that's not an easy thing to do. We are so enamored with our own position we cannot think of any possible argument against it. But notice the technique in successful debates, successful salesmanship, successful books—they had all taken into account the opposite point of view and had an answer for it. They were prepared to answer any question that required clarification, explanation, or further data. Whether you are trying to entice people to support your organization or accept your research plan, you need to plan ahead to win the argument.

The crux of the matter is that you have stimulated the argument and you are interested in winning. Winning doesn't just happen by itself. So if you are going to start an argument, be prepared to win it. You have the edge because the opposition is not prepared for an argument, nor does it have a vested interest in its outcome.

Let's say that you have already experienced losing your research argument, which went something like this: I want to study children's reactions to injections. Your instructor looks at you and says, "Well, that sounds like a reasonable enough topic, but why do you want to study it?" Somewhat taken back by being questioned at all, you respond with, "I'm in pediatrics, and I think it would be good to know." A pained expression comes over your instructor's face, perhaps even a sigh, and all of a sudden you feel pretty inadequate.

Suppose you had said, instead, "I'm on a children's unit, and I've noticed differences in children's reactions to injections. I have a hunch that there is a difference in boys' and girls' reactions after, say, about the age of 5 years because of the way children are socialized into sex-stereotyped role reactions to painful experiences. I'm not sure just when—what age, I mean—these differences begin to be noticed, nor am I sure if it has anything to do with previous experiences with injections. But it seems to me that if we could find out when those differences occur—if they do—and if there is any relationship among prior experience, age, and sex, we as nurses could then change our approach to giving children medications on the basis of these findings."

Result? Full approval and a go-ahead. Why? Because you thought out your rationale for why you want to do your study, you gave a personal observation to back up your idea, you suggested a theory to explain your observation, and you pointed out a use for the information that you might gather from your study. You won your argument simply because you answered all the questions. Your position was logical, sound, and thoughtful. Perhaps without knowing it, you incorporated all of the elements on problem selection. You spoke with authority.

Your argument also had a basic structure. You began with the general problem area that you wanted to study. Then you conceded that you didn't know all the answers (I have a hunch . . .), and, third, you pointed out the practicality of the project. This was your punch line, which you shrewdly left for the end. Strong arguments always include (1) central points, (2) concessions, and (3) the points in favor of the position.

The basic elements of the full problem follow the requirements for an argument. Your rationale for developing the question uses the style of arguments—the central issue you are dealing with, the many and diverse ideas or situations that could be explored through research, and your reason for settling on this particular project. Your argument is strengthened by your literature review. Each point you make in a concession, or in your favor, should have relevant, documented facts to substantiate your statements.

The conceptual or theoretical framework also follows the logic of argument, whether you integrate your framework into your rationale for developing the question or write it as a separate section. You will begin with your central point, make concessions to other relevant theories or concepts, and then point out exactly which theory or concept is most applicable to your study and why. Here, again, your literature review substantiates your basic framework.

Whether you are doing research on a theory, an observation, or a particular tool, use the psychology of argument in the development of your problem.

Strongest Argument Last

Imagine for a moment that you are the teacher of a research course, and all your students have handed in their problems for you to read. Which of the following problems would you ask the student to rewrite and which would convince you that the student had thought through and described the research problem well?

Problem 1

Recently bereaved widows have greater difficulty adjusting to the social problems of daily living than the literature on bereavement suggests. Most of the research and theory on bereavement deals with the phenomena of psychological adjustments to loss. Nurses need to know more about loss and grief. This study will add to the body of knowledge on loss and grief in widows.

Problem 2

Nurses are constantly interacting with patients who have suffered some form of loss—the death of a spouse or child, loss of a job, or loss of a limb. Most theories on loss are psychological explanations relating to grief or bereavement. Few studies have explored the relationship between a particular loss and the resulting daily social adjustments that must be made. Yet, a major area of nursing care is to assist the patient with problems of daily living and adjustment to the loss—not just to assist patients to cope psychologically without the lost object. Therefore, a study that focuses on the social adjustments to loss should provide nurses with some ways to assist the patient in adjusting to the social changes resulting from the loss. For this reason, this study will focus on the social adjustments of daily living that newly bereaved widows must make.

If you agree that Problem 2 makes the stronger statement, look at the structure of the problem again. Notice that it begins with a generalization and ends with a specific, from "loss" to "widows' daily adjustments to a loss." Then it builds to a climax, "Therefore, a study that focuses on . . ." and presents the final, irrefutable argument supporting the focus of this study. Finally, the problem deals with the usefulness of the data to be learned. The structure of the argument is maintained by listing concessions first and points in favor later. The movement in Problem 2 is from the problem area to the purpose of the study. In one paragraph, the skeletal outline for the entire research problem has been presented.

On the other hand, Problem 1 starts with the specific and ends with a generality; it makes the major point first and ends on a weak note. The same argument presented in Problem 1 is presented in Problem 2, but the ordering of the problem is different. Putting the strongest argument last leaves a stronger impression in the mind of the reader, who will have forgotten the first sentence by the end of the paragraph. The last sentence is the one the reader will remember, therefore, it should be the strongest.

Notice that Problem 2 is longer than Problem 1, even though both are single paragraphs. This result is due to the logic of the argument. When you begin your argument with your major point, it is difficult to create concessions and defenses afterward. If you start with the general problem, make concessions, and then build your defense from minor to major points, your argument is necessarily longer. But, because of its structure, you can easily check it to see that you haven't left anything out.

Read a good essay, article, or research report, and notice the way the author leads you from the general to the specific, from minor to major points, from concessions to defense. Remember that the advantage is always to the person who has the final, definitive argument.

Substantiate What You Say

By now, you should have your research question; a topic outline of your theories, concepts, or observations; working definitions of every major term in your question; and a one-paragraph statement of your entire problem area. In other words, you should have the skeleton of the final research problem for your written proposal. Before you proceed to write the full and final problem as an essay, however, you have one final area to check: your review of the literature. It is this step that substantiates your argument.

Look at Problem 2 again. Notice the sentences that begin with "Most theories on loss . . ." and "Few studies . . ." In your full and final problem, you can't get away with those statements just as they are. You have to justify those statements with facts. Here is where your review of literature comes in.

To be at this stage in your project where you have the skeleton for your final problem, you need to have done some reading. If you have bibliography cards or annotated references on everything you have read, you are now ready to build a case for your project.

Begin the process with your research question, which, after all, is the central point you are trying to make. Put it up somewhere in front of you so that you can refer to it frequently. Now reread your question. Which is the most central point you are trying to make in your question? Which is the topic of the question, the fulcrum around which all the rest of the question revolves? Underline that portion of the question. Take every other word or phrase and rank them under the central point in descending order of importance. Do your outline and definitions agree with this order? If not, look at your question again. Does it include your strongest argument? If not, you need to rewrite it. Your question must contain your strongest argument.

Now take your outline and arrange each point under the headings you made from your question. You are now restructuring your outline from the most relevant issues to the least relevant. You also have a reference for each point in your outline. Separate the pros and cons under each heading. Make sure that for each heading you have references both in favor of and against that point.

As you work with your question and your outline, you will begin to notice two things happening to your notes. One, you will find interesting, but irrelevant, pieces of information. Set those aside. You may need them later, but right now you are building your argument and don't need them. Second, you may find that some of your notes fit under more than one topic heading. That always happens. Cross-reference your topic headings so that you can easily find your notes. Sometimes a reading will give both the pros and cons for the subject. Don't throw them out. You can always use the same author or even the same reading in several different places.

You now have a topic outline of your problem from the strongest to weakest argument, with concessions and defense. And for each topic heading, you have a list of readings. Recheck your outline to see if there are any gaps in your argument. Does every heading in your outline have at least two contrasting subcategories? Does your argument include both pros and cons? Do you feel that you are an authority? Are you confident that you can defend your position from any point of view?

If you feel that you are being overwhelmed by reams and reams of paper, there is another way of developing the outline for your problem. Outline the central and substantiating areas of your question. Then sort or arrange your annotated references under the appropriate outline headings. Now sort or arrange each group of annotated references according to the major and minor points. Now place them under each heading according to the pros and cons. You now have your annotated references sorted into an outline.

If you sort or arrange your annotated references under each content heading, all you have to do as you begin your problem essay is to use your outline sorted as previously mentioned to develop your essay. This method saves wear and tear on your nerves and prevents the loss of any significant points you want to make.

The process of sorting or arranging your annotated references can be done by hand with handwritten pages or cards, or it can be done within a computer software program for word processing or referencing. These programs all offer you the opportunity to set up an outline for your project. The headings, previously described for your references, become the headings in the outline of your project.

The critical objective in this discussion is that you have ready references for every point you are making in developing your problem. You can quickly and easily substantiate your position with a quote, paraphrase, or reference to authors who have said things that back up what you have said. Because you have done your homework, you can make your point well—you have become an authority.

Bibliography

Chinn, P. L. (2008). *Integrated theory and knowledge development in nursing* (7th ed.). St. Louis, MO: Mosby Elsevier.

de Chesnay, M., & Anderson, B. A. (2008). *Caring for the vulnerable: Perspectives in nursing theory, practice and research.* Sudbury, MA: Jones and Bartlett.

Diers, D. (1971, November/December). Finding clinical problems for study. *Journal of Nursing Administration*, 15–18.

Flaskerud, J. H. (1984). Nursing models as conceptual frameworks for research. *Western Journal of Nursing Research, 6*, 153–155.

Hurley, B. (1978). Why a theoretical framework in nursing research? *Western Journal of Nursing Research, 1*(1), 28–41.

Martin, P. A. (1994). The utility of the research problem statement. *Applied Nursing Research, 7*(1):47–49.

McDonald, D., Monaco, A., Guo, R., Fiano, J., Matney, L., Turner, G., et al. (2009). The effect of personal relevance on learning stroke symptoms/ response. *Western Journal of Nursing Research, 331*(2), 141–152.

McEwan, M., & Mills, E. M. (2007). *Theoretical basis for nursing* (2nd ed.). Philadelphia: Lippincott Williams & Wilkins.

Meleis, A. I. (1997). *Theoretical nursing: Development and progress* (3rd ed.). Philadelphia: J. B. Lippincott.

Moody, L. E. (1990). *Advancing nursing science through research* (Vols. 1–2). Newbury Park, CA: Sage.

Musil, C., Warner, C., Zauszniewski, J., Wykle, M., & Sanding T. (2009). Grandmother caregiving, family stress and strain and depressive symptoms. *Western Journal of Nursing Research, 31*(3), 389–408.

Petty, R., Barden, J., & Wheeler, S. (2002). The elaboration likelihood model of persuasion health promotions that yield sustained behavioural change. In R. DiClemente, R. Crosby & M. Kegler (Eds.), *Emerging theories in health promotion practice and research. Strategies for improving public health*. San Francisco: Jossey-Bass.

Polit, D. F., & Beck, C. T. (2004). *Nursing research: Principles and methods* (7th ed.). Philadelphia: Lippincott.

Smith, M. C., & Stullenbarger, E. (1991). A prototype for integrative review and meta-analysis of nursing research. *Journal of Advanced Nursing, 16*(11), 1272–1283.

CHAPTER FOUR

Critical Review of the Literature

➤ TOPICS

Content of a Critique
What to Critique
How to Do a Critique
Guidelines for Critique of Published Research
Where Does the Critique Belong?
Bibliography

➤ LEARNING OBJECTIVES

- Describe the contents of a research critique.
- Understand how to do a good critique.

Although "literature" may conjure up romantic ideas that are the stuff of poems or novels, the term has a more limited focus when you are looking for information on your research topic and questions of interest. You will need to develop a search strategy to find relevant work that sheds light on your research area. Such a strategy will need to be both systematic and thorough to identify what you need to know. Although you may have burning questions that you would like to investigate, most people need to do a significant amount of reading to arrive at that stage. Whether or not you have arrived at a research question that you would like to pursue, you will need to find as much information about it as you can to learn what has and has not been undertaken by others. As you read, you will need to evaluate what you are reading and begin to integrate it into something meaningful that will help guide and direct your research.

A critical review of the literature does not necessarily imply criticism. It simply means taking an analytical approach to your reading. An analytical approach to any literature review implies purposive reading. You read the literature for a particular purpose. Because the ultimate aim of most research in nursing is to improve practice, a critical appraisal of the research literature is essential to evidence-informed practice. Thus, the first criterion for the critical review is *usability*, just as with research itself. Whether you plan to use the material for general background information or as a reference in your proposal, whether it is a research report or a theoretical one, it must have some practical value.

People often have less trouble determining the usability of theory than research. The theory feels right or explains something that is not fully understood. The usability of a research report is not as readily perceived. The findings may support your hypothesis, but whether or not you can use the report depends on your ability to understand the report and its conclusions.

Some feel defeated when asked to read research. "I just don't understand statistics," they say. But look again at the structure of the research plan. How much of the plan is statistical? Very little. The structure of the research report is exactly the same as that of the research plan, except that the report is written in the past tense. The statistics are only one part of research, and you can get help with statistics if you understand the rest of the report.

Another person will sigh and say, "But I just don't have a logical mind, so there's no point in my reading research." Nonsense. You may think differently from other people, but this doesn't make you illogical. Did it ever occur to you that perhaps the reason you couldn't understand the report was because the report was illogical? Just because research is published doesn't mean that it's well done or even well written. So don't decide you can't understand research until you've had a chance to evaluate the report.

Evaluating a research report for its usability is a simple matter of asking a series of questions. Research is usable only when the person who reads it knows its strengths and weaknesses on the basis of the critical review. The reader is also the person who will apply the findings. Applicability means more than use in further research. When reading research reports, look at your own professional practice—can this information be used in clinical practice, in educational settings, or in administrative functions?

When we know the side effects of a particular level of medication dosage, then we can reduce the amount if we wish to decrease the side effects. If we know that increased age affects length of convalescence, we can plan for longer periods of convalescence. If we know that nurses have difficulty providing care to certain types of patients, we can alter nurses' attitudes, patient type, or simply make everyone aware of the situation.

Finally, applicability means the use of research to further our knowledge base. Basic and applied research are both usable in nursing. Simply because research is usable does not make it applied. Basic research is also usable.

The second criterion for any research critique is *completeness*. The report must be comprehensive, addressing all your questions about the problem, the sample, the data collection technique, and the method of evaluating the data. As you read, are you still left with questions? Do you feel you don't quite understand the point being made? If so, the author probably left something out. A good way to check for completeness is to see if you can replicate the study. If you have to ask the author for more information, the report is incomplete.

Incomplete studies are easy to spot. Look for the key words: purpose, problem, hypotheses, definitions, sample, methods, analysis. Does the author give you complete information on each? Or are there omissions such as who forms the sample? Does the author mention only who is excluded? Does the author forget to tell you about the interview, if one was used? These and other gaps mean you cannot use the report as the basis for a similar research project, so its usability index goes down.

The third criterion of a critical review is *consistency*. Every area of the report must proceed logically. Can you follow the logical progression of ideas from problem to purpose, sample, data collection, analysis, and, finally, to the conclusions? Does the sample section follow from the problem? Is the data analysis consistent with the sample? Or were some of the research subjects thrown out without explanation? Whether you start with the conclusions and recommendations and read back or begin with the introductory matter, the relationship between each component of the research process needs to be clear and logical. If the report is inconsistent, it is incomplete and therefore not usable.

Your critique of the literature, therefore, is your analysis of its usability, completeness, and consistency. In your best judgment, and according to your own logic, you decide if what you have read will serve your purpose.

A final point needs to be made. Don't expect perfection! Nobody is perfect—not even published researchers. So don't throw the baby out with the bathwater when you are reading research. Evaluate the report with a critical eye. Look for ideas you can use; even a poor report might offer something useful. Look for ways to improve the research.

Content of a Critique

Despite everything you may have heard, read, or thought before, the purpose of a research critique is to determine whether the findings are usable for you. Because you are the person doing the reading, you decide whether you can use the research.

You may have noticed in your reading that some journals regularly publish a critical review or a critique along with the published research. These critiques are done by professionals who have an extensive understanding of research in the area. They bring up points and issues that may not have occurred to the average reader. These critiques have specific purposes because they (1) raise points that should be considered in further research on the problem, (2) provide an analysis of the entire research process for beginning researchers, and (3) offer information about one or more aspects of the research process that can be used by other researchers.

As a beginner, you are not expected to do such an extensive critique. But if you look over these critiques, you will observe that the same general questions are asked, and in the same order, as those discussed in the following pages. Only the detail is missing.

What to Critique

Unless a critique already has been presented in conjunction with a research report, you will be expected to critique every piece of research literature you read. Remember that you must be able to supply reasons for your choice of material and the way you use it in your proposal. Your critique should supply you with these reasons. No matter which aspect of your project you are attempting to substantiate with the literature, you will need a rationale for inclusion or exclusion of the relevant material. And your rationale is always based on your analysis of the literature.

Remember, all research is subject to a critique, including yours. The best research has been critiqued from the inception of the idea all the way through to the published report. But until you, the reader, have critiqued the report yourself, you have no way of knowing if it is, in fact, good research. Much of the information you need can be found in computer databases, such as CINAHL, MEDLINE, PsycINFO, Sociological Abstracts, Biological Abstracts, Dissertation Abstracts, and so forth. Search techniques often allow you to perform the same search on several databases. Identifying search terms is important, and don't hesitate to consult reference librarians because these individuals are intimately familiar with the headings that are indexed in various databases. Because you need to learn how to find articles relevant to your research question, librarians can be extremely helpful to you in doing so. However, they can't help you if you don't ask! Abstracts found in the databases often provide enough information to decide whether or not the article is usable. However, many databases now offer the full text of indexed articles. This allows you to review articles online as you search and can save you a great deal of time. With this in mind, let's move on to the actual technique of doing a research critique.

How to Do a Critique

There are several methods of doing a critique. Which one you choose depends on your background and experience. The more experienced you become in critiquing and the more you know about research, the more detailed you will become in your analysis. But when you are starting out, you simply need some basic guidelines to follow. You will be surprised at how adept you become at critiquing.

Before you make a decision about whether or not you can use an article, even before you read the paper all the way through, scan the conclusions and recommendations. Using your usability index, decide if you want to read the rest of the paper. If you can't use the findings or recommendations, you probably won't want to use the rest of the report. If you are looking for a particular research instrument, scan the section on methods or design to see if it is there. If you can't use the material, you will not be sufficiently interested in the full report to analyze its contents critically. So before you commit yourself to an article, scan it for usability and interest. A major failing in reported literature is the separation of the theoretical framework from the rest of the problem statement. It should be an integral part of the problem. When you see this format, separating the two, it is quite likely that the theoretical framework will prove to be meaningless for the study.

Another problem you may run into is the use of secondary sources in a literature review. If the secondary sources are inaccurate, then the current review will be as well. Always check original sources as the basis for a project.

After selecting an article, scan the entire article from beginning to end. Look for the key terms: problem, framework, purpose, design, sample, methods, findings, analysis, protection of human rights, and conclusions. They should be in approximately this order. Is each area of the report given a subheading that corresponds with each step in the research process? They usually aren't, in which case you should reread the report and highlight or underline each of the major topic headings on your copy of the article, whether online or on paper. If you cannot find a title to underline, then insert your own key term in the margin. This gives you an easy reference guide to all of the steps in the process.

Now scan the order of the headings. Do they follow the ordering you have learned? For example, can you find the introductory matter in the headings, or is it somewhere else? Whether you had to label the content yourself or the author provided the appropriate headings, you are looking for the logical progression of the material in the report.

Because you have a basic outline of the report's content, now look for gaps. Has any area been left out? Make a note of that to yourself. You may have missed it in your initial scan, or it may not be there. In either case, you will be looking for gaps and misplaced material as you continue your critique.

Now go back to the article and look at the section you have labeled as either the introduction or the problem. Read that section carefully and watch for three things: *clarity*, *significance*, and *documentation*. You will decide on the basis of these three items if the report is defective, substandard, or adequate.

A defective problem statement lacks clarity, significance, and documentation of earlier work. The writing style is ambiguous, unclear (you can't identify the point being made), and inconsistent. The research itself is meaningless, unsolvable, or trivial. Either the documentation is missing entirely or the references are incorrect. A substandard problem statement is either incomplete or unclear, of limited interest, or not fully documented. An adequate or standard problem statement, on the other hand, covers all the major research objectives. The writing style is clear. You know and understand what the research is about, and the progression of ideas is logical. The documentation of the problem seems to be reasonably complete and is used correctly. Finally, its significance is clear in that the problem needed solving and/or the results are reasonable.

To arrive at this evaluation of the problem, you must first identify it. If the author doesn't clearly label it, you must find it on your own, which means reading the report thoroughly. Use your outline of the article as your guide. If you find yourself reading about the sample or data collection, you have read beyond the problem. Go back to the introduction and look for the statement of the problem there. It might be stated as a question, a statement, or a hypothesis. You decide how well or how poorly it is stated—but first you have to determine what it is.

As you read this book, you are given certain rules of conduct about the research process and the writing of a proposal not found in previously published reports. In fact, some of the research articles you read will directly violate some of the principles you read here. Try to keep in mind that you are learning how to write a research proposal and how to plan a research project. The plan for the project and the final, written report do not always look the same.

A difference you may find between what you learn in this book and final, written research reports is the way in which the purpose of the study is written (see Chapter 5). Most published nursing research reports have hypotheses rather than purposes. You can find research reports with hypotheses at all levels of research design—some even write null hypotheses as the purpose of the study. No matter how the researcher has stated the purpose of the study, you need to determine whether or not the statement accurately reflects what you believe the research purpose to be.

The purpose of a study tells us the (1) aim of the study, (2) objective of the study, (3) intention of the study, (4) plan of the study, and (5) design of the study. Without a stated purpose for doing the study, we cannot know, for certain, what the study is about. We must guess or assume. The purpose of a study directs the researcher's and the reader's attention to what the study is about in one succinct statement. The purpose of a study follows the problem statement and, as such, is its culmination. After you have read the problem, the purpose should not come as a surprise to you. It tells you precisely what the study is about. In some research reports, the researcher will write both hypotheses and questions. This gives you a more specific idea of exactly what they are looking for in their research.

The discussion and conclusions in a research report must answer all the questions asked and tell you whether the hypothesis was supported or rejected and why. If there is no relationship between the stated purpose of a study and the conclusions, you have a faulty study. The purpose of the study tells the reader what the variables are and who the population is, and it indicates the methods or design used. If these three pieces of information cannot be extracted from a statement of purpose, it will be difficult for you, the reader, to critique the rest of the research report. For example, sometimes you will see a predictive hypothesis given as the basis for a descriptive study. We don't know if the hypothesis was really written before the study was conducted or if the hypothesis was written for the article after the researcher found some interesting things in a descriptive study.

When you read research studies with predictive hypotheses, look at each hypothesis and see if it incorporates a direct cause-and-effect relationship or a more remote cause-and-effect statement. If it is remote, then the assumptions linking one part to the other must be identified in the statement of the problem. Remember, predictive hypotheses are stated positively. A predictive hypothesis is also called the *research hypothesis*. A null hypothesis is stated in the negative indicating that there is no relationship between the variables. You learned about null hypotheses in statistics. People write a null rather than a research hypothesis at the beginning of a research report either because they don't know a research hypothesis is needed or they don't understand that the null hypothesis is the statistical hypothesis that is tested and is not normally written in the research report. You need to figure out for yourself what the researcher is trying to say.

The purpose of the study should be stated before a description of the study design is given. If you find the purpose hidden among the conclusions, the report is defective. If, on the other hand, the purpose is where it should be but is not as clearly expressed as it should be, the report is merely substandard. An adequate statement of purpose can be written as a question, a statement of relationships, or a hypothesis, but it must clearly describe what the study is all about.

Research designs are specific labels used by an author to designate a precise form of research process. The parts of the research design are the method of sampling, the process of data collection, and the method of data analysis. When the author of a research article labels the design, you can expect to see certain things in the research report. If you know what the author puts forward as the design, you can critique the study according to the author's statement. Sometimes the author is wrong and the editor of the journal and the reviewers are also wrong. The worst errors in design labels are in qualitative research approaches. Many authors and their reviewers mislabel their designs. The design of a study has a purpose and a direction. A research design is chosen because of the type of question the researcher asks and the level of knowledge about the topic to be studied.

Design choices should make logical sense. If you want to find out how people feel about things, an experiment is an illogical choice. If you want to find out what people do under certain circumstances, an interview or questionnaire is an illogical choice (they will tell you what they *think* they do, which is not the same thing at all). If you want to find out about the health of the population of a state or province, or even what the majority of that population thinks about healthcare cuts, interviewing a few nursing students at one school does not make sense. So the purpose of the study dictates the design, and the design dictates the sample, the methods of data collection, and the data analysis. Research must make logical sense.

In the same way as you addressed the problem, you will evaluate the research design as either defective, substandard, or adequate. You will be looking at the sample, the methods of data collection, and the analysis.

What do you need to know about sampling when you are reading a research report? First, you need to know the purpose of the sample. The general purpose of sampling is to represent the population as closely as possible. Samples are small portions of a population. A population is the group of people the researcher wanted to study. A *total population* is everyone in the world who meets the stated criteria. No researcher can possibly study a total population unless it is extremely small. A *target population* is the theoretically available group to whom the researcher wanted to generalize the results. Researchers usually sample from a theoretically available population to which they have access. This means that populations are (1) geographically available, (2) available by phone, (3) available through some address list, or (4) available through some secondary source. Usually, the researcher will report the way in which the sample represented the population from which it was drawn.

Next you need to ask, What is the size of the sample and what is its proportion of the population? Samples can range in size from one to thousands. They should be as large as possible given the time and resources of the researcher; given the amount of error the researcher is willing to accept (stated in the research report); and given the research design, which includes the number of variables being measured, the number of times each variable is measured, the type of variable being measured, and the type of measurement of each variable. How samples are selected will affect the sample size. The criteria for sample selection reflect the decisions made by the researcher on who will be included and who will be excluded from the study. Only those included in the study are said to represent the target population. The stated criteria, therefore, limit the generalizability of the findings to people having the same characteristics as the sample. If the purpose of the sample is not meant to statistically represent the population, then what is it meant to reflect? Next, you need to ask yourself, How was the sample selected? What were the criteria used for sample selection and what was the sampling procedure? Was it a probability or nonprobability sample?

Does the sample make sense in light of the research purpose? Samples should make sense in relation to the purpose of the study. Note the following:

- If there is no complete list of a population, a random sample is not possible.
- If each variable is measured many times, the sample can be smaller.
- If each member of the sample is measured only once, the sample should be larger.
- If the sample is measured with numerical measures, the sample should be larger.
- If the sample is measured with qualitative measures, the sample should be small.

Finally, as you review the research report, you will note the sampling procedure—whether the sample selection was through probability or nonprobability sampling. Probability sampling is recognized by terms such as the following:

Simple random sampling: Every member of the target population has a known probability of being included in the sample either through (1) a percentage of the population or (2) a predetermined number of subjects.

Stratified random sampling: Refers to the target population being stratified (divided) on some characteristic or variable. Equal numbers or percentages of subjects are drawn from each strata or group.

Cluster sampling: Refers to geographic stratification of the population.

Random assignment to groups: There are a preplanned number of subjects in each group. The method of assignment to groups is preestablished and, depending on the number of groups and the number of subjects in a group, can be established by computer assignment.

The second major sampling procedure is called *nonprobability sampling*, which includes *convenience* or *accidental* sampling (whoever is available and willing to be studied); *network samples* in which friends recruit friends into the sample; *quota samples* (also known as nonprobability stratified samples); and *systematic samples* in which every *n*th person or object is included. Systematic samples may have a random or a nonrandom start. All of these terms are discussed further in Chapter 8.

A defective sample does not represent the population in a logical manner. The sample may have nothing to do with the population. Or the sample may not be fully described. You may feel that the author selected a biased sample from the population. If the sample is meaningless, inconsistent with the problem, or biased, it is defective.

In a substandard sample, the author is unclear regarding either the population or the sample. The sample may be meaningful to the problem but not to the population. Or you may simply have a hunch that something is wrong within the sample.

An adequate sample is clearly specified, defined, and related to the particular population and problem being studied. It is representative of the population.

Data collection methods are based on the problem and the sample. Again, look for the clarity, significance, and documentation of the methods in relation to the adequacy of the report.

If the data collection methods have no relationship to the problem or the sample, or if they simply are not presented, they are defective. Phrases like an interview was conducted, a questionnaire was constructed, and available data were used are insufficient in themselves. Sometimes authors will actually use a method of data collection that is inappropriate to the labeled research design. This means either the author does not know the design or has simply failed to be clear. Remember, if you cannot use the information—if you cannot replicate the research on the basis of the information given—the report is defective.

Substandard methods give only partial information. You may have a general idea of what the author has done but not enough detail to use the information. If the author used a reference for the method, look that reference up. If the reference is unavailable from the usual sources and you have to write to the author, the report is inadequate. On the other hand, you may have full and complete information on the methods used, but you decide on the basis of your readings that only a partial or tentative solution can be achieved through this method.

An adequate or standard report on methods will tell you what, why, and how it was done in sufficient detail that you can make an informed decision about it. The method must be logically consistent with the problem and the sample. Look at the age of the report you are reading. Is it an old piece of research? Was any work done in that area prior to this research? If not, the relationship among the problem, sample, and method is critical. If the work is new, does the author rely on prior literature to establish the relationship among problem, sample, and methods? Or does the article deviate completely from established sequences? When the methods are irrelevant to the problem, the research is illogical and defective.

At this point in your critique, your analysis of data is rough and somewhat skimpy. Unless you understand statistics, you will have some difficulty with this part of the critique. Nevertheless, you should look at the clarity of the reporting style, the documentation of method, and the relationship between analysis and method.

Most research reports have tables of information, charts, and graphs. Can you find the sample adequately represented in the table? What about the methods—are they exemplified anywhere? If you were to develop an answer to the question based on the methods and sample, what would you include? See if the author has included this critical information.

A defective analysis does not answer the question that was asked. Such an analysis is unclear, ambiguous, unrelated to the data, or inconsistent with the rest of the research. A substandard analysis shows bias toward one aspect of the data over another or does not fully present an analytical tool. The adequate analysis, on the other hand, is comprehensible, responsive to the data, and congruent with all preceding material in the article.

Finally, you are ready to examine that aspect of the report that discusses the findings, conclusions, and usability of the research. You have read the report quite thoroughly to this point and can form an impression of the findings or conclusions. Are they clear? Relevant? Usable?

The findings and conclusions have to be generated from the research. If the researcher makes some assumptions or conclusions that have not been adequately substantiated elsewhere in the report, you may suspect bias. One small research project, as you know, will not solve global problems. So look for the type of generalizations made by the author. If they go too far beyond the research, the author probably is too egocentric. Or the conclusions might be too narrow or too specific. You are, after all, looking for some creativity from the researcher.

Defective conclusions are either too broad, too specific, or nonexistent. Substandard conclusions lack completeness. An adequate conclusion has a sense of finality and closure and is derived directly from the problem, and it accurately reflects the findings.

You now know this article backward and forward. You have an opinion of its value by the end of the report. Now let's see how objective that opinion is. Go back to the beginning of the report. Get out a pencil and paper. Start at the top left-hand side of the paper and list each of the major portions of the research report: *problem*, *sample*, *methods*, *analysis*, *findings* and *conclusions.* Across the top of the paper, list your headings: *defective, substandard,* and *adequate.* Now check off under which heading each section of the article falls. Add up the number of checks you have made in the *defective* column and multiply by 1. Add the checks in the *substandard* column and multiply by 2. Multiply the sum in the *adequate* column by 3. Total the scores. If you gave the report at least 12 points, it is adequate. If the report scored from 8 to 11, it is substandard. If the score falls below 8, you have a defective study.

Check your score against the impression you had after you had thoroughly analyzed the article. Do they agree, or is the score totally inconsistent with your impression? If they are similar, you have just verified the reliability of your perception. But, because feelings and impressions are not always reliable indicators of how good each aspect of the report is, use your objective scoring method until your feelings and the scores agree consistently.

Guidelines for Critique of Published Research _____

Another method of critiquing a published research report is to evaluate the study based on the following questions:

1. What is the research question on which the problem for this study is based? (Restate the question according to the level of design.) Is the problem clear and logically stated? Is it *appropriately* supported by the literature?

2. Research design:

   a. Sample: What is the target population? What are the criteria for inclusion? How is the sample selected? What is the sample size? Are these four elements of sample appropriate to this design? Was an appropriate power analysis provided?

   b. Methods: What are the variables under study? What methods were used to collect data for the study? Were issues of reliability and validity of measurement adequately addressed? Are the procedures adequately explained? Are the methods the most appropriate ones that could have been selected?

   c. Data analysis: Did the data analysis provide an answer to the research question? Is there sufficient power to support statements made about the relationship(s) between–among independent and dependent variables? Are the analysis techniques appropriate and properly conducted?

    d. Internal validity: Could there be an alternative explanation for the relationships observed (or not observed) among the variables? If so, what might these be?

    e. External validity: Would the findings be applicable to other settings, times, people, places?

3. Evidence-informed practice: How can the findings of this study be applied to nursing practice, nursing education, or nursing administration without further research? (Acknowledging that all studies are flawed, and assuming that this study is no more flawed than most, how could you see the results in practice? Remember that if we refuse to use the findings because there were flaws in the study, nursing practice will not move forward. Be specific about what can and cannot be implemented from this study.

4. What is the next logical research question that arises from this study? (Remember that all research raises more questions than it answers, and assume that the researcher will do replication studies.)

Where Does the Critique Belong?

It may surprise you to find out after all this work that the critique doesn't belong anywhere. The critique is a basic part of your development as an authority in this area of research. You won't find critiques at the end of research proposals as appendixes. You won't include your critique as part of your proposal. But you will use the results of your critiques throughout your research plan, data collection, analysis of data, and final written report. As specific entities, they don't belong anywhere. As a process critical to your development as a researcher, they belong everywhere all the time.

The process and the end result are different. Your critiques are a part of the process of building your proposal. Thus, you will cite either in your bibliography or in your list of references every adequate piece of research you have actually used to develop your proposal. You will reference inadequate or substandard reports only when they are all that is available, specifying how they were inadequate and why you used them anyway. To do all this with reasonable veracity, you must have thoroughly appraised what you read.

No one can, or will, do this for you; it is your responsibility. The results, however, are worth it.

Bibliography

Avis, M. (1994). Reading research critically. II. An introduction to appraisal: Assessing the evidence. *Journal of Clinical Nursing, 3*, 271–277.

Beyea, S. C., & Nicoll, L. H. (1997). Qualitative and quantitative approaches to nursing research. *AORN Journal, 66*(2), 323–325.

Carr, L. T. (1994). The strengths and weaknesses of quantitative and qualitative research: What method for nursing? *Journal of Advanced Nursing, 20*, 716–721.

Cooper, H. M., & Hedges, L. V. (1994). *The handbook of research synthesis.* London: Sage.

Coopey, M., & Nix, M. P. (2006). Translating research into evidence-based nursing practice and evaluating effectiveness. *Journal of Nursing Care Quality, 21*(3), 195–202.

Coughlan, M., Cronin, P., & Ryan, F. (2007). Step-by-step guide to critiquing research. Part 1: Quantitative research. *British Journal of Nursing, 16*(11), 658–663.

Cronin, P., Ryan, F., & Coughlan, M. (2008). Undertaking a literature review: A step-by-step approach. *British Journal of Nursing, 17*(1), 38–43.

Dickinson, F. (2004). Assessing the state of the art: Doing a literature review. *Midwifery Matters, 101*, 6–7.

Dornan, T., Peile, E., & Spencer, J. (2008). On "evidence." *Medical Education, 42*, 232–234.

Duffy, J. R. (2005). Critically appraising quantitative research [Electronic version]. *Nursing and Health Sciences, 7*(4), 281–283.

Dyer, I. (1997). The significance of statistical significance. *Intensive and Critical Care Nursing, 13*, 259–265.

Frame, K. (2003). Reading nursing research: Easy as ABCD. *Journal of School Nursing, 19*(6), 326–329.

Gerrish, K., Ashworth, P., Lacey, A., Bailey, J., Cooke, J., Kendall, S., et al. (2007). Factors influencing the development of evidence-based practice: A research tool. *Journal of Advanced Nursing, 57*(3), 328–338.

Giuffre, M. (1994). Reading research critically: Threats to internal validity. *Journal of Post Anesthesia Nursing, 9*(5), 303–307.

Giuffre, M. (1995). Reading research critically: Assessing the validity and reliability of research instrumentation—Part 1. *Journal of Post Anesthesia Nursing, 10*(1), 33–37.

Giuffre, M. (1995). Reading research critically: Assessing the validity and reliability of research instrumentation—Part 2. *Journal of Post Anesthesia Nursing, 10*(2), 107–112.

Harrell, J. A. (1995). Reading research reports: Should I apply the findings to my practice? *Tar Heel Nurse, 57*(2), 26–27.

Hek, G. (1996). Guidelines on conducting a critical research evaluation. *Nursing Standard, 11*(6), 40–43.

Hinshaw, A. S., & Schepp, K. (1984). Problems in doing nursing research: How to recognize garbage when you see it! *Western Journal of Nursing Research, 6*(1), 126–130.

Houser, J. (2008). *Nursing research: Reading, using, and creating evidence.* Sudbury, MA: Jones and Bartlett.

Lobiondo-Wood, G., & Haber, J. (2010). *Nursing research: Methods and critical appraisal for evidence-based practice* (7th ed.). St. Louis, MO: Mosby.

Loiselle, C. G., & Profetto-McGrath, J. (2007). Canadian essentials of nursing research (2nd ed.). Philadelphia: Lippincott and Williams.

Luker, K. (2007). Assessing the quality of research: A challenge for nursing. *Nursing Inquiry, 14*(1), 1.

Miracle, V. A. (2004). Making sense of conflicting research findings. *Dimensions of Critical Care Nursing, 23*(5), 230–233.

Mulrow, D. (1994). Systematic reviews: Rationale for systematic reviews. *British Medical Journal, 309*, 597–599.

Norbeck, J. (1978). The research critique: A theoretical approach to skill development and consolidation. *Western Journal of Nursing Research, 1*(4), 296–306.

Summers, S. (1991). Defining components of the research process needed to conduct and critique studies. *Journal of Post Anesthesia Nursing, 6*(1), 50–55.

Supino, P. G., & Borer, J. (2007). Teaching clinical research methodology to the academic medical community: A fifteen-year retrospective of a comprehensive curriculum. *Medical Teacher, 29*, 346–352.

Volmink, J., Siegfried, N., Robertson, K., & Gulmezoglu, A. M. (2004). Research synthesis and dissemination as a bridge to knowledge management: The Cochran Collaboration. *Bulletin of the World Health Organization, 82*(10), 778–783.

CHAPTER FIVE

Stating the Purpose of the Study

➤ TOPICS

Level I: The Purpose Written as a Declarative Statement
Level II: The Purpose Written as a Question
Level III: The Purpose Written as a Hypothesis
Examining the Components of a Hypothesis
The Significance of the Statement of Purpose
Stating the Purpose of the Study: A Summary
Bibliography

➤ LEARNING OBJECTIVES

- Describe how the statement of purpose relates to the question at all three levels.
- Outline the components of a hypothesis.
- Understand the significance of the statement of purpose.

You might wonder why you must state the purpose of the study when the question has already been developed into the problem and supported through logical argument? Of what use is a statement of purpose?

The research question itself directs the development of a research proposal, yet the question often does not appear in the final proposal. It leads instead to the development of the purpose of the study. The question becomes the purpose. If the purpose is clearly written, it says exactly what you intend to do to answer your question. The purpose first includes what you will do to collect data (for example, observe and describe, listen and describe) or what variable you will observe or measure (for example, age, occupation, self-image). Second, it includes some information about where the data will be collected (the setting of the study). Third, the purpose should identify the subjects of the study. The stated purpose of a study comes after the written research problem and is a normally stated as a one-sentence encapsulation of your proposed study. The question you wrote initially included what you were going to study (your study variables) and who you were going to study (your population). The statement of the purpose of the study expands on the question to include where, when, and sometimes how.

The statement of purpose, therefore, includes what and who you plan to study, plus where, when, and how you plan to do the study. The what, where, when, and who of the purpose are stated in such a way that the research design follows logically.

The three ways of stating the purpose of a study are (1) a declarative statement, (2) a question, and (3) a hypothesis.[1] The appropriate method depends on the level of the question and the extent of the existing knowledge about the problem.

Level I: The Purpose Written as a Declarative Statement _____

When your knowledge about the research topic is limited because little or no research has been done, your study will focus on a search for information. At the simplest and most basic level, your initial question begins with what. These questions are exploratory. For example:

> What are the behaviors exhibited by mothers and infants during the first week of the infant's life?
>
> What are the characteristics of nursing students who fail state board examinations?

Because these questions have a what stem, we can assume there is either no literature available that answers the specific question, no theory to explain it, or no previous research on which to base a study. Therefore, to answer these questions requires an exploration of the topic in great depth and detail. Instead of starting with concepts and a conceptual framework, you will develop concepts as your end product. Now, how does the statement of purpose differ from the original question?

---

[1] The idea for stating the purpose depending on the level of the study was adapted from Wandelt (1970). Wandelt related these differences to the level of knowledge and available theory about the topic.

The statement of purpose states exactly what you intend to do, and where and when you intend to do it and with whom, to answer the question. Purposes written as declarative statements always result in description.

The question, What are the ambient levels of noise in neonatal intensive care units (NICUs), and what factors contribute to these levels? (Darcy, Hancock, & Ware, 2008) exemplifies the type of Level I question that had to be explored and described to understand whether or not noise is present in the environment where premature infants receive care. If ambient sound levels exceed those designated as safe by the American Academy of Pediatrics and the Environmental Protection Agency, patients may be being exposed to harmful physiological effects of noise as documented in the literature. In that premature infants lack fully developed neurosensory systems, it has been suggested that exposure to continuous and unpredictable noise can interfere with this developmental process.

This study is an important first step in determining the nature of the care environment in NICUs. Without the knowledge and understanding of the results of this study, namely that there were excessive levels of noise in the ambient environment of the NICUs studied and the nurses' perceptions of its causes, it would not be possible to develop a plan to control for high levels of noise.

A possible next step might be the development of a comparison between the impact of sound levels upon the heart rate and blood pressure of premature infants being cared for in control NICUs, where steps were employed to reduce levels of ambient sound, with several standard NICUs, where acoustic levels were not subject to such control measures. In developing measures to control acoustic levels, the perceptions of nurses relative to the causes of the high levels of sound in the original study would be used.

The exploration of the nature of the acoustic environment may lead to the emergence of new concepts, but no predictions are possible from this kind of data, only descriptions and classifications. Therefore, the purpose states what the study will describe, including what will be done, where, when, and with whom.

The next question, What are the characteristics of nursing students who fail state board examinations? came from a nurse educator who had been puzzled about why some students fail and others do not. She, the teacher, did not know enough about the characteristics of those students to ask a Level III why question. Although theories existed to explain failure among students, the nursing students did not seem to fit those theories. No description could be found of students who failed state boards.

The appropriate purpose of this study, therefore, is to explore and describe. The purpose would be stated as follows:

> The purpose of this study is to describe the characteristics of generic nursing students at X School of Nursing who failed state licensing board examinations between 2005 and 2010.

The setting and the sample are described briefly in general terms; specifics are given later in the proposal. All Level I statements of purpose are written exactly the same way because their purpose is always to provide a description.

Sometimes, Level I studies are explorations of a single process or single process variables with the express intent of exploring the variable in depth and describing the process as completely as possible. These studies all begin with a what question on one variable or one concept, such as coping strategies, or other social–psychological processes that have not previously been described in the population of interest. For example:

> The purpose of this study is to identify and describe the social–psychological processes nurses use in a Level III neonatal intensive care unit (Hutchinson, 1986).

Often studies at this level will look at a single concrete variable in a population under two different circumstances. First, the variable may have been studied before in other populations but not in the present one. Second, the population may be well known, but the variable has been unexplored. For example, many studies have documented the behaviors of people dying of cancer. However, the efforts of dying people to prepare family members for life without them may not have been studied. This is an unexplored variable. In another case, a variable that is well studied, such as coping mechanisms, may not have been examined in certain populations, such as military families. These situations are both appropriate cases for Level I studies.

Level II: The Purpose Written as a Question

When you know what you will be observing but cannot predict the findings, your purpose is stated as a question. How much knowledge is enough but not too much? How can you tell if your study should be at this level? Let's look at some sample questions:

> What is the relationship between age and rate of learning in autotutorial settings?

> What is the relationship between ethnicity and suicide rate?

These questions start with concepts about which the researcher obviously has some knowledge because the question asks about relationships between concepts or among ideas within a concept. The immediate difference between these questions and the exploratory kind is that these begin with a concept.

The concepts from which the first question emerges are maturation and learning. These concepts have to be discussed during the development of the problem to clarify the frame of reference. You know that the concept of maturation was based on Erikson's stages of development, and the concept of learning stemmed from stimulus–response theory. However, nothing in the literature gives any basis for predicting the effect of maturation on learning; therefore, the question asks, What is the relationship?

This question raises another point. Maturation was described in such a way that the age of the individual represents the level of maturation. Other aspects of maturation that might be measured by psychological or physiological variables are not considered in this study.

One of the effects of the statement of purpose is that it limits the study. This prevents you from being sidetracked. Therefore, the statement of purpose should be as specific as possible to make the rest of the proposal easier to develop.

The purpose of the study derived from a Level II question would look like this:

> The purpose of this study is to answer the question, Is there a significant relationship between age and rate of learning pharmacology among staff nurses in an autotutorial program at the Queens Hospital?

The difference between this purpose, written as a question, and the initial research question is that the answer will be yes or no as determined by the data. Because the significance of the findings will also be determined, the answer to this level of question always requires statistical analysis. This level of purpose leads to a descriptive design, but one that is testing the relationship between two known variables, rather than exploring the unknown as was the declarative statement.

Let's look at another example of purpose stated as a question.

What is the relationship between ethnicity and suicide rate?

This question deals with two concepts: ethnicity and suicide. Both may be studied alone or in combination with other variables. In this case, they are being examined together to determine if they vary together. The question is a simple one, asking if ethnic groups differ with regard to suicide rate. The literature tells you that in traditional Japanese society, hara-kiri or seppuku was practiced as an honorable form of death for a warrior. You might speculate, therefore, that the Japanese American would have a higher suicide rate than other groups if traditional values about suicide were retained. Other ethnic groups might have different values that would affect suicide rates. This is an appropriate question for Level II, and the purpose would be stated as follows:

> The purpose of this study is to answer the question, Is there a signifi-cant relationship between ethnicity and rate of suicide among adults between the ages of 30 and 60 years in X community in 2010?

The answer will be that there is, or is not, a statistically significant dif-ference in the suicide rates among ethnic groups in X community.

As a statement of purpose at Level II, your question changes from What is the relationship? to Is there a significant relationship? Why couldn't you have written your question this way in the first place? The reason is a matter of emphasis. First, notice the difference between the three levels of questions: (1) what? (2) what is the relationship? and (3) why? Questions 1 and 2 begin with what because they are descriptive studies. When the purpose of the study is stated, however, it is written differently because it evokes a different answer. As a final example of the difference between the original question and the final statement of purpose, notice the difference in the complexity of the two.

Level II Question

What is the relationship between a patient's length of stay and the need for social support of the patient's significant others?

Level II Statement of Purpose

The purpose of this study is to answer the question, Is there a statistically significant relationship between a critical care patient's length of stay in an adult medical, surgical, coronary, or combined intensive care unit and the need for social support of significant others at the University of Iowa Hospitals and clinics, VAMC, and Mercy Hospital in Iowa City?[2]

At Level I you cannot predict the answer because you will explore a new area of research. At Level II, however, you know exactly what the content of the answer will be because the purpose has limited the scope of the

---

[2] Margo Halm, graduate student, University of Iowa.

study. The statement of purpose at Level II specifically excludes everything except the variables to be studied. The description provided by the answer will be narrow in focus and will describe the statistical relationship between the variables. When you originally asked the question at Level II, you were not sure if this relationship was already known. Asking a What is the relationship? question emphasizes the descriptive nature of Level II studies and facilitates searching the literature for related studies. It leaves the issue of prediction for Level III.

Look back at the questions and purposes on pages 82–84. Note that two of the variables are age and ethnicity. Both variables are mentioned first in their individual questions, and both can be assumed to come first in time; we may even be able to predict that as age increases, the rate of learning will also increase. So why are we maintaining that these are Level II questions? Why not Level III? The reason is very simple. All Level II studies are descriptive studies—they are designed to describe the relationship among variables—and all Level III studies are experimental studies in which the investigator manipulates the independent variable. Neither age nor ethnicity can be directly manipulated by the investigator. You can create a sample based on different age groups or different ethnic groups, but this is not manipulation—actually changing something. You can change the temperature of water, you can show different movies, you can teach different content using different techniques, but you can only observe the effects of age and observe the effects of ethnicity as they occur naturally. You cannot age a person, and you cannot change his or her ethnic identity—these are inherent human qualities that are not amenable to experimental manipulation.

It is equally impossible to do Level III studies when manipulation of the independent variable might cause harm to the subject. Even if you know a great deal about a disease process, you cannot (ethically) cause that disease in human beings to have a Level III study. The best you can do at Level III is a laboratory experiment using tissue cultures or animal subjects. These studies are difficult to generalize to human subjects. Although you may know a great deal about the variable and its effects, you cannot write the question or study it at Level III with humans.

Level III: The Purpose Written as a Hypothesis

When you have enough information to predict the outcome of your study and you intend to test the significance of your prediction, your question is stated at Level III as a hypothesis.

A hypothesis is simply an assertion of a specific relationship between two or more variables. Hypotheses are possible only in studies based on conceptual or theoretical frameworks. They are supported by an argument developed during the definition of the problem. Although hypotheses are sometimes referred to as hunches, in reality they are carefully thought out proposals that can be supported by theory and previous research.

The term *hypothesis* in this text is used interchangeably with predictive hypothesis, in which the exact relationship between two variables is predicted. A predictive hypothesis specifies which variable is the cause and which is the effect, or which is independent and which is dependent. We believe the predictive hypothesis is preferable to the simple statement of a relationship between two variables found in some literature, such as, There is a relationship between gender and successful weight loss among dieters. The latter sounds like a statement of fact and may lead the researcher to feel that the point has been proved before the study has been done. We believe that predictive hypotheses are precise statements of relationships that should not be made unless they can be supported through the literature. If you cannot predict the direction of the relationship, go back to Level II to identify and describe it first.

Hypotheses are predictions of causal relationships between variables that must be tested. At this level of study, your focus becomes quite narrow. At Level III, the independent variable or cause is the one that you, the researcher, manipulate. You are fully responsible for this variable because it is under your full control. Without a good idea of what the result will be, it is unethical to inflict your independent variable on people. The result is the dependent variable. That is why predictive hypotheses must be developed from previous research findings and from the theoretical answer to the why question. There is always a great deal of information available about the variables in Level III studies. Without sufficient data, it would be impossible to predict cause-and-effect relationships. Consider the following Level II question:

> What is the relationship between ethnicity and suicide rate in Los Angeles County in the year 2009?

The answer is that Japanese Americans had a significantly lower incidence of suicide in Los Angeles than any other ethnic group.

A search of the literature, however, did not reveal a theory to explain this finding; therefore there is not enough information to write a predictive hypothesis that would meet ethical guidelines. Likewise, you could not ethically manipulate ethnicity and suicide in an experimental design.

Here is another finding from a Level II study:

Nurses who work for 10 years or more in long-term psychiatric facilities are significantly more authoritarian (as measured on an authoritarianism scale) than are medical–surgical nurses who work for the same length of time.

Think about the two variables in this study. If you asked why the relationship exists, you would have difficulty predicting a cause or effect from the answer. Which is the causal variable? We don't know which came first, authoritarianism or choice of psychiatric nursing. Does the psychiatric setting foster authoritarianism, or does authoritarianism influence the choice of nursing specialty? When your knowledge is still too general to predict exactly how one variable influences another, you are not ready to write a predictive hypothesis.

Extensive research and theory on teaching and learning by nurses have been effectively used in the clinical setting. You can predict, for example, that any structured teaching program is more effective than no teaching program for all patient populations and for all types of knowledge. Because there has been extensive research on these theories, they can be safely tested on patient populations. Varying levels of prediction are possible, however, based on the level of knowledge gained from patient teaching studies. For example, take the following hypothesis:

Diabetic patients who receive structured group teaching about their diabetes will have a significantly lower readmission rate than will diabetic patients who receive standard teaching on a nursing unit.

In this situation, you are trying to demonstrate that there is a direct relationship between structured teaching and readmission rates on the basis of a series of assumptions: structured teaching improves knowledge, which improves understanding, which improves adherence, which improves health, which decreases the need for hospitalization. The predictive hypothesis was written to indicate that the investigator knew about teaching–learning theory and was applying it to a specific patient population. You can see from the hypothesis that only structured versus unstructured teaching and readmission rates will be measured in the diabetic studies. The assumptions themselves are not being tested in this study. They are accepted as true. If you cannot support these assumptions through the research literature, you need to go back and test each one before measuring the effect of teaching on readmission rates. When you write a predictive hypothesis, you need to be able to list the assumptions underlying the prediction you have made regarding your independent and dependent variables. These assumptions are then supported in your theoretical framework.

Because each investigation builds on previous results, each subsequent patient teaching study should become more precise than the previous one. Precision, in this case, means a narrower focus on patient teaching. When you have established that structured teaching affects other variables, such as readmission rate, you refine structured teaching into narrower units, such as contrasting group teaching with individual teaching or comparing multimedia instruction with a lecture format. The hypothesis would be written like this:

> Patients who receive structured group teaching will have a significantly higher level of knowledge than patients taught by any other method.

To test this general hypothesis, a series of more specific hypotheses are written:

- Patients who receive structured group teaching will score higher on the posttest than patients who receive standard teaching on a nursing unit.
- Patients who receive structured group teaching will score higher than patients who receive structured individual teaching.

You might consider a series of teaching strategies to test the question, Is structured group teaching more effective because of the teaching strategy or simply because the teaching is structured? Hypotheses could be written to test specific teaching techniques, such as the use of videotape versus lecture, videotape versus printed material, or other combinations of teaching methods.

To carry this study further, assume you found that structured teaching plus interpersonal interaction produced better learning. Now you want to find out if knowledge about diabetes affects patients' adherence to the treatment prescribed after discharge. Your hypothesis would read like this:

> Patients with greater knowledge of diabetes will have a significantly higher rate of adherence to the treatment regimen upon returning home than patients with lesser knowledge of diabetes.

As you can see, with these predictive hypotheses you always provide at least one comparison group. Your specific hypothesis includes a prediction for what will happen to each set of comparison groups.

An entirely different study could begin with the following general hypothesis:

In hospitals where nurses have received assertiveness training, the nosocomial infection rate will be significantly lower than in hospitals where nurses have not received that training.

In this situation you assumed that assertiveness training produces assertive nurses, that assertive nurses will be more likely to demand that their patients' visitors follow rules of cleanliness, and that following rules of cleanliness leads to fewer nosocomial infections.

Once again, this example consists of a chain of assumptions or connections to explain the cause-and-effect relationship between nurses' assertiveness and hospital infections, which are not directly tested in this study. Support is either found for each of these assumptions in the research literature or it will be necessary to test each assumption before embarking on the study as proposed. The first step would be to test the effectiveness of assertiveness training in producing assertive nurses. The next step would be to test the relationship between assertiveness and patient protectiveness. In this case, the hypothesis might read as follows:

Nurses who receive an assertiveness training program will have a significantly higher patient protectiveness rating than those who do not receive the training.

At this point, you may find you can support the rest of your assumptions from your own previous research findings or from the published research literature. In other words, you are able to demonstrate that patient protectiveness leads to following rules of cleanliness and that good aseptic technique reduces the incidence of nosocomial infections. Now you are ready to test directly the relationship between assertiveness and nosocomial infections in the first hypothesis:

In hospitals where nurses have received assertiveness training, the nosocomial infection rate will be significantly lower than in hospitals where nurses have not received that training.

Depending on the level of knowledge about a topic and the amount of research that has preceded your work, the specificity of your hypothesis will vary. In studies based on physiological measures, for example, the hypotheses are very specific. Nursing research on human behavior is generally less specific. The following hypotheses were written for a study to test the effect of ice water on the blood pressure and pulse rate of healthy subjects (Siegel & Sparks, 1980):

> Subjects who consume ice water will have significant increases in systolic and diastolic blood pressure and pulse rate compared to the same subjects who consume comparable volumes of room temperature tap water.

To test this general hypothesis, the following specific hypotheses were developed:

- Subjects who ingest 240 cc of ice water within 5 minutes will have a significant increase in systolic blood pressure compared with the same subjects who consume 240 cc of room temperature water within 5 minutes.
- Subjects who ingest 720 cc of ice water within 10 minutes will have a significant increase in systolic blood pressure compared with the same subjects who consume 720 cc of room temperature water within 10 minutes.

These hypotheses were repeated using diastolic blood pressure and pulse rate as the dependent variables. As you can see, three independent variables were tested: amount of water, temperature of water, and time taken to drink the water. There were three dependent variables, as well: systolic blood pressure, diastolic blood pressure, and pulse. The investigators were interested in grouping these independent variables in different ways to test their influence on the three dependent variables. This study could have been carried on until all possible combinations of the three independent variables had been exhausted.

Examining the Components of a Hypothesis

Because Level III studies are designed to test theory, the way the hypothesis is written will greatly affect the study design. Writing the hypothesis correctly will save effort later.

The way hypotheses are written is similar to that of the examples we have considered in the preceding pages. For example:

> Nurses who receive assertiveness training will have significantly higher patient protectiveness ratings than those who do not receive the training.

The first clause of a hypothesis will identify both the sample and one position of the independent variable. In the previous hypothesis, this clause is "nurses who receive assertiveness training." Nurses is the sample, and receiving assertiveness training is one position of the independent variable.

The next clause specifies the direction the dependent variable is expected to take as a result of the independent variable. In the example, this clause is "will have significantly higher patient protectiveness ratings." The dependent variable is patient protectiveness ratings, and the direction in which it is expected to change is significantly higher. The last clause of the hypothesis provides the other position of the independent variable. In this case, "those who do not receive the training" specifies the group that will provide the comparison as another position of the independent variable.

A well-written hypothesis will contain all three clauses. The first describes the experimental group, the second specifies the expected result, and the third describes the comparison group. Here is another example:

Clause 1: Subjects who ingest 720 cc of ice water within 10 minutes

Clause 2: will have a significant increase in systolic blood pressure

Clause 3: compared with the same subjects who consume 720 cc of room temperature water within 10 minutes.

Dividing your hypothesis into three components and checking that each component includes the necessary information will make writing the hypothesis easier.

The Significance of the Statement of Purpose

When your statement of purpose has been written as a declarative statement, question, or hypothesis, your decision about where your question belongs in the research literature, as well as the degree of sophistication of the study, is final. You are now committed to a particular plan of action.

Stating the Purpose of the Study: A Summary

1. The purpose of a study should include:

   a. What you intend to do to collect the data

   b. Where you intend to collect the data

   c. Who are the subjects of the data collection

2. Purposes can be written as statements, questions, or hypotheses.

3. Writing the purpose as a statement (Level I questions):

Example: The purpose of this study is to explore and describe the value orientations of Hutterite women in western Canada.

Example: The purpose of this study is to explore and describe coping strategies used by intensive care nurses.

4. Writing the purpose as a question (Level II questions):

Example: The purpose of this study is to answer the question, Is there a significant relationship between perception of postoperative pain and length of convalescence among abdominal surgery patients at Waverly Hospital in eastern Oregon?

Example: The purpose of this study is to answer the question, Is there a significant relationship among health problems, health services sought, and types of abuse among battered women in Pennsylvania?

5. Writing the purpose as a hypothesis (Level III questions):

To write the purpose as a hypothesis, you need to include three clauses:

   a. The first clause gives the first position of the independent variable plus the sample.
   b. The second clause gives the dependent variable.
   c. The third clause gives the second (contrast) position of the independent variable.

The research hypothesis (written as the purpose of the study) is always written positively. The null hypothesis (there will be no relationship between the independent and dependent variables) is used only for statistical data analysis purposes.

Example: The purpose of this study is to test the following hypothesis: Nurses who receive assertiveness training will have significantly higher patient protectiveness ratings than nurses who do not receive assertiveness training.

Example: The purpose of this study is to test the following hypothesis: Decubitus ulcers treated with topical regular insulin will have a significantly faster rate of healing than decubitus ulcers treated with any other method.

Example: The purpose of this study is to test the following hypothesis: Persons with Type II diabetes who have a greater knowledge of their disease will have a significantly higher rate of adherence to the treatment regimen than persons with lesser knowledge of their disease.

Bibliography

Brockopp, D. Y., & Hastings-Tolsma, M. (2003). *Fundamentals of nursing research* (3rd ed.). Sudbury, MA: Jones and Bartlett.

Darcy, A. E., Hancock, L. E., & Ware, E. J. (2008). A descriptive study of noise in the neonatal intensive care unit ambient levels and perceptions of contributing factors. *Advances in Neonatal Care, 8*(3), 165–175.

Hutchinson, S. A. (1986). Creating meaning: Grounded theory of NICU nurses. In W. C. Chenitz & J. M. Swanson (Eds.), *From practice to grounded theory: Qualitative research in nursing* (p. 192). Menlo Park, CA: Addison-Wesley.

Larson, R., & Farber, B. (2002). *Elementary statistics: Picturing the world* (2nd ed.). Upper Saddle River, NJ: Prentice Hall.

Lobiondo-Wood, G., & Haber, J. (2010). *Nursing research: Methods and critical appraisal for evidence-based practice* (7th ed.). St. Louis, MO: Mosby.

Polit, D. F., & Beck, C. T. (2004). *Nursing research: Principles and methods* (7th ed.). Philadelphia: Lippincott.

Siegel, M. A. & Sparks, C. (1980). The effect of ice water ingestion on blood pressure and pulse rate in healthy young adults. *Heart and Lung. 9*(2), 306-309.

Wandelt, M. (1970). *Guide for the beginning researcher*. New York: Appleton-Century-Crofts.

CHAPTER SIX

Defining Your Terms

➤ TOPICS

Types of Variables
Defining the Independent Variable
How Variables Are Measured
Terms That Need Definition
Writing Operational Definitions: A Review
Bibliography

➤ LEARNING OBJECTIVES

- Define operational definitions.
- Differentiate independent from dependent and intervening variables.
- Discuss the types of scales for measurement of variables.
- Choose an appropriate scale for your variables.
- Understand how the definition and measurement of variables relates to the level of the question.

Because the research question is the guiding force behind a research project, there must be links at every stage of research that all stem from the question. One such link is created when you define the terms in your question. Often the terms we use can mean many different things, but now is the time to put into words just what you mean by the terms in your question. You will then be able to cast away all the other meanings you might have chosen, but did not, and focus in on exactly what you want to study.

In our discussion about writing a research question, the question was divided into its component parts: the stem question and the topic. The stem question directs the research process, and the topic is the actual focus of the study. The same stem and topic are then used to formulate the purpose of the study. The literature review is done in relation to the topic—who has studied it, what was said about it, how the variables were measured, and whether or not the variables you are using have been put together in the same way before. The information you find on the topic helps you to determine the exact purpose of your study. Now you need to be more precise about the variables themselves.

Recall that we defined a variable as anything that varies or any property that takes on different values. Before you can define your variables, you must decide exactly what you want to know. Suppose you are interested in anxiety. You know that anxiety can be short term or long term, acute or chronic, normal or abnormal, perceived by an observer or reported by an individual, manifest or latent, mild or severe. The aspect of anxiety in which you are interested and the ways in which it varies is what you want to measure. The aspect of anxiety that you measure and the method you use constitute its operational definition. Operational definitions describe what you are going to measure and how you will measure it. The process of developing operational definitions involves deleting all aspects of the variable except those in which you are interested and then specifying how it will be measured.

As an example, your definition of anxiety might read, vague feelings of alarm that persons report when faced with a stressful situation; or it could read, behavioral manifestations of persons subjected to stress, which can be identified by grimaces, muscle tensing, and palmar sweating. Still another definition might say, a trait possessed by all persons to some degree, which is reflected in their responses to questions about their view of life in general.

Each definition measures a completely different concept of anxiety. The first measures people's reports of how they feel. The second measures an observer's perception of the individual's behavior. The third requires that the researcher infer how the individual feels from his or her responses to questions. None of these is a perfect measure; none is better than the others; however, one of these may seem to be a good fit for what you want to know about anxiety. If not, you will want to look at other ways to define it.

Your operational definition must specify what you want to study and how you want to study it, and nothing more.

During the development of the problem, you dealt with the whole realm of literature and theory about anxiety. You decided which frame of reference you wanted to assume. Now you must eliminate everything except that which fits your frame of reference and represents what you will be measuring. In other words, the operational definition isolates the central component of the variable under study and excludes all other components of that variable.

Theoretically, your operational definitions can be anything you want them to be, as long as they are consistent with your conceptual–theoretical framework (if you have one). They should have logical, empirical meaning and should define your concepts explicitly and precisely. In addition, they should relate directly to the theory on which they are based.

For example, Halbesleben et al. (2008) defined nurse burnout as psychological response to work-related stress, consisting of emotional exhaustion, depersonalization or pulling away from those associated with the job, and a belief that one is not as good at the job as one formerly was. Burnout was measured by the Maslach Burnout Inventory (Halbesleben et al., 2008, p 365). This operational definition clearly specifies the definition of the concept and puts it into the context of the theoretical framework of the study, which proposes that the negative impact of burnout is that nurses with burnout are less likely to invest energy in new nurse–patient relationships, and this can adversely affect patient care.

Operational definitions of terms, therefore, first define the term and then state how the term will be studied in this particular research project. Just as the definition is written in the context of the study, so is the operationalization of the definition. Usually, your operationalization refers to the method you will use to collect the data on that variable and can be either a single method or multiple methods. Let's say you wanted to study patients' attitudes toward bed baths. You know that such attitudes are feelings, beliefs, or ideas about bed baths, but how do you intend to find out about those feelings? Generally you will ask patients about their attitudes. But you can ask directly or in a questionnaire—either one is appropriate. Your operationalization of attitudes is to state whether you plan to interview or use a questionnaire.

Similarly, if you are studying stress, you can operationalize your definition by using an interview, questionnaire, observations, or even physiological measures such as blood pressure, urinalysis, or pulse rate. But however you decide to study stress, state it briefly as the operational part of your operational definition of the term. And that's what is meant by an operational definition of terms: (1) what you intend to study, specifically, and (2) how you intend to study it.

The rest of this chapter will focus on how precisely you want to study or measure your terms and what these terms mean. If your study is at Level I, you will be doing an exploratory or descriptive study, and your findings will describe your variable in great detail. At Level I you are not concerned with precision of measurement. But, as you proceed through Level II and Level III studies, the requirement for precision of measurement increases, so that at Level III your operationalization must be precise and clear.

Here is how it works.

After completing the literature review on your topic and learning all you can about your variable(s), you made your final decision as to the level of knowledge about the topic and the level of design you were determined to use. On the basis of this decision making, you wrote the purpose of your study as a statement (Level I), as a question (Level II), or as a hypothesis (Level III). From your review of literature and your statement of the purpose of your study, you are now ready to develop operational definitions of terms for your variables, concepts, or topics.

> Level I: The purpose of this study is to explore and describe the reasons parents give for taking their children to alternative healthcare centers for treatment of leukemia.

In this purpose, the variable you need to define is reasons. The rest of the purpose is either the sample or the dependent clause describing reasons. But your study is about people's reasons for their behavior. Therefore, you will need to define what you mean by reasons, in the context of the rest of the purpose. For the preceding study you may define reasons as statements made by parents to explain their process of decision making in relation to their child's health care. To operationalize this definition, you simply need to add how you intend to elicit those statements. The operational definition then becomes statements made by parents to explain their process of decision making in relation to their child's health care as elicited by a semistructured interview. Another example might be:

> Level I: The purpose of this study is to explore and describe the types of medication errors made by medication nurses at Mercy Hospital.

Here you will define what you mean by types of medication errors and how you intend to measure them. You could say that types of medication errors are descriptions of a situation in which a medication was given to a patient, later discovered to be an error. This definition could then be operationalized by adding as written on incident reports over a six-month period and filed in the office of the chief nursing administrator.

At Levels II and III, the operational definitions become even more specific.

> Level II: The purpose of this study is to answer the question, Is there a significant relationship among ethnicity, maternal diet, and

full-term newborn birth weight at Community Hospital in Las Cruces, New Mexico?

In this purpose, three variables need operational definitions. The following examples are simply one way of studying these variables. Ethnicity is defined as self-identification of cultural background, ethnic identity, or national origin as checked off on the admission sheet of Community Hospital. Diet is defined as the adequacy of diet (inclusion of major food groups as recommended by the Canada Food Guide) consumed each day as recorded in a food diary kept by pregnant women from the beginning diagnosis of pregnancy to birth of the child. Determination of adequacy made on a three-point scale by a registered nutritionist. Newborn birth weight is defined as the weight in grams of a full-term infant (whose mothers participate in the study as recorded immediately after birth in the neonates' charts at Community Hospital).

Another example might be the following:

Level II: The purpose of this study is to answer the question, Is there a significant relationship between obesity and heart disease among adults in greater Chicago?

For the purpose of this study, heart disease could be defined as a diagnosis of some form of heart ailment (as given in the cardiology diagnostic manual) listed on the final diagnosis page of all patients' charts for 2009 at hospital X. Obesity could be defined as the weight of an individual listed on the chart at time of admission that is 15% or more over the ideal weight, as defined by insurance standards.

At Level III, terms are much more specific because you know so much more about them. For example, because a great deal of research and theory has been done on vitamin C, we can write a hypothesis for an experimental study.

Level III: The purpose of this study is to test the following hypothesis: periodontal patients who receive 1000 mg of vitamin C daily will have a significant reduction in calculus compared to patients who receive no vitamin C.

The independent variable here is vitamin C, which can be defined as a vitamin supplement synthetically produced by brand X and given daily to experimental groups of patients in amounts of none, 1000 mg, 2000 mg, or 3000 mg for a period of 12 months. The dependent variable, calculus formation, can be defined as the formation of calculus that is manually removed by a dental hygienist or dentist during routinely scheduled dental hygiene visits, graded, and recorded on patients' charts every three months for a period of 12 months.

When you have written your purpose and have operationally defined your terms, you will have a clear idea of what your research study is about. The rest of your research plan is simply filling in the details.

Types of Variables

When the research plan hypothesizes relationships between variables, it is necessary to clarify expected relationships by categorizing them as independent or dependent. The terms come from experimental research, where an independent or experimental variable is introduced into a controlled setting, and the result is measured. This result—the response to the independent variable—is the dependent variable. Changes in the dependent variable are considered to be caused by the introduction of the independent variable. When the hypothesis does not predict a causal relationship but simply an associative one, as you may see in the literature, the independent variable can still be identified as the one that came first in time and is thought to be affecting the response or dependent variable. For example, in the finding, turnover of staff nurses was significantly higher in units where the leadership style was authoritarian, a relationship was found between turnover of staff and authoritarian leadership. No direct cause-and-effect relationship is specified because too many other possible variables could be working with authoritarianism to bring about turnover. The hypothesis, however, implies that authoritarianism is affecting turnover. Therefore, authoritarianism is the independent variable and turnover is the dependent variable.

One easy way of differentiating between independent and dependent variables is to remember that independent means standing alone and dependent means relying on something.

Two other types of variables need to be considered in research at Levels II and III. Intervening variables are those thought to affect the relationship between the independent and dependent variables. In Level III studies their action must be highly controlled or accounted for. Extraneous variables are all those that are not of direct interest to the researcher but that could affect the variables measured. When hypotheses are tested, the major purpose of the research design is to control the extraneous variables so that the effect of the independent variable on the dependent variable can be estimated. In testing the effect of authoritarian leadership on nursing staff turnover, some extraneous variables would need to be controlled, such as nurses' age, educational background, marital status, and number of children. Other possible extraneous variables would be things like the staffing mix, the severity of illness of patients, and the nature of the relationship between nurses and physicians. All of these variables could affect turnover.

Defining the Independent Variable

In research, the independent variable is the cause or influencing variable by which the subgroups in the sample are distinguished. In other words, the researcher must be able to divide the sample into alternative groups based on this variable. For example, authoritarian–nonauthoritarian and smoking–nonsmoking are both instances in which the independent variable is divided into two categories. Or you might wish to establish more than two categories: light, medium, and heavy smokers, based on the number of cigarettes smoked per day. In some studies, the independent variable may be divided into numerous precise classes, such as multiple dosage levels of a drug or exact monthly income. In defining the independent variable, the researcher decides on the categories for the sample. In doing this, there are three important objectives to keep in mind.

First, the various subdivisions or categories of the variable must be clearly distinguished from one another, and they must be mutually exclusive. There may not be a single case in which a subject would easily fit into more than one category at a time. The number of cigarettes per day constituting a medium smoker must be clearly distinguishable from that constituting a light smoker. The method of measurement for the categories must be clearly defined so that others who read the study can replicate the results. If the number of cigarettes is to be counted for a week and then divided by seven days, the procedure must be clearly stated and understood.

Second, the distinction between the categories should mean something in terms of the research problem. If age categories are developed to test the idea that children of different ages respond differently to health teaching, then the age categories must have some meaning in light of developmental theory. It is not enough just to set age categories by five-year increments; the categories selected must relate to the theory behind the study.

Third, the definition of the independent variable must remain constant during the data collection, as well as during the analysis of the data. If a nursing intervention is introduced to reduce pain in postoperative patients, and, part way through the study, it becomes apparent that the intervention is not working, it may not be increased or decreased, nor may it be changed to another intervention to improve the results. A study that shows no difference between the intervention and nonintervention groups makes an important contribution to nursing theory.

A more subtle alteration in the definition of the independent variable can occur in this example. If several members of the nursing staff are required to carry out the intervention, perhaps even the entire staff of a particular unit, it may happen that some nurses do not follow the protocol of the study unless the researcher is actually present, or some nurses may carry out the intervention using much better technique than others, unbeknownst to the researcher. When this happens, an alternative version of the independent variable is present, and its effect is being combined with that of the true variable. If the researcher is unaware of the problem, the relationship that emerges between the independent and dependent variables might be a spurious one.

The definition of the independent variable is critical to studies in which the purpose is stated as a question or a hypothesis. When a study is testing the independent variable as the cause or the dependent variable as the effect of the independent variable, then the description and definition of the independent variable are mandatory. On the other hand, in exploratory studies all variables are assumed to be independent. This is simply due to the lack of knowledge about the variables (see Table 6-1). Therefore, when a variable's status is unknown, the variable is treated as if it were independent.

TABLE 6-1
Definition of the Independent, Dependent, Intervening, and Extraneous[1] Variables

Independent Variable	Intervening Variable	Dependent Variable
Stands alone	Comes between the independent and dependent variables	Is affected by the independent variables
Cause	May interfere	Effect
Comes first	Comes between	Comes later or last
	Can mask the effect of the independent variable	

[1] *Extraneous* variables are variables you feel may influence or mask the dependent variable and is another name for an intervening variable. Unlike independent variables, extraneous variables are not of primary importance to the study, however they may be interesting or helpful in understanding the findings.

How Variables Are Measured

Variables are measured according to what you want to know about them as well as the amount of knowledge available from the literature. There are levels of measurement used in data collection, and these are nominal, ordinal, interval, and ratio scales. Each type of measurement dictates the way you collect your data and, subsequently, the way you analyze your data. So it's best to know, right at the beginning, exactly what these terms mean, how they are used, and what they do to the rest of your research plan. Although there are four levels of measurement, only the first three will be discussed in detail. Because there is little significant difference, for research, between interval and ratio scales, these levels of measurement will be discussed together.

The way you study your variable depends on what you want to know. Your choice of measurement scale depends on the answer you want from your data. If you want great precision, you will choose an interval (or ratio) scale. If you want to rank people or things in some order, you need an ordinal scale. If you simply want to categorize and count things and neither precision of measurement nor ordering from small to large or bad to good are possible, you will choose the nominal scale.

There are other reasons for choosing a particular scale or scales to measure your variables. One reason has to do with the variable itself. Religious affiliation is measured on a nominal scale made up of categories into which people can be placed. Similarly, membership in a political party is measured only in nominal scales because Republican, Democrat, or Independent is a named category with no numeric significance. Other variables are numeric scales, such as distance, temperature, and time. As numeric scales, distance can be given in precise measurement of miles or kilometers; time can be given in hours and minutes; temperature can be precisely calibrated in degrees. Each of these scales can be manipulated mathematically. Yet, at the same time, each of these three variables can be viewed nominally or ordinally. Time can be viewed as morning or afternoon; temperature can be given as cold or hot. How and when you will use a nominal or a numeric scale depends on your particular study and what you want to know. That is why your literature review is so important; you will discover the level of measurement of your variables in previous studies so you can decide how to measure your variables in this study.

Another factor in choosing how to measure your variables depends on how you collect your data. If you plan to use unstructured observations, your data will be either nominal or ordinal. If you use unstructured questionnaires, interviews, or projective tests, your data will still be at the nominal or ordinal level. If, however, you plan to use hospital records on blood gases, urinalysis, or EKGs, you will find that you have precise numeric scales to work with.

So your choice of measurement is dependent on your level of study, how you want to collect your data, and how your variables will occur naturally.

Finally, your choice will depend on the degree of precision you need to answer your original question.

Nominal Scale

When objects, events, or people are classified into two or more categories, and there is no difference in size or magnitude of the categories, then the variables are measured on a nominal scale. A nominal scale is a qualitative scale in that the qualities of a variable are examined rather than its quantities. The classic example of a nominal scale is the variable gender. Everyone can be categorized as male or female. There is no magnitude to maleness compared with femaleness. They are contrasting categories, labeled with a descriptive title.

The only specified relationship between the categories in nominal scales is that they are different from each other; they contrast with each other. There is no suggestion of any magnitude or quality differences. Nominal scales can have as few as two categories or many categories, as in a taxonomy of diagnoses. The categories must be exhaustive so that all variations of the variables can be classified somewhere. When developing your categories, you must exhaust the possibilities as to where your sample will fall on that variable. If you planned to collect data on marital status and left out the category single, you would lose part of your sample. What of the people who are never married as opposed to those who were formerly married but are now divorced and are, therefore, single again? When you decide to use a nominal scale, you should have a good idea of the possible categories.

Finally, nominal scales demand a system of classification that is mutually exclusive. Each person must fit into one, and only one, category of a given variable. There must be no question where each person fits. A person cannot be part Republican and part Democrat. A person must be one or the other. If you are a Republican, you are not a Democrat or an Independent. If you are a nurse, then you probably are not an engineer or an accountant. If you are looking for the presence or absence of a particular trait, a person who has a little of that trait is classified along with the person who has a lot of it. Nominal scales do not allow for a little bit versus a lot because there is no magnitude to a nominal scale.

Ordinal Scale

Ordinal scales differ from nominal scales in that they rank a variable on a scale of increasing magnitude. Ordinal scales, like nominal scales, are generally named categories that, in addition, follow a particular ordering system. For example, to measure age on an ordinal scale, you can develop categories such as young, middle-aged, and old. The magnitude alters with the age of the individual because an old person is older than a middle-aged person, who is older than a young person. You do not attempt to specify how much older an elderly person is than a young person. The number of years is not relevant here; what is relevant is the system of ranking. Just as with a nominal scale, the ordinal scale categories must be mutually exclusive. An individual cannot be rated as both young and middle-aged. The difference between the categories must be clearly established so that every person in the sample falls into only one category.

Many nursing studies use ordinal scales. In attitudinal research, people are asked to rank their opinions (on the basis of whether they agree or disagree with a statement) on a scale from strongly disagree to strongly agree, with several points in between (the classic Likert scale). We can measure the success of nursing interventions by the level of comfort or discomfort expressed by the patient or by the degree of learning that has occurred. Any variable that can be ranked from none to a great deal can be measured on an ordinal scale.

Interval (and Ratio) Scale

In contrast to nominal and ordinal scales, the interval (and ratio) scale is a quantitative numeric scale. Its significant feature is that the numbered intervals between points are equidistant, whether those intervals are measured in miles, centimeters, pounds, or degrees. (There is little significant difference, for research, between interval and ratio scales. The only thing you need to remember is that ratio scales have an absolute zero, and interval scales do not. Otherwise, the scales are treated identically in data analysis.) The intervals can be added or subtracted to provide each subject with a score on the variable being measured. The scores can then be analyzed statistically to determine whether subjects are significantly different from one another.

Interval scales are used when precise information about variables is needed. You must know enough about the variable to develop a precise form of measurement. Therefore, the use of interval scales for variables that are being explored for the first time must be ruled out.

Most nursing research utilizes nominal and ordinal scales, the most commonly used scales in behavioral and social research. Increasing use is also being made of interval and ratio level data, especially in nursing research that involves biological and physical sciences. Later you will see how the measurement scale of your variables affects the possibilities for data analysis.

Let's look at an example.

If you wanted to do a study on runner's fatigue and you decided to test fatigue levels by the presence of blood in the urine, you could set up your study on the basis of a nominal scale: the presence of blood in the urine versus no observable blood in the urine. This scale would not measure the amount of blood in the urine or the degree of fatigue expressed in terms of severity of bleeding. What is desired in this case is a mutually exclusive statement on the presence or absence of blood, so a nominal scale is used.

If you want to measure the presence of blood on an ordinal scale, you could rank the amount of blood by the color of the urine—from none (clear yellow), to a little (pink), to moderate (light red), to much (bright red), to a lot (dark red). Now there is magnitude to the measurement of blood in the urine, although it is not known how much blood is classified as moderate versus a little.

Using this same example, an interval scale also could be used. Here you would test samples of urine for the number of red blood cells present, a precise measurement of the amount of blood. Now you can describe subjects by the precise amount of hematuria each one has. (With this example, you can trace the development of knowledge about the variable through the levels of measurement. If there were no precise way to measure blood in the urine other than gross observation, you would not be able to use a numeric scale.)

You may wonder what scaling has to do with operational definitions. Every variable in the written purpose must be defined according to a nominal, ordinal, interval, or ratio scale. The way you define your variable is the way you will measure it. The way you plan to measure it determines the methods of data collection you will use. This decision, in turn, requires certain forms of data analysis. Therefore, when you define your terms according to a particular scale, you determine the rest of your study.

At Level I exploratory levels of research, you have either one variable or one sample that you intend to explore and describe. Because you probably know little about either, you may not know whether an interval or ratio scale should be used. You must know something about your variable to determine if it can be studied quantitatively, but you must know a great deal to be able to choose an appropriate numeric scale. As a result, Level I studies generally use either a nominal or an ordinal scale. When exploring at the most elementary level, you may start with no scale at all. An initial content analysis of the data may produce categories that can then be used as a nominal scale. After that, individuals can be classified according to whether or not they possess the characteristic or variable. The researcher answers questions like, Does the variable exist? What is it? When does it exist? Where is it? Who has it? How often does it occur? Each of these questions can be answered by a word or a name of something; therefore, a nominal scale is appropriate.

In Level II studies where you are looking at the relationship between two or more variables, you need to decide which scale would be most appropriate for each variable (because you can study each variable on a different scale) so that you can plan your data analysis.

For example, if you were looking at the relationship between distance running and hematuria, you would be at Level II. Although you have a hunch that increased running causes bloody urine, you cannot prove it. First you must do a descriptive survey of runners to see if there is a relationship between running and hematuria. Using the same example—the purpose of this study is to answer the question, Is there a significant relationship between the number of miles run each week and the amount of hematuria among marathon runners?—you will count the number of miles per week per runner from zero (the runner may not have run at all for a week) to the highest number achieved by one of the runners for 1 week. You will take urine specimens daily to perform blood counts. These data also will range from zero to the highest actual number for any one runner in one week. You will have two ratio scales because both variables have absolute zeros.

Had your purpose been to test the relationship between miles run per week and the presence or absence of blood in the urine as reported by the runner, you would have had a ratio scale for number of miles and a nominal scale for presence or absence of blood in the urine.

If you wanted to conduct a Level III study, you would first verify the relationship between running and hematuria. Your hypothesis would predict that hematuria occurs, for example, when an individual runs more than 50 miles each week or that the amount of hematuria for a runner will progressively increase in weekly increments from 100 miles per week as the base.

In this case you state that the amount of running causes hematuria and that a specific number of miles run is necessary for such a physiological condition to occur. You also state that the more one runs, the more blood will be found in the urine. You must have a physiological theory of distance running related to hematuria to hypothesize that increased running causes more blood in urine. To make this prediction you have to know that excessive running causes hematuria, that running is the independent variable, and that hematuria is the dependent variable.

Hypotheses predict relationships, thus you, the researcher, must know which variable is the cause and which is the effect. Every study has an independent variable—one you assume is independent because there are no others (Level I); one you think is independent, but you are looking for proof (Level II); and one you know is independent and can be manipulated (Level III). The level of knowledge about your topic indicates which variables are independent and which are dependent. If you are testing at Level III, your knowledge also tells you which variables are intervening or extraneous.

When defining your terms, keep in mind how you intend to measure your variables and whether the variable is dependent, independent, or extraneous. Remember, also, to define your terms according to the needs of your study. Here is an example:

> Level I: The purpose of this study is to explore and describe the characteristics of runners at the Boston Marathon Club.

The critical term to define is characteristics. They could be defined as traits, qualities, or properties that distinguish an individual or a group, such as standard demographic data that are descriptive of certain classes of people—age, gender, marital status, education, and occupational status—as well as number of miles run per week, type of clothing worn, time of run, and so on. Most of these characteristics are nominal. Your definition of runners probably would include a minimum number of miles run per week and the speed of the run. In another example:

> Level II: The purpose of this study is to answer the question, Is there a significant relationship between miles run per week and weight loss among distance runners in Denver?

Here you could define weight loss as none, little, and much, or under 5 lb, 5 to 10 lb, or according to the actual number of pounds lost. (Of these three definitions of weight loss, the last is a numeric scale and the first two examples are ordinal.)

For a Level III study predicting that successful dieting is accompanied by regular exercise, successful dieting might be defined as weight loss of 10 lb or more that was not regained 1 year following the end of the dieting program. In this case the scale would be a nominal scale of yes or no—if the individual was successful or not. Regular exercise must be defined according to what constitutes exercise and what is meant by regular exercise.

In a Level I study, the only term needing definition is the variable or concept under study. So when your purpose is to explore and describe the strategies used by frail older widows to allow home care providers access to their homes, the only variable to be defined either conceptually or operationally is strategies to allow access to their homes. Although frail older widows needs definition as well, this is better dealt with in the section on sample (Porter, 2007). If you have a Level I study, you will define only one variable or concept in the statement of purpose. In a research proposal, the sample is not defined under definition of terms but instead in a section called sample.

Many people planning a Level I study define their sample under definition of terms simply because this group of people has never been studied or because study of them has been so variable. Homeless men are a good example of a population that has no real parameters. When a national census is taken, it is difficult to establish how many members of the population are homeless when the criteria for inclusion in the census requires a home address. In the same way, a study dealing with menopausal women would require a definition of the sample simply because there are no census data describing this group of the population. A review of the literature on successful dieters, for example, revealed that there was no consistency as to what was considered to be successful versus unsuccessful. To plan a study of these populations requires the researcher to set up the parameters for who will qualify for the study.

Where do these definitions belong when you are planning your research? At the very beginning of your thinking and planning process, when you are writing out your question and your working definitions, you need to define your target population (see Chapter 8). You need to consider the criteria for those who will be included in your study group and for those who will not. Try to use mutually exclusive characteristics to describe your study population. Then, when you write the proposal itself (see Chapter 13), you will describe these characteristics in the section on target population. The criteria for the selection of particular characteristics has already been discussed in your problem simply because you need to talk about the people you want to study before you actually study them. In the chapter on definition of terms, therefore, you will not find a section to describe your sample as part of the definition of terms.

Terms That Need Definition

The purpose of your study states exactly what you intend to measure. Because of the specific nature of the purpose, every variable should be operationally defined. The economy of words in a statement of purpose necessitates operational definitions.

This chapter has focused on the operational definitions of the independent and dependent variables as the critical issues for the project. Remember, in a descriptive study, all variables are assumed to be independent; therefore, all variables need definition. In an experimental design, you, as investigator, are theoretically in complete control of the independent variable; therefore, you must know everything you can about it. Your study describes the effect of the independent variables on the dependent variable. You also need to define the possible intervening or extraneous variables to show your reader that you have considered them.

Writing Operational Definitions: A Review

1. First, write out what the term (or variable) means in relation to the purpose of the study. This is the conceptual definition of the term.

   Example: The purpose of this study is to explore and describe <u>successful dieting programs</u>. (The terms to be defined are underlined.) Dieting programs: Fee-for-service regimens established to assist persons to lose weight.

   Successful: A dieting program that has a high percentage of clients who were able to achieve their goal weight and keep that weight off for one year or more.

2. Second, write out how you intend to study that definition or how you intend to measure the variable. This is the operational part of the operational definition of the term.

   Example: The purpose of this study is to explore and describe <u>successful dieting programs</u>. (The terms to be defined are underlined.)

   Dieting programs: Fee-for-service regimens established to assist persons in losing weight, as listed in the Yellow Pages of the telephone directory of Greater Boston.

Successful: A dieting program that has a high percentage of clients who were able to achieve their goal weight and keep that weight off for 1 year or more as measured by the successful dieters questionnaire sent to all program participants in the previous year.

3. Combine both parts of the definition to form the operational definition of the term or variable.

    Example: Successful dieting program: Fee-for-service regimen, established to assist persons in losing weight, that has a high percentage of clients who were able to achieve their goal weight and keep that weight off for one year or more as measured by the successful dieters questionnaire sent to all program participants from programs listed in the Yellow Pages of the Greater Boston telephone directory.

4. Operationally define every major variable in your purpose whether the purpose is written as a statement, a question, or a hypothesis.

5. Your sample should not be operationally defined.

6. Additional examples of operational definitions:

    Purpose of the study:
    The purpose of this study is to explore and describe the value orientations of Hutterian women in western Canada.

    Definition of terms:
    Value orientations: A 23-item ordinal scale instrument designed to elicit an individual's beliefs about the best way to solve four basic common human problems.

    Purpose of the study:
    The purpose of this study is to answer the question, Is there a significant relationship between level of stress and coping strategies in hospitalized patients?

    Definition of terms:
    Level of stress: The number and intensity of events, perceived by the patient as causing strain or tension, that occurred during the past 12 months as measured by the Holmes and Rahe Significant Life Events scale.

    Coping strategies: A person's customary pattern of adapting to or dealing with perceived stressful events as measured by a rating scale evaluating both the number of strategies and the frequency with which the individual uses them.

Purpose of the study:

The purpose of the study is to test the following hypothesis: Nurses who have had assertiveness training will have significantly higher patient protectiveness ratings than those who do not have assertiveness training.

Definition of terms:

Assertiveness training: A program designed to increase an individual's ability to select assertive behaviors when faced with a conflict situation. The experimental group will receive a four-day program in assertiveness training.

Patient protectiveness rating: A nine-item ordinal scale to measure a nurse's feelings of responsibility for preventing harm from occurring to the patient.

Bibliography

Halbesleben, J. R. B., Wakefield, B. J., Wakefield, D. S., & Cooper, L. B. (2008). Nurse burnout and patient safety outcomes: Nurse safety perceptions versus reporting behavior. *Western Journal of Nursing Research, 30*(5), 560–577.

Lobiondo-Wood, G., & Haber, J. (2010). *Nursing research: Methods and critical appraisal for evidence-based practice* (7th ed.). St. Louis, MO: Mosby.

Polit, D. F., & Beck, C. T. (2004). *Nursing research: Principles and methods* (7th ed.). Philadelphia: Lippincott.

Polit, D. F., Beck, C. T., & Hungler, B. P. (2001). *Essentials of nursing research: Methods, appraisal and utilization* (5th ed.). Philadelphia: Lippincott.

Porter, E. J. (2007). Actions taken by frail older widows to allow home care providers access to their homes. *Current Neurovascular Research, 16*(1), 44–57.

Summers, S. (1991). Level of measurement: Key to appropriate data analysis. *Journal of Post Anesthesia Nursing, 6*(2), 143–147.

Waltz, C. F., Strickland, O. L., & Lenz, E. R. (1991). *Measurement in nursing research*. Philadelphia: F. A. Davis.

Wandelt, M. (1970). *Guide for the beginning researcher*. New York: Appleton-Century-Crofts.

CHAPTER SEVEN

The Research Design: Blueprint for Action

➤ TOPICS

Designing Your Study from the Question
Characteristics of Research Designs
Issues of Control
Descriptive Designs
Experimental Designs
Controlling Unwanted Influences
Level of Study and Degree of Control
Bibliography

➤ LEARNING OBJECTIVES

- Understand the purpose of the research design.
- Describe characteristics of research designs.
- Discuss issues of control in research designs.
- Review the relationship between the level of the study and the research design.
- Describe the essential features of an exploratory descriptive design.
- Describe the essential features of a descriptive survey design.
- Describe the essential features of an experimental design.
- Discuss the various means to control unwanted influences in research designs.

Up to this point, you have explored the process of deciding what to study. You have learned how to choose a topic and establish an appropriate question to ask about it.

Now that you have a good idea of what you want to study, you are ready to decide how to study it. The remaining chapters will take you through the process and help you decide how to study it. You are ready to take the work you have already done—your stem question, your topic, your operational definitions, and your statement of purpose—and lay them out into a working plan, a blueprint for action.

As with any blueprint, you start with an overall picture of the design before you go on to show close-up pictures of each section. In that way, you won't get bogged down in details before you have visualized the end result. If you tried to design a kitchen by starting with a detailed plan for the spice cupboard and then tried to fit the rest of the kitchen around it, you would be in trouble. Similarly, the research plan will suffer if you start by minutely describing the sample before you know what the overall plan is to be. The result would be a research design planned to fit the sample instead of a sample selected to meet the needs of the design.

The purpose of a research design is to provide a plan for answering the research question. The major concern within the blueprint, or plan, is to specify the control mechanisms you will use in your study so that the answer to the question will be clear and valid. The concept of control in research is an extremely important one, and the extent to which you can achieve control depends on the level of your study. Control refers to the control of the variables under study and other variables that may possibly affect the study. Control is attained by (1) allowing for no variation, (2) specifying the variation to be allowed, or (3) distributing the variation equally. Laboratory settings, for example, provide for control by allowing no variation. Homogeneity of the sample allows for no variation on some characteristics, and matched samples ensure that some characteristics are identical. Randomization distributes the variation equally among study groups.

In experimental studies, control is a major requirement; the only thing that is allowed to freely vary in the pure experiment is the dependent variable. The experimenter manipulates (controls) the independent variable and observes the effect on the dependent variable while everything else is kept stable. Extraneous variables are controlled only if the groups are formed by random assignment and are kept intact. Any other form of group assignment or any dropout from the group diminishes control over extraneous variables. Variables are said to be distributed normally among groups or throughout the sample by either random assignment to groups, in experimental designs, or by the use of probability samples in comparative and correlational designs.

Another type of control is to build extraneous variables into the design. This is accomplished in one of two ways: either by writing the variable into the study as part of the purpose as an alternate independent variable or intervening variable; or by collecting data on the variable and then analyzing it at the end of the study during the data analysis. When variables are built into the design, they should be included in the discussion of the problem and definition of terms, there needs to be literature review on all variables that are to be measured in the study, and there needs to be discussion on how the data will be collected and analyzed. When data on extraneous variables are collected as demographic data, they can later be treated as intervening variables during data analysis. In this way, their effect on the dependent variable can be calculated and separated out from the effect of the independent variable.

Allowing for no variance is accomplished with homogeneous samples in which everyone is alike on one or more dimensions. When everyone in the sample is the same gender, or has the same disease, or is of the same racial or ethnic group, it is a homogeneous sample on that variable because that particular variable is not allowed to vary or is specified as having no variance.

Variables on which data are collected, analyzed, and simply described at the end of the study are considered to be neither intervening nor extraneous; these are usually demographic variables used to describe the sample and would include things like age, gender, socioeconomic status, occupation, education, and marital status.

Designing Your Study from the Question

All research designs fall into one of two main categories: descriptive or experimental. The choice of which to use is made during the development of the problem. Descriptive designs result in a description of the data, whether in words, pictures, charts, or tables, and whether the data analysis shows statistical or merely descriptive relationships. Experimental designs result in inferences drawn from the data that explain the relationships between the variables. If the topic is appropriate for Level I or II, the design will be descriptive; if your study is at Level III, it requires an experimental design.

What questions invariably lead to descriptive designs; why questions are always experimental. Thus, the choice of design is made when the question is finalized; it can then be given a name and be developed into a detailed plan of action.

The design is a set of instructions to the researcher to gather and analyze data in certain ways that will control who and what are to be studied. Unwanted or extraneous variables can thus be controlled, the variance of specific variables is enhanced, and the possibility of error in measurement is minimized. In other words, the design makes it possible for you to isolate the variables you are interested in from all other variables and to measure them accurately so that your data are reliable and valid.

The design chosen must be the best way to answer the question, that is, it must fit the level of the question. Variables about which little is known need to be questioned at a basic level, and the answer will be a description of those variables.

The design always builds on previous findings. When the specific variables you are interested in have been the subject of Level I research, you would normally move on to study them at Level II. The only exception to this rule is the replication study. If you feel the results of previous research require further support, your study may replicate the previous research, following the design exactly as it was in the original study.

Characteristics of Research Designs

When you read research studies that specify the design being used, you can make judgments about the adequacy of the design to answer the question, and you can evaluate the study in relation to its goodness of fit with the requirements of the design. When a research report does not specify the design being used, then you have to guess what the researcher intended to do and then evaluate the study in relation to your best guess. Obviously, it is easier to evaluate a study when the writer tells you in advance the name of the design rather than your having to figure out the type of design being used. To help you select a design that meets the requirements of your stated purpose and evaluate studies more easily, the following areas need to be considered.

The Setting for the Study

Will your study be conducted in a laboratory setting or field setting? When you are planning a study, the setting in which it will be conducted is a first order of decision making. If your study will be conducted in a laboratory, you will have far greater control than if your study is conducted in a natural setting. If you are doing research in a laboratory but do not build in the controls that are usual to this setting, then you are wasting your setting because you could have done the study anywhere.

Laboratory studies are designed to be more highly controlled in relation to both the environment in which the study is conducted and the control of extraneous and intervening variables. You are familiar with physiological laboratory experiments, chemistry and physics experiments, as well as psychological and microbiological experiments. All are laboratory experiments designed to control the possibility of extraneous variables influencing the effect of the independent variable on the dependent variable. In the laboratory setting, it is possible to control environmental variables, such as temperature, humidity, light, and sound, as well as physiological variables such as nutrition and hydration of the subjects during the experiment.

All other studies not conducted in laboratories are called field studies, which simply means they occur somewhere other than in a controlled laboratory setting. Field studies occur in natural settings and use a variety of methods, such as field experiments, participant observations in villages or hospital units, interviews in the home or office, questionnaires sent to research subjects, and, in fact, anything at all that does not occur in a controlled laboratory setting.

Timing of Data Collection

What type of study do you plan to conduct in relation to time? Will you look into the past, study present behaviors, or predict future events? There are several design labels that describe the timing of your data collection. Those looking at events that are underway or expected to occur in the future are called prospective or longitudinal studies. Those focusing on events that have occurred in the past are called retrospective, ex post facto, or historical studies. Those in which data collection is strictly in the present time are called cross-sectional studies. You may find these labels useful in designing your study because they may help you to clarify how the timing of your data collection fits into your design. They are also terms that you will see in the literature, and an understanding of how they are meant to be used will help you in critiquing research reports.

Of the three labels for studies that focus on events in the past, the first is the retrospective study. This term is used by epidemiologists to describe a cause and effect study in which the effect is known (such as lung cancer) and the cause is sought by examining past events. Social scientists use the label ex post facto to describe this same type of study. In other words, a phenomenon that occurs in the present is thought to have a cause that can be found (retrospectively) in the past. Many early studies of diseases (such as alcoholism, obesity, lung cancer, and diabetes) were retrospective (or ex post facto) studies.

Historical studies, on the other hand, are often descriptive studies that ask people to recall events, other people, and memories from the past, or they refer to written historical documents and artifacts to reconstruct past events.

Studies that look to the future are called prospective or longitudinal studies. These terms generally mean the same thing, but epidemiologists are apt to use "prospective," whereas social scientists use "longitudinal," to describe studies that are designed to follow the subjects for a period of time, obtaining repeated measurements, and establishing changes in the variables over time. In this type of study, the sample is chosen on the basis of the presence of a presumed causative (independent) variable. The sample is followed to find out if the dependent variable occurs and/or changes over time. Prospective or longitudinal studies can be very expensive. They can require a considerable investment of time because the researcher must wait for the presumed effect to occur and therefore must be prepared to follow the subjects for long periods, sometimes many years. The strength of these designs is that they have more control over extraneous variables than do retrospective studies.

Cross-sectional studies collect data one time only and are meant to obtain a cross-section of the population at a given moment in time. The result is a measurement of what exists today, with no attempt to document changes over time either in the past or the future.

The decision you make as to whether you will do a retrospective or a prospective study is based on whether you are looking for causes in the past (retrospective) or present-day causes for future effects (prospective); or looking for descriptions of events and things that occurred in the past (retrospective) or following people into the future to describe events as they occur (prospective); or using one measurement time to describe what exists today (cross-sectional).

Sample Selection

The type of sample you will use for your study is an important part of the design. Two main points to think about are, first, whether or not it will be a random sample, and second, the degree to which the sample you want is accessible to you.

In sample selection, a random sample complies with the principle of randomization, which assumes that every member of a population has an equal chance of being selected for the sample. When this principle is followed, we expect that individuals with certain distinguishing characteristics—male or female, high or low intelligence, religious or not religious, and so on—will, if selected, be counterbalanced in the long run by the selection of other members of the population with the opposite quantity or quality of the characteristic. The major benefit of a random sample is that it gives an accurate picture of the overall population. Also, a random sample is required for certain statistical tests that might be needed to analyze the data from a study.

When you are selecting a random sample from a population, the idea is to have distinguishing characteristics randomly distributed in the sample so that the sample is representative of the population. In other words, the distribution in the sample approximates that in the population. In experimental research, when subjects are randomly assigned to groups, the principle is used to ensure that these distinguishing characteristics will be equivalently distributed among all the study groups so that the groups themselves can be considered equivalent at the beginning of the study, before the experimental treatment has been started. The purpose of randomization is to distribute extraneous or intervening variables throughout the sample in such a way that no particular group is favored over another.

Randomness is generally associated with generalizability. The degree to which the sample represents the population affects the degree to which the study can be generalized to the same population. These ideas will be discussed in further detail later.

Accessibility of the sample refers to whether you can reasonably expect to find enough individuals, animals, events, or units of the population that meet the criteria for your study—that is, you can be reasonably sure they are available to you. If you are looking for people with a relatively rare characteristic, you need to have an accessible target population that is large enough for your study. For example, your sample might require people with rare diseases or characteristics not commonly found in large numbers in the general population, such as people with Bilharzia, or triplets, or people who have been married more than five times. Because these are difficult-to-find populations, your ability to do the study may be inhibited.

Type of Data to Be Collected

In general, all data can be categorized according to whether it is collected as qualitative (qualities) or quantitative (numeric). All studies are categorized according to the type of data collected and will emphasize one over the other. Qualitative data have names or labels rather than numbers. Any attribute or variable having a number is called quantitative. Within quantitative data, there will be differences in the scale used to measure the variables (nominal, ordinal, or interval–ratio). These scales, which we have discussed elsewhere, vary according to how precisely they are able to measure a variable. Normally higher level designs require higher level scales of measurement.

Issues of Control

Before discussing the individual research designs for each level of research, there are two concepts basic to the idea of control that you need to consider. These are internal and external validity.

Internal validity is defined as the extent to which the results of the study can actually be attributed to the action of the independent variable and not something else. In this case, validity refers to the truth of the findings as determined by the purity of the design. Internal validity is determined by the way the experimental and control groups are formed in an experimental design. If the investigator is able to say with perfect certainty that all groups were equal at the beginning of the study, and no other variables were allowed to interfere with the independent variable, then any change in the dependent variable can be attributed to the effect of the independent variable. The study then has internal validity. That means there is no possibility that another, perhaps unknown independent variable is the actual cause of the change observed in the dependent variable. The degree to which that perfect certainty is compromised indicates the degree to which the study does not have internal validity. How much control can you plan to have over your experimental variables? Is this to be a relatively uncontrolled field experiment or a highly controlled laboratory experiment? With all of the methods you plan to use, be sure that nothing can interfere with the action of your independent variable to attain internal validity.

External validity refers to the degree to which the findings of the study are generalizable to the target population. The key issue here is the degree to which the sample represents the population. Random sampling is intended to produce a representative sample, providing the sample size is large enough to incorporate all the relevant extraneous variables. If the sample is not representative, then the results do not generalize and you can only describe what you have found in your sample. If you did generalize on the basis of a nonprobability sample, people would accuse you of making a quantum leap from the data to the conclusions. The reason for using random sampling is to promote the external validity of your results. Here the focus is on the degree to which your sample represents the target population accurately, so that the results you obtain can be applied to the entire target population. Chapter 8 discusses in detail the strategies for attaining external validity through obtaining random or representative samples.

Descriptive Designs

No matter what method is chosen to collect the data, all descriptive designs have one thing in common: they must provide descriptions of the variables to answer the question. The type of description that results from the design depends on how much information the researcher has about the topic prior to data collection. Look at the design in the same way that you looked at the question. Level I questions, with little or no prior knowledge of the topic, lead to exploratory descriptive designs. Level II questions, where the variables are known but their action cannot be predicted, lead to descriptive survey designs.

Exploratory Descriptive Designs

At this level, the design is one of two basic models: exploratory or descriptive. Exploratory studies provide an in-depth exploration of a single process, variable, or concept, such as bereavement or role conflict. Descriptive studies examine one or more characteristics of a specific population, such as the health beliefs of aboriginals in Canada or the health concerns among new immigrants from Southeast Asia. Level I studies always involve one variable and one population.

When the purpose of a study is exploration, a flexible research design that provides an opportunity to examine all aspects of the problem is needed. As knowledge of the variables increases, the researcher may have to change direction. Ideas occur as data are collected and examined. The key to a good exploratory design is flexibility.

We emphasize throughout the book that the research process is dependent on what is known about the topic. The word "exploratory" indicates that not much is known, which means that a survey of the literature failed to reveal any significant research in the area. Thus, you cannot build on the work of others; you must explore the topic for yourself.

Even though we talk about the exploratory study as an entity in itself, it should be remembered that it is an initial step in the development of new knowledge. Because of the flexibility of this type of design, very few, if any, variables are under the researcher's control. They are said to be under the control of the situation—in other words, observed as they happen or as the researcher comes upon them. As a result, no inferences can be drawn from the data. The data may lead to suggestions of hypotheses for further study or to an idea for a conceptual framework to explain the action of the variables, but the exploratory question must be followed by higher-level questions if new knowledge is to be gained.

There are many areas in nursing that have not previously been studied. Questions about these areas will lead you to conclude that exploratory studies are required to build a beginning base of knowledge through description. For example, a research question might be, What are the reactions of patients to being transferred from room to room during hospitalization? This is a Level I question. If the literature review reveals no information on this topic, the purpose of your study will be to explore and describe patients' reactions to being moved from room to room during a hospital stay. In this type of study, you may not ask, What is the *effect* of moving patients from room to room? To ask questions about effect, you must know the cause and have sufficient information to predict the effect; or you may know the effect, in which case you must be able to predict the cause. Either option requires a lot of information. You do not have this type of information in the present example. You have no idea whether moving patients has an effect on anything at all. And if there is an effect, you have no idea of its extent. Perhaps it will be temporary annoyance, a mild disorientation, a severe setback in convalescence, an increase in sensory disturbances, or a loss of social relationships—the list of possibilities could fill volumes. To find out what the patients' reaction actually is, you will have to explore all these possibilities. That means asking open-ended questions and being prepared to shift gears, depending on the patients' initial response. You will need to observe patients being moved and describe what you see; you will need to interview patients and families and ask what their reactions are; you will want to question nurses, unit secretaries, physicians, family members, and others who are in contact with the patient to see what their experiences have been. Your methods and questions will change depending on what you find out as you go along. Thus, it is imperative that the design be flexible.

The results of this study will provide detailed descriptions of all the observations made by the researcher, arranged in some kind of order. Conclusions drawn from the data include some educated guesses or hypotheses for further study. A relationship between the observations made and a concept such as territorialism might be proposed. Or perhaps a relationship with systems theory might be seen. Further research would be required to test these proposals. This is the purpose of exploratory research.

The basic exploratory design requires the personal involvement of the researcher with a small number of people (usually less than 25); uses purposive or theoretical sampling; occurs in a small, circumscribed geographic setting; and uses either field notes or audiotaped transcriptions of interviews. The strongest exploratory design is based on repeated interviews, observations, or both of the same people or phenomena. In this design, more than any other, the data control the investigator, and not the reverse. Underlying this design are the following assumptions: the topic has never been studied before, the people in the sample have personal experience in or knowledge about the topic, and the participants are able to talk about the topic.

The exploratory design is also known as qualitative research when the samples are deliberative or convenient; questions and observations are qualitative; and the analysis of data is via verbal description and, perhaps, preliminary or tentative theorizing about the findings. Examples of exploratory–qualitative designs include ethnomethodology and ethnography. Other qualitative designs, such as grounded theory or phenomenology, do not fit the model of an exploratory design as we use it here because they have unique philosophic bases that are quite different from the scientific paradigm used in this book. Exploratory designs, by their nature, are not replicable.

Exploratory designs, as opposed to descriptive designs, include a beginning exploration of an idea or concept; an attempt at discovery rather than description; an attempt to find meaning in the data; and an immersion in the area studied.

Descriptive studies differ from exploratory studies in several ways. They are studies of known variables in unknown populations, whereas the exploratory study collects in-depth data on a single abstract concept or process variable. In the descriptive study, there may be literature on the variables but the variables have not been studied in a particular population. For example, in Brink's 1984 study of the value orientations of the Annang of Nigeria, the tool used to measure value orientations had been used previously in a comparative study of five cultures in the United States (Kluckhohn & Strodtbeck, 1961), but nothing was known about this variable for the Annang. For this study, a tool was available to measure a known variable in an unknown population. Some flexibility is built into a descriptive study because there is little information on the population, and available tools may prove inadequate to measure the variables; but descriptive studies do not have the degree of flexibility found in exploratory studies.

Another descriptive design is the census or population study. This descriptive design is used in the collection of census data every ten years by the US Census Bureau. Similar studies are carried out in Canada and other countries. In this type of descriptive study, the total population is surveyed using structured data collection methods. In this instance, the purpose is to compile a complete description of the population to record changing trends in population characteristics over a specific period. Each census, however, is an individual descriptive study. The purpose is not to look for relationships among variables but rather to provide a descriptive database for the population. These studies do not have a theoretical or conceptual base. The Higher Education Research Institute at UCLA collects annual data on college freshmen. National norms are reported and compared to previous reports from this same survey. New areas are added from time to time. For example, in 2008, an election year, particular attention was paid to variables like political awareness (HERI, 2008). Census studies will always be fairly structured in design compared to exploratory studies. They usually have large samples (or total populations), and the type of data to be collected will always be predetermined. The usual form of data collection is structured questionnaires, although there may be some open-ended questions to account for areas in which the researcher may be unsure of the potential responses.

The results of a descriptive study will provide detailed information on the variable(s) under study. No relationships among variables are predicted in these studies, although comparisons over time or among whole populations are frequently made during a secondary analysis, and associations between demographic characteristics and the study variables are often sought.

The purpose of the purely descriptive design is to describe a single variable or a single population. The basic assumptions of this design are that (1) the variable exists in the population; (2) the variable may have been studied in other populations (in other words, there is a literature base for the study) but has not been studied in this population; (3) the variable is a new variable, such as a new form of influenza not seen previously or a new population discovered somewhere in the world that requires a complete description; (4) although a theoretical or conceptual framework may form the basis for the study, the intent is not to theorize or conceptualize; (5) in the absence of a theoretical or conceptual framework, a thorough rationale for the study is required based on the known research or literature on the variable; (6) if the population parameters are known, a probability sample is the basic sampling frame; (7) if the population parameters are not known, population characteristics from other studies on the same (or similar) variable can be used; and (8) the purpose of the study is to describe the variable as it exists in the specific population. Data are controlled through the sample selection methods and the conditions under which variables are observed and measured.

Several types of descriptive designs usually are associated with a specific discipline, such as ethnography (anthropology), census studies (government), demography (sociology), and ethology (the observation of animal behavior). Each design has its own rules, although all must meet the criteria for a descriptive design.

Methods of data collection in descriptive designs include observation (both participant and nonparticipant observation); questioning in the form of either interviews or questionnaires; physiological measures; and available data, such as artifacts and written records. The level of measurement can be either quantitative or both quantitative and qualitative. Data analysis involves, therefore, verbal description of the findings, content analysis to organize the findings into a framework, and descriptive statistics, as in measures of central tendency.

Sampling includes the total available population, as in census studies, probability sampling techniques, and convenience sampling through (1) formal interviewing of key informants, (2) informal interviewing with available subjects, and (3) participant observation. Remember that sample size and data collection methods for Level I studies have an inverse relationship. In other words, the smaller the sample size, the larger the number of unstructured questions that can be used. Because of the vast quantity of data produced by unstructured questions, the larger the sample size, the smaller the number of unstructured questions that can be used in data collection.

In single method (i.e., questionnaires) descriptive studies (such as census studies and demographies), questionnaires and interviews usually have face and content validity. In ethnographic studies, validity of data in an unknown culture is established through triangulation of data collection methods, such as interviews, with observation and available data. In single method descriptive studies (i.e., interviews), face and content validity of the data is established through repeated interviews. In historical research, the document review is the literature review. The study involves making connections among pieces of data according to chronology. Each piece of data must be validated (contextually, comparatively, and by the source).

Descriptive designs differ from correlational designs by studying only one variable or one population, making no attempt to find statistical relationships, having either or both qualitative and quantitative data, using data collection instruments whose validity may not be well developed, and by not requiring a conceptual framework at the beginning of a study.

These designs are most useful when the variable has not been described for the population or when population parameters have not been established. It is, however, unethical to use these designs when the instrumentation is neither valid nor reliable or when there is no possibility of producing usable results. It is impossible to use a descriptive design when the variable does not exist in the population or when the population refuses to be studied.

Both exploratory designs and descriptive designs meet the criteria of a Level I study based on little prior knowledge of the variable or the population under study. Neither design is looking for cause-and-effect relationships but instead are studies of single variables or single populations.

Descriptive Survey Designs

The primary designs at Level II are the correlational and comparative surveys. The major differences between them stem from the level of knowledge of the topic. Correlational designs have a conceptual base and are looking for cause-and-effect relationships in the results but often cannot specify the direction of the relationship at the beginning of the study. In contrast, comparative designs can specify cause and effect at the beginning of a study and are based on a theoretical framework. Both the comparative and correlational designs are based on an accurate description of the variables as they occur naturally. The major difference between the comparative and the experimental design, and the reason the comparative design is placed at Level II, not Level III, is that the independent variable is not manipulated.

Questions at Level II ask, What is the relationship between or among variables? You know what the variables are, and you know how to measure them, so you are beyond the scope of an exploratory study. The variables you are interested in have been studied before, either independently, as in an exploratory study, or with other variables, so that there is sufficient information to ask a question about the relationship between them. You are able to relate the variables in your study to a concept or conceptual framework so that the study builds on previous work. The major consideration is accuracy in the measurement of the variables.

Designs for studies at Level II require a descriptive survey. The design dictates how the variables are to be measured in testing their relationship. In this design, the variables are partly controlled by the situation, as they are in exploratory designs, but they are also partly controlled by the investigator, usually by the method of choosing a sample for the study. For example, in a study of the relationship between educational level of nurses and ability to make sound judgments about patient care, the investigator controls the first variable by selecting a sample of nurses with all types of educational backgrounds. The judgments of these nurses are then analyzed. The nurses' judgments will be examined in relationship to their educational level. The purpose of the study will be accomplished by seeing if the occurrence of sound judgment is related to educational background.

Surveys cover all types of studies in which a group of people are studied on two or more variables. Some descriptive surveys look at a specific population, such as nurses, to see whether their attitude toward some issue, such as abortion or women's rights, is related to their age or educational background. Others take two or more groups, such as men and women or urban and rural, and see if they differ on some variable, such as life expectancy or the incidence of a particular health problem. Still others take a small patient population, such as renal dialysis patients, and study their coping mechanisms in relation to their acceptance or rejection of a transplanted kidney. All of these are descriptive surveys. Just as with exploratory designs, the answer is in descriptive form, but the description is of the relationship between the variables rather than of the variables themselves.

Many research questions ask about variables that cannot be subjected to experimental manipulation, either because the variables cannot be manipulated or because to look at them outside their natural setting would be meaningless. For example, in looking at factors leading to mental illness, it would be unethical to isolate a single factor, such as poverty, and manipulate it to see if it results in mental illness. An experimental design would require that subjects be assigned to groups and required to live at different levels of poverty. After the specified length of time had passed, the groups would be examined to see if mental illness had developed. The absurdity of such an approach is obvious.

Rather than using experimentation to discover the causes of mental illness, you start with the effect and select a sample of mentally ill patients. Then you look for variables that might be related to mental illness. You might find a significant relationship between poverty and mental illness.

You might also establish that poverty precedes mental illness in time. However, you might discover that well-to-do persons are less likely to be diagnosed as mentally ill even when they have the same symptoms as persons at the bottom of the poverty scale. The type of health care available to persons of different economic levels is different, as are educational opportunities and many other factors. Thus poverty cannot be isolated as the single cause of mental illness. Other variables cannot be controlled or ruled out as possible causative factors either. This is the chance you take when trying to establish causality: alternative explanations are always possible in descriptive surveys. Subjects differ on many factors, only a few of which can be controlled.

Although absolute proof of causality cannot be established in a descriptive survey, it is possible to accumulate extensive evidence to support causality. Much of the research on cigarette smoking and lung cancer was done using descriptive surveys. No experimental research has been or will be done with human subjects to see if lung cancer can be caused by introducing cigarette smoking. But, by showing that cigarette smoking is the one variable preponderant in persons with lung cancer, support grows for the theory that the disease can be caused by smoking.

Many variables of interest to nursing researchers cannot be experimentally manipulated. Attitudes, beliefs, or behaviors are concepts that are often thought of as causal in health, illness, response to treatment, and other effects. The descriptive survey can be of great value in the study of these variables.

Correlational designs are studies of the relationship of two or more variables. An outcome variable may be known, but the causative variable is unknown or thought to be a combination of several variables. Two variables may be known to coexist, but research has not shown any relationship between them or established the direction of their relationship. In other words, you may not know if the variables are positively or negatively correlated. These are field studies that may be cross-sectional, prospective, or retrospective. The concept of control in these studies will focus on reliability testing of data collection instruments and sample selection procedures. The central issue in correlational designs is to establish generalizability to the target population or external validity.

The purpose of correlational designs is to establish definitively the strength and direction of the relationship between two or more variables based on the findings from previous research. These designs are different from comparative designs because they do not require a theoretical framework or explanation; they only look for relationships among variables.

They may not be able to establish (from the literature) which variable is independent and which is dependent at the beginning of the study. They require large probability samples. They are similar to comparative designs in that there is no control over the independent variable; in other words, there is no manipulation, and they require reliable and valid measurement of variables based on previous research literature on the study variables.

All correlational designs demand a conceptual framework or an explanation of why the researcher thinks these variables are related to one another and how. The basic assumptions of the design are that the variables exist in the population; the sample represents the population (probability sampling); the variables can be measured accurately, on a numeric scale; and there is no manipulation of variables.

Variations of the classic design include systematic or convenience samples (which must provide detailed information on the population), time series, and designs that are either retrospective or prospective. Data collection methods must be quantitative, with reliable and valid measurements. Each subject is measured more than once (multiple measurements on each subject). Because of the type of data collected and the size of the samples, data analysis usually involves multivariate statistical techniques, such as correlational analysis, regression analysis, and factor analysis.

Researchers generally use correlational designs when they are not sure if the variables are related to each other, when they think the variables are related to each other but are not sure how they are related, or when they think variables are related to each other but do not know how strong that relationship really is. It is unethical to use correlational designs when the instrumentation is neither valid nor reliable and when there is no possibility of producing usable results. It is impossible to use correlational designs when there has been no previous research on the variables, when variables cannot be measured numerically, or when the sample is too small.

When critiquing correlational designs, you should focus on the sampling strategies used as well as the measurement of variables.

Comparative designs are usually field studies in which the independent variable already exists and the sample is selected on the basis of the independent variable. For example, the sample is divided into groups at the beginning of the study based on the age of the subjects. The comparative design is distinguished from the quasi-experimental design by not having researcher manipulation of the independent variable.

The comparative design, like the correlational design, is a descriptive design because it does not control or manipulate the independent variable. Therefore, a comparative design cannot prove or disprove theory. It does, however, provide information about naturally occurring phenomena in a way that is impossible for experimental designs. To use this design, it must be possible to find naturally occurring groups that differ on the independent variable.

Just like the experimental design, the comparative design must have the following characteristics: (1) at least two known and previously studied variables: an independent variable that is believed to be causative and a dependent variable that is believed to be the effect; (2) the dependent variable is the only variable that is measured; (3) the design is theory based; and (4) the design uses a predictive hypothesis rather than a simple statement of relationship.

Unlike the experimental design, (1) the independent variable is observed as it occurs naturally in the population; (2) the independent variable cannot be manipulated in reality or ethically; (3) the design cannot test theory directly; (4) the design is based on a research question, such as, What are the differences between groups when the groups represent different positions of the independent variable? and (5) the design attempts to represent the population through probability sampling.

The classic comparative design is similar to the experimental design with two groups: a treatment group and a control group. After the change or intervention has occurred naturally, the dependent variable is measured with either a ratio or interval level measurement tool, which has been previously tested and found to be both valid and reliable. An example of a two-group comparative design would be the classic study of smokers versus nonsmokers (the independent variable) on their length of life (the dependent variable), based on the predictive hypothesis that nonsmokers would live longer than smokers. The study would have been designed on the basis of findings from a correlational survey answering the question, What is the relationship between smoking and state of health?

The comparative design has more than one form. The study can be retrospective if the sample is selected on the basis of the dependent variable. The sample could have consisted of individuals with a variety of cancers (the effect or dependent variable). Their past histories would have been examined for their smoking history (the assumed cause or independent variable). Another variation could be a time series comparative design in which an effect had been noted in a hospital chart (e.g., staphylococcus infection) as occurring on a specific date in the patient's stay. Multiple observations are made before and after the onset of the infection. A third variation could be the study of existing multiple treatment groups, such as nursing management systems in the same or different hospitals compared to one or more patient outcomes.

In the comparative design, control over the data is accomplished through the sample selection methods, the conditions under which variables are observed and measured, and by the statistical techniques used to analyze the data.

There are several sampling issues in comparative designs. The most desirable sample is the stratified random sample, a probability sample based on a known population. The second option, based on unknown population parameters, is the quota or nonprobability stratified sample drawn on the independent variable. Samples may be either proportionate to the total population or groups of equal size. The third and most common sampling type is the convenience sample: runners versus nonrunners, normal weight versus obese subjects. If the samples are not representative of the population (i.e., probability sampling), then the groups must be equivalent on all relevant variables except the independent variable.

When collecting data for a comparative design, all quantitative methods of data collection are acceptable. At this level of design, the reliability and validity of the measurement instruments are critical because the validity of the results will depend on accurate discrimination between groups. The best measurements are on ratio or interval scales. A nominal or ordinal scale can be used if it is a numeric scale. It is always best to use known data collection instruments that have been previously tested.

Data analysis procedures involve looking at the differences between two groups. If we assume probability sampling and interval–ratio levels of measurement, then the t-test is the appropriate test because it compares the mean scores on both groups and examines the probability that this magnitude of difference could have happened by chance. If we used multiple groups, and the independent variable was categorical, then the ANOVA is appropriate. This tells us if multiple group means are statistically different from one another. If we have only one independent variable, then we can use the one-way ANOVA. If the independent variable is quantitative, such as annual income, and the dependent variable is also quantitative, use a regression analysis.

Experimental Designs

All experimental designs have one central characteristic: they are based on manipulating the independent variable and measuring the effect on the dependent variable.

Control is achieved in experimental designs by eliminating all sources of variation except that which the researcher introduces. In a study designed to measure the outcome of an intervention, for example, everything that happens to the subjects during the study must be equivalent for both the experimental and control subjects except the fact that the experimental subjects receive the intervention and the controls do not. This ensures that differences between these groups, following the intervention, can be attributed to the effect of the intervention.

Even with perfect control of the independent variable, however, the assumptions of cause and effect cannot be met unless the experimental and control groups are equivalent to each other before the intervention is imposed. Extraneous differences between the groups could affect the outcome of the experiment, which would then falsely be attributed to the success or failure of the intervention. These extraneous variables are considered to be controlled when the sample is randomly assigned to the experimental and control groups, and the groups remain intact for the duration of the experiment. Other forms of assignment to groups and large dropout rates diminish the confidence of the investigator in the results of the experiment.

Another type of control is achieved by building extraneous variables into the study as independent variables and therefore being able to measure their effect on the dependent variable(s). This method is generally used in Level II studies where random assignment to groups is not possible. Each additional variable added to the study will increase the cost of the research; therefore, adding variables must be done with care.

The classic experimental design consists of an experimental group and a control group with a before and after measurement of the dependent variable. First the dependent variable is measured in both groups. Then in the experimental group, the independent variable is introduced. Nothing is changed for the control group. After the specified time has passed, the dependent variable is measured on both groups again. The prediction is that the dependent variable in the experimental group will change in a specific way and that the dependent variable in the control group will not change.

	Independent Variable	Dependent Variable
Experimental Group	Changed	Measured
Control Group	Unchanged	Measured

When data are analyzed, only the measurements on the dependent variable for the two groups are contrasted.

For example:

Independent Variable	**Dependent Variable**
Preoperative teaching	Postoperative pain, medication consumption
No teaching	Postoperative pain, medication consumption

A number of variations are possible. First, there are designs in which there is one control group and two or more experimental groups, and the independent variable is manipulated in several different ways. For example:

Independent Variable	**Dependent Variable**
Usual preoperative teaching	Postoperative pain, medication consumption
Structured preoperative teaching	
Lecture–Discussion	Postoperative pain, medication consumption
Videotape–Discussion	Postoperative pain, medication consumption

The hypothesis would predict which of the three teaching methods would be most successful (that is, the group with the lowest pain medication consumption postoperatively). The point is to contrast the three groups.

Another more sophisticated design would pretest all three groups on the content to be taught. After the teaching (manipulating the independent variable), the subjects would again be tested on the same content (the dependent variable). The scores for each subject before and after the teaching would be compared. The differences among groups would then be placed side by side to see which teaching method was most effective. Following the surgery, pain medication consumption would be compared among all groups (the second dependent variable). Each subject would be examined in relation to knowledge and consumption of pain medication. With the addition of pain medication consumption as a dependent variable, knowledge of the subject would become an intervening variable between preoperative teaching and medication consumption. The design would look like this:

Pretest	Experiment Teaching	Posttest	Surgery	Medication Consumption
O_1	Group 1	O_2	Control	O_3
O_4	Group 2	O_5	Exp 1	O_6
O_7	Group 3	O_8	Exp 2	O_9

We simply have added several other variables to the classic experimental design and measured them as well, as in the first design. In addition, we have added groups to the design and tested and compared them as well.

Each group is tested or observed (O) three times: pretest, after the teaching program, and after the intervening variable of surgery. Group 1 is the control group and does not receive any form of experimental teaching. Following the teaching, each group is tested on their knowledge base (second set of Os). The third set of Os follows the surgery and tests the amount of medication consumed. Subjects therefore can be compared to themselves, to others in their group, and to other groups.

The most critical characteristic of experimental designs is investigator manipulation of the independent variable; it is always manipulated, altered, or changed in some way in the experimental group. In true experiments there is always a control group and random assignment of subjects to groups. The theoretical base for the study predicts the direction of the change in the dependent variable as a result of the introduction of the independent variable. The distinguishing feature between true experiments and quasi-experiments is that the quasi-experiment does not have random assignment to groups and/or does not have a control group.

Features of the True or Classic Experiment

- Subjects are randomly assigned to groups (R).
- The experimenter manipulates the experimental variable (X).
- There are at least two groups: experimental (X) and control (C).

The control group is used to measure the dependent variable when the independent variable has not been applied. The experiment is based on the assumption that there will be a difference in measurement of the dependent variable depending on the manipulation of the independent variable.

The following are some examples of experimental designs where R = random assignment to groups; X = experimental group; C = control group; O = measurement or observation before or after the experimental manipulation.

After-Only Design

R $\quad\quad\quad\quad$ X $\quad$ O_1
R $\quad\quad\quad\quad$ C $\quad$ O_2

In the After-Only design, there are two groups, random assignment to both groups, experimental manipulation of one group, no manipulation of the other group, and both groups tested.

Before-After Design

R $\quad\quad\quad\quad$ O_1 $\quad$ X $\quad$ O_2
R $\quad\quad\quad\quad$ O_3 $\quad$ C $\quad$ O_4

In the Before-After design, both groups are tested at the same time on the dependent variable both before and after the experimental manipulation in the experimental group.

Solomon Four Group Design

R $\quad\quad\quad\quad$ O_1 $\quad$ X $\quad$ O_2
R $\quad\quad\quad\quad$ O_3 $\quad$ C $\quad$ O_4
R $\quad\quad\quad\quad$. $\quad$ X $\quad$ O_5
R $\quad\quad\quad\quad$. $\quad$ C $\quad$ O_6

In the Solomon Four Group design, the After-Only and the Before-After designs are combined into one design. The rationale for this combination is that subjects have been known to do better on a measurement the second time they are tested no matter what has happened between testing periods. There is some learning that occurs simply with familiarity with the measuring instrument or the experience itself. For this reason, this design compares the scores of groups who have not had a pretest (After-Only) with the scores of the two groups who have been pretested. In this way the two experimental groups are contrasted and the two control groups are contrasted to verify the difference in the posttest as a result of the pretest. Then the After-Only groups are contrasted and the Before and After groups are contrasted on the dependent variable. Finally the two experimental groups together are contrasted with the two control groups' scores.

Although this may sound like a pointless exercise, it really isn't. Remember that the true experimental design is expected to be the most highly controlled laboratory study possible. As a result, a number of statistical analyses are required in all types of combinations to test the hypothesis.

Quasi-experimental designs are based solely on experimenter manipulation of the independent variable and lack at least one characteristic of the true experiment.

Features of the Quasi-Experiment

- Experimental manipulation of the independent variable
- No random assignment to groups, and/or
- No control group(s)

The quasi-experimental design looks much like the previous experimental designs; simply remove the R for random assignment to groups and the same type of experiments are possible. Instead of random assignment, you may substitute matched groups or you may have convenient groups. A quasi-experimental design without a control group might look like this:

$$O_1 \ O_2 \ O_3 \ O_4 \ X \ O_5 \ O_6 \ O_7 \ O_8$$

In this example, the experimental group serves as its own control in a time series design with one or more measurements before the experiment and one or more measurements after.

Sometimes a true experimental design is simply not possible to carry out. Many nursing studies are forced into quasi-experimental designs by the nature of the study or the natural clinical setting. A study of a new nursing intervention on an inpatient unit might use a quasi-experimental time series design like the previous one to test the old intervention over time before instituting a new one and then testing the new one over time. Or if two nursing units were fairly similar in their type of patient population, the two units might be used for comparison, each using a different nursing intervention. Both units would serve as a comparison group for the other in Before-After designs without random assignment to groups.

The limitations of the experimental design are that some variables are simply not amenable to manipulation (such as age, gender, and ethnicity). Other variables (such as smoking to cause cancer, use of a placebo in place of a contraceptive device, nontreatment of a disease for which a cure is known) are not experimentally ethical. Sometimes experiments are impractical, sometimes they seem artificial or contrived, and sometimes the Hawthorne effect (discussed later in this chapter) causes people to change their behavior.

A major purpose of the experimental design is to eliminate alternative explanations or hypotheses to account for the findings. It is the controlled setting, the contrast groups, and the control over the experimental variable that allow for acceptance or rejection of the hypothesis being tested. Although the experiment may have turned out correctly, there is still the outside chance that something other than the experimental variable caused the effect in the dependent variable. As a result, we always hold that we tentatively accept the findings in the light of current evidence, always subject to change with new knowledge.

Controlling Unwanted Influences

To obtain a reliable answer to the research question, the design must indicate how it will control or eliminate possible unwanted influences. The amount of control that the researcher has over the variables being studied varies, from very little in exploratory studies to a great deal in experimental design, but the limitations on control must be addressed in every research proposal.

These unwanted influences stem from one or more of the following: extraneous variables, bias, the Hawthorne effect, and the passage of time. These four will be discussed in turn, along with some suggestions for controlling their effects. You will need to identify those that seem relevant to your question and show how you will control their effects.

Extraneous Variables

As explained in Chapter 6, extraneous variables are variables that can interfere with the action of the ones you are studying. They could as easily have been chosen as independent variables had you been interested in them because of their known effect on your variables. Because they are not part of your study, their influence must be controlled.

In the research literature, you will see extraneous variables also referred to as intervening, environmental, organismic, confounding, or demographic variables. Each term, however, defines a slightly different class of extraneous variables. Intervening or confounding variables, found in Level III experimental designs, directly affect the action of the independent variable on the dependent variable. They must be controlled in the design even though they are not of prime interest to the researcher because they will affect the results of the experiment. Environmental variables are those that occur in the study setting. They include economic, physical, and psychosocial variables. Organismic variables refer to person characteristics, such as physiological, psychological, or demographic variables. Demographic variables are descriptive characteristics, such as age, gender, marital status, and education.

Your literature review should help you determine which extraneous variables might be present in your study. As an example, look at the question, What are the relationships among style of leadership, educational opportunities on the job, and the job satisfaction of staff nurses? Many factors are known to influence job satisfaction. Why not choose age, marital status of the nurse, the amount of independence on the job, or the level of education of the nurse as independent variables? Any of these could qualify, but, because you are not interested in them, they are not directly a part of your study. They are extraneous to your study, and you want to be sure they do not interfere with the relationship between style of leadership and job satisfaction and between educational opportunities and job satisfaction.

Extraneous variables usually are not a problem in Level I studies. Because you are studying only one variable in depth, these variables are assumed to be independent. They could all be extraneous variables as well. That is why an exploratory descriptive study explores in depth: all variables must be accounted for and taken into consideration to be described adequately.

At Level II, when you do not know which variables are independent and which are dependent, you must assume that there may be variables that have not been accounted for that may be related to the dependent variable. Some variables have been shown to be related to one of your variables in other studies. These are known extraneous variables and must be considered when designing your study, so that their effect on your variables can be controlled. At Level II, it is sometimes difficult to establish which one is the independent variable, even after confirming that there is a significant relationship between two variables. Unless you can demonstrate that one variable precedes the other in time, it may be impossible to determine which is the independent variable. Therefore, it is important to control extraneous variables when you can identify what they are, so that you can isolate the relationship between the ones you are interested in studying.

At Level III, where you are predicting the relationship, you must be very careful to control all possible extraneous variables that might intervene in your test. These variables can be identified from the literature on your topic.

Methods of controlling extraneous variables include randomization, homogenous sampling techniques, matching, and building the variables into the design.

Randomization

Theoretically, randomization is the only method of controlling all possible extraneous variables. The random assignment of subjects to the various treatment and control groups means that the groups can be considered equivalent in all ways at the beginning of the experiment. It does not mean that they actually are equal for all variables. However, the probability of their being equal is greater than the probability of their not being equal, if the random assignment was carried out properly. The exception lies with small groups where random assignment could result in unequal distribution of crucial variables. If this possibility exits in your study, perhaps one of the other methods of control would be more appropriate. In most instances, however, randomization is the best method of controlling extraneous variables.

The principle of randomization applies to both Level II and Level III studies. In Level II studies, a random sampling technique results in a normal distribution of extraneous variables in the sample, which approximates the distribution of those variables in the population. Probability theory demonstrates that this will happen in 95 random samples out of 100 from the same population. The purpose of randomization at Level II is to ensure a representative sample so that your result can be generalized from the sample to the population.

At Level III, randomization comes into play when you randomly assign subjects to experimental and control groups, thus ensuring that the groups are as equivalent as possible prior to the manipulation of the independent variable. Random assignment ensures that the researcher was not biased in putting certain people into the experimental groups. Instead, each subject had an equal chance of being in any of the groups at the beginning of the assignment process.

Here is one method of random assignment. This method is called systematic assignment to groups with a random start and is used when the sample is expected to arrive sequentially, such as patients do in an emergency room on any given day. When the first patient who meets the criteria for the sample arrives, that person is randomly assigned to one of the groups. This assignment can be done by flipping a coin or by drawing a number out of a hat. If the study has four groups, and the first patient is assigned to group 2, the next patient goes to group 3, the next to group 4, the next to group 1, and so on. With this method, you make no choice as to which group a patient will be in, and the groups will be of approximately equal size at any given time during the study. This is important if you expect it to take a long time to fill the groups to the desired size.

If all the subjects are available at the beginning of the study, you can place tickets in a box with group numbers representing the way you want the subjects distributed (that is, 30 subjects per group divided into four groups), and then have each subject draw a number. If you use this method, and subjects arrive sequentially over a long period, you might end up with one group filling sooner than the others, which could introduce some bias into your study.

Whichever method is used, every precaution must be taken to remove subjectivity from the assignment of subjects to groups. Clinical studies, for example, have been seriously affected by having professional staff reassign subjects away from the protocol. A research colleague once reported having to cancel a clinical experiment because the nursing staff, believing that the experimental variable was highly successful, began assigning patients who they felt would benefit from it rather than following the protocol for random assignment. Such decisions should not be made by clinical staff, so the research design must be carefully monitored to make sure the system is carried out.

Homogeneous Sample

One simple and effective way of controlling an extraneous variable is not to allow it to vary. Choose a sample that is homogeneous for that variable. For example, if you are concerned about the effect that the patients' cultural backgrounds might have on your study of pain, choose a sample from only one cultural group, such as all Asian Americans or all Mexican Americans. In this way, you have eliminated the possible effect that the subjects' cultural backgrounds might have on their responses to pain because they all represent the same culture. This method has one serious drawback, however: the ability to generalize the findings is limited. As you might expect, if you study only Mexican Americans, then your results apply only to Mexican Americans and not to African Americans, Asian Americans, or Native Americans. If the sample is limited to one age group, the results apply only to that age group because the relationship you find between your variables might be different for other age groups. You will not know; you can only guess.

For example, in the example on job satisfaction, the sample could be limited to nurses with bachelor's degrees or to nurses older than 50 years of age. On the other hand, the study could be of nurses on night shift or nurses who are in critical care units. The sample is being made homogeneous for certain variables and not others. Kang, in her study of uncertainty and health locus of control in patients with atrial fibrillation, sought to have a homogeneous sample on the variable of diagnosis, choosing only participants diagnosed with atrial fibrillation within the previous six months. Excluded were people diagnosed more than six months ago, those with any disease other than atrial fibrillation within the previous three months, and anyone with a terminal illness. Thus Kang attempted to control for the potential effect of duration of diagnosis, as well as that of a new diagnosis and/or the effect of expected death on the participant's perceived uncertainty (Kang, 2009).

Matching

When randomization is not possible, or when the experimental groups are too small and contain some crucial variables, subjects can be matched for those variables. The experimenter chooses subjects who match one another for the specified variables, such as gender, age, and diagnosis. One of these matched subjects is assigned to the control group and the other to the experimental group, thus ensuring the equality of the groups at the outset. In survey designs, comparison groups can be created through matching, allowing theory to be tested without experimentation.

Costanzo et al. examined whether cancer survivors showed impairment, resilience, or growth responses in four domains—mental health and mood, psychological well-being, social well-being, and spirituality— compared to a sample matched on age, gender, and educational level who reported no cancer. All participants in this study were part of a large survey in the United States. Cancer survivors were a subset of this large sample. Matching individuals were identified by a computer program, and two individuals were randomly selected from this group for each cancer survivor (Costanzo, Ryff, & Singer, 2009).

The process of matching can be time-consuming and often introduces considerable subjectivity into sample selection. If you use matching, limit the number of groups to be matched and keep the number of variables for which the subjects are matched low. Matching with more than five variables becomes extremely cumbersome, and it is almost impossible to find enough matched partners for your sample. Matching may be used in all research designs (besides Level III) when you are looking at certain outcomes and want to have as much control as possible.

Building Extraneous Variables into the Design

When extraneous variables cannot be adequately controlled by randomization, they can be built into the design as independent variables. They would have to be added to the data collection plan and tested for significance along with your other variables. In this way, their effect can be measured and separated from the effect of the variables you wanted to study initially. Particularly in experimental designs, but also in descriptive surveys, the effect of these variables can be removed statistically from the total action of the variables. This method adds to the cost of the study because of the additional data collection and analysis required. Therefore, it should be used with caution.

In exploratory descriptive studies where the nature of the variables is not known, extraneous variables are said to be built into the design. The purpose in these studies is to identify the relevant variables and assess their relationship in the data analysis. Therefore, it is essential that you treat all variables as independent during the data collection so that no data that later might point to relationships among variables will be overlooked. The separation of extraneous variables from independent and dependent variables is part of the analysis of data in exploratory research.

Bias

Bias results from collecting the data in such a way that one answer to the research question is given undue favor over another. Bias can be introduced into a study at any point, from the initial writing of the research question to the conclusions of the research report, and must be constantly guarded against when you are developing your research project. All researchers are biased in relation to their own studies as a natural outcome of their intense interest in their research topics. We all know how we would like our studies to come out and what we think we will find when we collect and analyze the data. We are therefore obligated to avoid influencing the outcome in any way, even unconsciously. The results must be an objective reporting of the real situation. Because most researchers are scrupulously honest in the accuracy with which they handle their data, we will only deal with the two areas where bias can easily be introduced (even by the most honest researcher) if care is not taken. These are during the sample selection and data collection phases of the project. (The other area of concern is the interpretation of data, which we do not deal with in this book, but you need to be aware of it when you are critiquing research reports.)

Because you know what you would like your results to be, you want to avoid unconsciously swaying the study in that direction. During sample selection, if you are not able to use random sampling techniques, it is too easy to acquire a biased sample if you are not careful. Always take precautions to maintain objectivity whenever you can, and use methods to predetermine who will be in your sample; do not wait until you are face to face with potential subjects to decide. For example, if your plan is to interview hospitalized patients on a particular unit, choose the room numbers you will visit from an available list, and then ask all patients in those rooms to be interviewed. If an interviewer arrives on a nursing unit to select patients without these kinds of guidelines, he or she may end up choosing patients who look as if they would enjoy being interviewed—a biased sample! Another biased sample could result from asking a staff member to recommend some patients for interview because you would not know the staff member's criteria for the recommendation. Any time random selection is not possible, make your choice of subjects as objective as possible by reducing the number of choices available to you by setting predetermined guidelines.

Bias during the data collection phase of research means that the researcher is either influencing the responses of the subjects in some way or is selectively recording data according to conscious or unconscious predispositions.

In the first case, the subjects' responses are influenced in any one direction by the way in which data collection is approached. This is easiest to do in an interview, where subjects can be given the impression that one response will be received more favorably than another or that one response represents the best choice. Careful training and monitoring of interviewers is required to prevent undue influence from affecting interview responses.

The second case refers to selective recording of data by the researcher. This can occur in observational studies and in reviewing audiotapes, audiovisual tapes, and written documents, even when structured tools are used to record the data. Selectively focusing on some parts of the data and overlooking significant opposing views can be easily done by persons eager to prove a point. Everyone must guard against this happening by building in checks and balances—such as having an impartial colleague periodically work along with the researcher. Other checks and balances are discussed in Chapter 10, in the sections on reliability and validity in participant observation. You cannot completely eliminate bias from an exploratory study because of the essential flexibility of the design. You can, however, plan for as much objectivity as possible and keep in mind the limitations of this design when drawing conclusions from your data.

In other levels of designs—descriptive survey designs and experimental designs—the elimination of bias from the data collection becomes more critical. The influence of the investigator's bias in an exploratory study, though difficult to eliminate, can at least be described along with the data. If, however, inferences are to be drawn from the data, there is no room for bias. Therefore, every precaution must be taken to prevent influencing the data collection process.

The Hawthorne Effect

The Hawthorne effect refers to the effect that the knowledge of being the subjects of a research study has on the subjects' responses. In experimental studies, care needs to be taken that the resultant changes in the dependent variable can be attributed to the independent variable and not to the special attention given to the subjects in the experimental group. When testing the effect of nursing interventions, it may be wise to equalize the amount of nursing time spent with patients in both the experimental and control groups to rule out the possibility that the patient is responding to the interaction with the nurse rather than to the intervention. The control group can be thought of as a placebo group in which nursing interaction is provided without the experimental variable.

In the early stages of nursing research, many studies capitalized on the Hawthorne effect without realizing that they had done so. These early clinical studies used a two-group experimental design in which the control group received the usual nursing care and the experimental group received the full force of a deliberate nursing intervention. In every case, the experimental group was significantly different from the control group. Because of the Hawthorne effect, these studies did not prove anything except that deliberate nursing actions do make a difference. They did not prove which interventions were better than others.

To minimize the Hawthorne effect in experimental designs, or at least to account for it, try to use more than one experimental group and preferably those who are competitive with the point you are trying to make. For example, in a patient teaching study, have several experimental groups who receive different teaching methods, or have a group that receives individualized attention from a nurse for the same length of time as the experimental group that receives the experimental variable. Otherwise, you will prove, once again, that people appreciate being noticed, even as research subjects.

Time

This category is used to cover those factors resulting from the fact that life goes on during the research process. Events that occur just before or during the study period can affect the responses of subjects, yet have nothing to do with the study—for example, an earthquake, a race riot, or a movie on television. These events can produce changes in attitudes, feelings, and behavior; if the researcher is unaware of their effect, they can lead to erroneous conclusions. Interviewing patients about sensory disturbances during the aftermath of an earthquake would produce some interesting data. But the data would be related to the earthquake rather than to being a patient. If you are questioning people about controversial issues to assess their attitudes, it would be wise to check the television schedule for the week of your data collection to avoid coinciding with a special program on your topic.

Developmental or maturation processes also can influence the variables you are planning to measure, particularly if your subjects are very young or very old. This is of special concern when it is necessary to have a long interval between data collection times. The use of control groups may be necessary to rule out the possibility of developmental changes. A special counseling program for disadvantaged students, for example, is expected to ease the students' adjustment to nursing school. A control group would give substance to the fact that the special counseling program did ease adjustment and that the students' adjustment was not due simply to the social experience that the school provides.

Level of Study and Degree of Control

In Level I studies, where as much flexibility as possible is encouraged, the concept of control of the variables in the design has little relevance. What is needed at Level I is the concept of control of external influences on the research process itself. Here you are concerned with the biases of the researcher and how to control or minimize them. You are expected to keep a journal of events that occur when you are doing exploratory research so that you can account for possible alterations in the study that may be related to these events. The Hawthorne effect occurs in Level I studies when the subjects react to being studied. It is controlled over time, when the presence of the investigator becomes so familiar that the subjects become unaware they are being observed.

At Level II, you are more concerned with controlling extraneous variables in the design and conduct of the study. When you are looking for significant relationships between two or more variables, you must be sure you have accounted for all other variables that might influence the interaction of the variable you are studying. These are accounted for by random sample selection and by collecting data on key extraneous variables so that their effect can be measured. At Level II, you are not as concerned with the bias of the investigator because the objectivity of the structured data collection methods tends to minimize investigator bias.

In experimental studies at Level III, you must be careful to control extraneous variables that occur as a result of time, the Hawthorne effect, or sampling. To accomplish this control, you attempt to keep the experimental conditions identical for the various groups in your design. You begin by randomly assigning the sample to the groups so that they will be equivalent at the beginning of the experiment. In addition, you may select a relatively homogeneous population to begin with so that some extraneous variables do not have to be considered. Next, make sure that the treatment of the groups throughout the collection of the data continues to be the same in every respect except for the application of the independent variable. Data on the dependent variable are collected in the same way from all groups. An excessive dropout rate from one of your groups may be an indication that the experimental conditions are not being maintained for all groups and that some subjects are dissatisfied with their role in the study.

In summary, the research design provides the blueprint for the research plan specifically in terms of the control mechanisms that will be used to provide a clear and accurate answer to your research question. The level at which you can study a given research topic is based on the level of knowledge already in existence about that topic. This will also affect the degree of control you can achieve over the variables in your study. To gain sufficient depth of information, the flexibility that is required for a Level I exploratory study will limit the degree of control over the study conditions. To achieve maximum control, every detail of a study must be planned in advance. Therefore, at Level I, control is limited to the choice of the initial sample and most commonly results in a homogeneous sample.

At Level II, the major concern is to maximize the external validity of the results; therefore, the critical control mechanism is the random selection of subjects from the population. When this is not possible in a Level II study, it is always considered to be a serious limitation in the design. Also at this level, you will be concerned with maintaining consistent conditions throughout the study so that bias in data collection will be minimized.

Experimental designs require maximum possible control over extraneous and intervening variables so that internal validity can be maximized. You want to be able to say with some assurance that the results are an accurate reflection of the action of the independent variable. Thus random assignment to groups is essential, as is maintaining consistent study conditions for all groups. When planning a Level III study, your goal is to be able to foresee every detail of the design so that unwanted influences can be avoided.

Regardless of the level of study you are planning, the design phase will require significant time and effort on your part to think through the elements that will be required to provide the answer to your question. This time is well spent, however, in terms of the time and effort it saves later when you are carrying out the steps in your plan.

Bibliography

Allen, D. (2004). Ethnomethodological insights into insider-outsider relationships in nursing ethnographies of healthcare settings. *Nursing Inquiry, 11*(1), 14–24.

Ameringer, S., Sertin, R. C., & Ward, S. (2009). Simpson's paradox and experimental research. *Nursing Research, 58*(2), 123–127.

Becker, H., Roberts, G., & Voelmeck, W. (2003). Explanations for improvement in both experimental and control groups. *Western Journal of Nursing Research, 25*(6), 746–755.

Behi, R., & Nolan, M. (1996). Causality and control: Threats to internal validity. *British Journal of Nursing, 5*(6), 374–377.

Brink, P. J. (1998). Exploratory designs. In P. J. Brink & M. J. Wood (Eds.), *Advanced design in nursing research* (2nd ed., pp. 141–160). Thousand Oaks, CA: Sage.

Brink, P. J., & Wood, M. J. (Eds.). (1998). *Advanced design in nursing research* (2nd ed.). Thousand Oaks, CA: Sage.

Brink, P. J., & Wood, M. J. (1998). Correlational designs. In P. J. Brink & M. J. Wood (Eds.), *Advanced design in nursing research* (2nd ed., pp. 160–167). Thousand Oaks, CA: Sage.

Brink, P. J., & Wood, M. J. (1998). Descriptive designs. In P. J. Brink & M. J. Wood (Eds.), *Advanced design in nursing research* (2nd ed., pp. 287–307). Thousand Oaks, CA: Sage.

Brown, S. R., & Melamed, L. E. (1990). *Experimental design and analysis.* Newbury Park, CA: Sage.

Buckwalter, K. C., & Maas, M. L. (1998). Classical experimental designs. In P. J. Brink & M. J. Wood (Eds.), *Advanced design in nursing research* (2nd ed., pp. 21–62). Thousand Oaks, CA: Sage.

Campbell, D. T., & Stanley, J. C. (1963). *Experimental and quasi-experimental design for research.* Chicago: Rand McNally.

Christie, J., O'Halloran, P., & Stevenson, M. (2009). Planning a cluster randomized controlled trial: Methodological issues. *Nursing Research, 58*(2), 128–134.

Cook, T. D., & Campbell, D. T. (1979). *Quasi-experimentation: Design and analysis issues for field settings.* Chicago: Rand McNally.

Costanzo, E. S., Ryff, C. D., & Singer, B. H. (2009). Psychosocial adjustment among cancer survivors: Findings from a national survey of health and well-being. *Health Psychology, 28*, 147–156.

Creswell, J. W. (2007). *Designing and conducting mixed methods research.* Thousand Oaks, CA: Sage.

Dillman, D. A. (2009). *Internet, mail, and mixed-mode surveys: The tailored design method* (3rd ed.). Hoboken, NJ: Wiley.

Fink, A. (2009). *How to conduct surveys: A step-by-step guide.* Los Angeles: Sage.

Gerrish, K., & Lacey, A. (Eds.). (2006). *The research process in nursing.* Malden, MA: Blackwell.

Higher Education Research Institute (2009). Retrieved November 1, 2009, from www.heri.ucla.edu/cirpoverview.php

Hertzog, M. A. (2008). Considerations in determining sample size for pilot studies. *Research in Nursing and Health, 31*(2), 180–191.

Holloway, I., & Freshwater, D. (2007). *Narrative research in nursing.* Malden, MA: Blackwell.

Kang, Y. (2009). Role of health locus of control between uncertainty and uncertainty appraisal among patients with atrial fibrillation. *Western Journal of Nursing Research, 31*(2), 187–200.

Mahoney, E. K., Trudeau, S. A., Penyack, S. E., & MacLeod, C. D. (2006). Challenges to intervention implementation: Lessons learned in bathing persons with Alzheimer's disease at home study. *Nursing Research, 55*(2S), S10–16.

McCann, T., & Clark, E. (2003). Grounded theory in nursing research: Part 2—critique. *Nurse Researcher, 11*(2), 19–28.

McGahee, T. W., & Tingen, M. S. (2009). The use of the Solomon four-group design in nursing research. *Southern Online Journal of Nursing Research, 9*(1). Retrieved December 23, 2009, from http://snrs.org/publications/SOJNR_articles2/Vol09Num01Art14.html

Menard, S. (Ed.). (2008). *Handbook of longitudinal research: Design, measurement, and analysis.* Burlington, MA: Elsevier.

Monsen, E. R. (2003). *Research: Successful approaches.* Chicago: American Dietetic Association.

Munhall, P. L. (Ed.). (2007). *Nursing research: A qualitative perspective* (4th ed.). Sudbury, MA: Jones and Bartlett.

Kluckhohn, F. R. & Strodtbeck, F. L. (1961). *Variations in value orientations.* New York: Row, Peterson and Company.

Nieswiadomy, R. M. (2008). *Foundations of nursing research* (5th ed.). Upper Saddle River, NJ: Pearson/Prentice Hall.

Polgar, S., & Thomas, S. A. (2008). *Introduction to research in the health sciences.* New York: Churchill Livingstone Elsevier.

Polit, D. F., & Beck, C. T. (2010). *Essentials of nursing research: Appraising evidence for nursing practice* (7th ed.). Philadelphia: Wolters Kluwer Health/Lippincott Williams & Wilkins.

Pollner, M., & Emerson, R. M. (2001). Ethnomethodology and ethnography. In P. Atkinson, A. Coffey, S. Delamont, J. Loftland & L. Loftland (Eds.), *Handbook of ethnography* (pp. 118–135). London: Sage.

Roper, J. M., & Shapira, J. (2000). *Ethnography in nursing research.* Thousand Oaks, CA: Sage.

Shadish, W. R., Cook, T. D., & Campbell, D. T. (2002). *Experimental and quasi-experimental designs for generalized causal inference.* Boston: Houghton Mifflin.

Stein, K. F., Sargent, J. T., & Rafaels, N. (2007). Intervention research: Establishing fidelity of the independent variable in nursing clinical trials. *Nursing Research, 56*(1), 54–62.

Strauss, A., & Corbin, J. M. (1990). *Basics of qualitative research: Grounded theory procedures and techniques.* Newbury Park, CA: Sage.

Sue, V. M. (2007). *Conducting online surveys.* Los Angeles: Sage.

Tabachnick, B. G. (2007). *Experimental designs using ANOVA.* Belmont, CA: Thomson/Brooks/Cole.

Waltz, C., & Bausell, R. B. (1981). *Nursing research: Design, statistics and computer analysis* (chap. 8–11). Philadelphia: F. A. Davis.

Whitmer, K., Sweeney, C., Slivjack, A., Sumner, C., & Barsevik, A. (2005). Strategies for maintaining integrity of a behavioral intervention. *Western Journal of Nursing Research, 27*(3), 338–345.

Wood, M. J., & Brink, P. J. (1998). Comparative designs. In P. J. Brink & M. J. Wood (Eds.), *Advanced design in nursing research* (2nd ed., pp. 143–159). Thousand Oaks, CA: Sage.

Yin, R. K. (2001). *Case study research: Design and methods* (3rd ed.). London: Sage.

CHAPTER EIGHT

Selecting the Sample

➤ **TOPICS**

Types of Samples
Sample Size
Level of Study and Sample Selection
Bibliography

➤ **LEARNING OBJECTIVES**

- Identify the defining characteristics of probability and nonprobability samples and outline the specific types of samples that fall into each of these categories.
- Explain the factors to consider when developing a sampling plan for probability and nonprobability samples.
- Describe the relationship between the level of the study and the type of sample needed for a study.

When you stop to think about the population for your study, you will realize that by now you have already given considerable thought to this topic in the process of developing your question into a research problem and in planning the design for your study. All along you have had a picture in the back of your mind of the group of subjects that would provide the data for your study. Usually, in nursing research, the subjects are people, but they can also be events, animals, cells, cultures, places, or objects. For simplicity's sake, in this discussion, we will proceed as though the subjects were always people.

151

The *total population* (or universe) can be defined as everyone in the world who meets the criteria for the people you are interested in studying. To decide who makes up this group, you need to look back at the purpose of your study. Perhaps you have said you would be studying pregnant teenagers, or preterm infants, bereaved widows, people with diabetes, hospitalized inpatients, or the general public. Now is the time to describe these people as fully as possible in relation to who they are, where you will find them, and when they will be found. Your total population could be all members of a village or tribe, all citizens of a town or city, all members of the United Nations, all individuals with breast cancer, all members of a single racial or ethnic group in the United States, or all students in baccalaureate nursing programs. Some of these represent very large groups of people; others are quite small. As you begin to describe your total population more fully, you will begin to eliminate some people as possible subjects. Perhaps you will be studying pregnant teenagers but are only interested in girls between the ages of 10 and 14 years who are in their first trimester. Now you have narrowed your focus considerably and have eliminated most of the pregnant teenagers in the world from eligibility for your study. Or perhaps you now realize, because of the conceptual framework you have used for your study, that you really want to concentrate on girls who reside in juvenile detention centers. This has further delineated your population. Now your total population looks like this: pregnant girls, ages 10 to 14 years, in the first trimester of pregnancy, who are incarcerated in juvenile detention centers in the city of Los Angeles. This is the group from which you would like to sample and to whom you would like to generalize your results, so you have answered the who, where, and when part of the definition of your population. You can now call this your target population.

The *target population* is always the theoretically available group to whom you expect to generalize your results. Sometimes this group is identical to the total population with which you started. For example, if your total population had been the current active members of the West Coast Cocker Spaniel Club, your task would now be simple. To answer the questions of where and when, you would obtain a mailing list of the current members from the club secretary and could draw your sample from that list at any time during the current fiscal year. Your total and target populations are identical. The same would be true if your task were to conduct the United States census in 2000. Your total population would be everyone residing in this country at the time of the census in 2000, and your target population is this same group.

This was not true for the population of pregnant teenagers that we previously described. It took several steps to get from the universe of pregnant teenagers to the target population that represents the group you really want to study. Even now, however, the target population of pregnant teenagers in juvenile detention centers in one city is too complex for you to handle, and so you begin to limit, or target, your study to an even more accessible group. The total population of pregnant teenagers becomes more specifically targeted to one juvenile detention center in your city to which you have access. Remember, the target population is the group that is theoretically available to you and to which you plan to generalize your results. The more you limit, or target, this population, the smaller the group to whom you can generalize in your final analysis. One specific juvenile detention center in your city is not representative of your original total population, and so you must change your idea of the total population to include inmates of just one juvenile detention center.

Some of the considerations you will make in targeting your population stem from your own resources. Can you get to the population after you have defined it? Are the subjects in your geographic location or do you have funds and transportation to get to them? Can you get permission to study the subjects you have targeted? Your study population is dependent on your resources, including the amount of time and money you have available to do research. If you want to study current college presidents, the total population in the world is very likely too much to handle, so you may limit your target population to US college presidents and sample from that group. You may decide on eastern college presidents or presidents of colleges in your own state. Each subsequent geographic narrowing targets the population further, and with each narrowing you further limit the group to whom you will generalize your results. At the same time, you are making your sample selection more and more reasonable. Think of targeting as narrowing or limiting the total population into something reasonable.

One further consideration needs to be made when you are finalizing the definition of your target population, and that is to *make sure the population will be accessible to you when you get ready to select your sample and collect your data.* This is the single most serious problem facing any researcher. Nothing is more discouraging than finding that the subjects you need are either not accessible or not available when you need them. Sometimes it is a problem of getting permission to access the subjects. Several students recently tried to access a population of AIDS patients for research and found that these patients are very protected by the organizations responsible for their care. Although as nursing graduate students they could get permission to give nursing care through a home health agency, they were not allowed to collect data for research. For your own population, you must give serious consideration to whether or not you will have permission to study them when you get to them. If the target population is not accessible to you, you cannot proceed.

The question of availability must also be considered. Are you sure there will be enough subjects available from which to draw your sample? How many pregnant girls are there at juvenile detention centers between the ages of 10 and 14 years at any given time? Perhaps even the entire population will not provide you with enough data to do your study. These are questions that can be investigated before casting your target population in cement. It is much better to discover these kinds of problems during the process of defining your population rather than after the study is under way.

When you have completely defined your target population, you can choose your sample from that group. The population is the group of people you are interested in studying. The sample merely represents them. Be as detailed as you can about who qualifies to be in the population, and your sample selection will be easier.

If you plan to replicate another study, remember that the population in your study must closely approximate the population used in the original study. The setting in which you find the subjects will be different, but all other aspects of the original population should be identical. For example, if the original study used nurses from two-, three-, and four-year programs; any age, gender, race, or ethnic background; working at UCLA Hospital within three years after graduating from nursing school, your replication study must use a population as close to this one as possible. Perhaps you are doing the study in Seattle and want to use nurses working at the University of Washington Hospital. This change is acceptable provided that you keep the other characteristics of the population the same.

When you replicate a study done by another researcher, you cannot possibly use the exact target population the other researcher used because you are not in the same place at the same time. In a sense, the difference in time and location validates the findings. In multiple concurrent replication studies (Brink & Wood, 1979) and clinical trials, the replication of a research project occurs simultaneously in multiple settings. Several investigators conduct the same study, using the same design, at different locations. Each can generalize only to the target population in the local setting. However, the total population can be expanded through comparison of the concurrent replication studies.

Where your subjects will be found is a major element in your population description. If you are interested only in ICU nurses at Battleground Hospital, say so. If you are interested in nursing staff or patients at a particular nursing home or day care center, specify where the population will be found. Populations must be defined according to location as well as to the time when the study will be done.[1]

Types of Samples

After you have set up the criteria for inclusion in your sample by describing the population in detail, you must determine whether yours will be a *probability* or *nonprobability* sample (see Table 8-1). In probability sampling, each element in the population has a known probability of being included in the sample. In nonprobability sampling, this probability is unknown. Some individuals may have no chance of being included, whereas others are sure of being subjects in the study, but these chances are not known to the researcher.

With probability sampling, the sample is much more certain to be representative of the population, making it possible to estimate the degree to which the findings differ from those that would have been obtained if the whole population had been studied. In addition, it is possible to calculate the necessary sample size for the margin of error you are willing to accept.

Nonprobability sampling, on the other hand, may or may not accurately represent the population. It is usually more convenient and economical and allows the study of populations when they are not amenable to probability sampling or when it is not possible to locate the entire population.

Probability Samples

The probability sample reduces the possibility of bias in sampling and ensures a more representative sample because the probability of each person in the population being selected for the sample is known. There must be an available list of all members of the population from which the sample can be drawn. This available list of the population is the single most important criterion in determining whether probability sampling is possible for a given study. If it is, then one of the three types of random sampling

---

[1]The research proposal must identify the specific population to be studied, even though you may not be specific later in a published article, to protect the anonymity of the subjects.

TABLE 8-1
Sample Selection

Probability Sampling	**Nonprobability Sampling**
Assumptions	
A complete list of all members of the target population is available.	No list of all members of the target population is available, or availability is expected to be sequential.
The researcher knows the probability of each subject being in the sample.	There is no way to estimate that all members of the population have some chance of being in the sample.
Systematic Sampling with Random Start	**Nonprobability Systematic Sampling**
Obtain a list of the population.	No list of the population is available.
Begin sampling with a random start.	Begin with the first available subject.
Select every *nth* subject from the list until a predetermined number has been reached.	Select every *nth* subject until enough subjects have been obtained.
Simple Random Sampling	**Convenience Sampling**
A specified percentage or number from the population is determined in advance.	A minimum number of subjects (or time frame) is determined in advance.
All members of the population are assigned a number (such as a Social Security number).	Every person who meets the criteria is asked to participate.
From a table of random numbers, select from the population until the sample size is reached.	The researcher goes to the setting and selects the sample from persons who meet the sample criteria.
Each member of the population has a known chance of being selected.	The actual population is unknown; other terms for convenience sample are available sample, accidental sample, deliberate sample, and chance sample.
Stratified Random Sampling	**Quota Sampling**
Divide the population into strata based on the sample criteria.	Make up a list of the criteria needed to divide the sample into groups (such as age, gender, education).
Draw a predetermined number from each group using a simple random sampling technique.	Decide on the number from each group you want in the sample, then go to the setting and select a convenience sample until you have filled your quota in each group.
Cluster (Multistage) Sampling	**Network Sampling**
List the relevant geographic locations of the populations (states, counties, cities).	Locate an individual or group that meets the sample criteria who agrees to be in the study (or a person known by persons who meet the sample criteria).
Draw a simple random sample from that list until your predetermined number is reached.	Obtain from the first and each subsequent member of the sample the names of (or a method of contacting) other individuals who meet the sample criteria.
List the sample according to the next relevant criterion (such as schools or healthcare facilities).	Continue the previous steps until the predetermined number has been reached or until all contacts are exhausted.
Draw a simple random sample from the new list until the predetermined number is reached.	
Repeat the previous steps until all relevant criteria have been exhausted. At the last stage, list all members of the population and draw a simple random sample to the predetermined number.	

can be used. If there is no list, a nonprobability sample is required. Sample size is discussed later in this chapter.

Simple Random Samples

The basic probability sampling design is the simple random sample, which gives every element in the population an equal chance of being selected. First draw up a numbered list of the population. Then refer to a table of random numbers. Beginning at some arbitrary point on the page, move up or down the column of random numbers one by one, counting off enough to complete your sample size. Now look for numbers from your population list that correspond to the random numbers, and they become your sample. Tables of random numbers can be found in many statistics books and provide a good method of taking simple random samples. There are also computer programs that will generate random samples for you.

Examples of population lists that can be used by nurses for simple random samples are members of a state or national nursing organization; all students enrolled at a university; all nurses with a current nursing license; all members of the county heart association; all babies born in the county or state during a given day, month, or year; all nursing schools accredited by the National League for Nursing; all hospitals with more than 200 beds that are licensed in a given city or state; all records of patients who were admitted (or discharged) with a given diagnosis within the last year at a given hospital; or all incident reports related to medication errors within a hospital or series of hospitals. There are many more possibilities; the key element is that a list of all members of the population must be available.

The following are some examples of how to draw simple random samples. Remember that in a simple random sample each element in the available population should have an equal chance of being selected.

- Example 1: From an available population of all inpatients at Walter Reed Army Hospital on December 1, 1988, and using the last four digits of the patient registration number, begin at the top of the fifth column of a table of random numbers and proceed down the page until 50 numbers have been selected. Select 10 more numbers to serve as replacements. Alternatively, using the last four digits of the patient number, use a computer program to generate a random sample of patients.
- Example 2: From an available population of all students in a research class at Azusa Pacific University, all students in the class who agree

to participate in the research project will pull a slip of paper out of a box. Thirty percent of the slips of paper will state, "You are a member of the sample!" Five percent of the slips will state, "You are an alternate." The rest of the slips will be blank. There are just enough slips for the number of students in the class. As each student selects a slip, the content of the slip is recorded. During the selection process the probability of each student being in the sample or an alternate can be calculated. Again, the alternate list is used for replacement purposes and is used from first to last.

- Example 3: From a target population of all currently registered graduate nursing students at the University of Alberta, and using a table of random numbers, select 10% of the listed registration numbers on February 4, 2010. An alternate list will be established by selecting a further 5% at the same time as replacements for those in the first list who decide not to participate in the study. Alternates will be approached in the order in which they were selected from the table of random numbers.

If a simple random sample is both possible and appropriate to your study, there is no better method of selecting subjects. Objectivity can be obtained and much bias eliminated, thus strengthening the results of the study.

Stratified Random Samples

This method is based on the same principle as the simple random sample, except that before the sample is drawn, the population is divided into two or more strata or groups. A simple random sample is then taken from each group. For example, if having equal numbers of men and women is vital to your study, you can divide the population into two groups according to gender and then draw an equal number of subjects from each group. Remember that the variable chosen as a criterion for stratifying a sample must be important to the purpose of the study.

In a study of the relationship between educational preparation and nurses' behavior, a stratified random sample would be very appropriate. If a simple random sample of nurses is taken, the proportions of subjects from each type of educational background will not be equal. In fact, some might be missing altogether. Therefore, it makes sense to first divide the population into strata according to educational preparation and then draw random samples from each group. The probability of being selected can be calculated for each element in the population, even though it may not be equal among groups.

Like simple random samples, this method requires a complete list of the population. It also requires information on the criterion for stratification. So if you plan to stratify by educational preparation, your list of the population must include information about educational preparation. The ease with which you can obtain the necessary information about the sample may help you decide whether to use stratified random sampling. Stratified sampling simply allows you to control the size of the sample from each stratum but does not increase the validity of your answer.

The whole point of stratifying a sample is to make sure that certain characteristics of a population are in the study. If you were interested in a study of diabetic behavior and you wanted to be sure that you had specific groups included, such as type of diabetes or age of onset (childhood or adult), you would want to stratify your sample on that basis. This way, you are sure that specific characteristics will be present in the sample. Sometimes studies are stratified by gender to be sure of equal representation.

Sometimes the question is asked, Should I use equal numbers in my strata or should I use percentages of my population? The answer is up to you. Do you want to have a particular number of subjects in your final sample, or is the total sample size irrelevant for your study (outside of the computation of error and levels of confidence)? In other words, it makes no significant difference whether you use 10% or a total of ten in each stratum as far as the sampling technique is concerned. It makes a difference in relation to your computation of the size of the final sample you wish to have. Frequently, too, the difference will be determined by the number of strata and their complexity.

If you were studying the nutritional status of school-aged children (K–6), you might want to be sure you include both boys and girls as well as the major ethnic or racial groups represented in your school. First you stratify your school by grade:

K   1   2   3   4   5   6

Then you stratify by gender:

K	1	2	3	4	5	6
M F	M F	M F	M F	M F	M F	M F

If you want to include ethnic or racial groups, you would have to decide which ones you want to be sure to include. If your school has a substantial proportion of children who are black (B), Hispanic (H), and white (W), you might want to be sure each major group is represented, so your stratification plan would look like this:

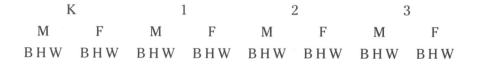

	K		1		2		3
M	F	M	F	M	F	M	F
B H W	B H W	B H W	B H W	B H W	B H W	B H W	B H W

This is the way you plan out your stratification procedures prior to doing any form of data collection. As you can see, the more you stratify, the more complex your sample becomes. The only reason for stratification in a study of this nature is to ensure representation of the major elements in the population. Otherwise, if you had simply drawn a simple random sample of all children in the school, your final sample may not have had any kindergarten children, or may have had an overrepresentation of Hispanic children, or may not have had enough boys. You could have stratified on grade level, on gender, or on ethnic group, but if you wanted to ensure representation of ethnic groups and genders at each grade, this is the way you would have to plan your sample.

Cluster Samples

In large-scale surveys, when the population represents broad geographic areas or large numbers of people, simple random samples and stratified samples can be very expensive. A nationwide sample of nurses might necessitate sending interviewers to scattered localities across the country, and the expense could become prohibitive. A cluster sample would reduce the expense while allowing the results to be generalized. The *cluster sample* method is also called *multistage* sampling because the process of sampling moves through stages until the final sample has been selected.

Starting with the overall population for the study, such as all nursing students in the state, you would proceed as follows: Prepare a list of counties and draw a random sample. Prepare a list of nursing schools in those selected counties and take a random sample of the schools. Then prepare a list of students from these schools and make a random selection of a sample of students. This three-stage process yields a representative sample of nursing students in this state, yet the location of the students is limited first to the counties selected and then to the schools selected from those counties. The savings in time, travel, and expense can be enormous by using cluster sampling.

As with simple and stratified random sampling, cluster sampling requires that lists of elements in the population be available. In cluster sampling, however, complete lists of the final subjects are not necessary until you reach the final stage. Then, you need only obtain complete listings of the elements needed for that stage.

Nonprobability Samples

The use of nonprobability samples is often a necessity in nursing research, as in other disciplines. Some populations do not have lists available. For example, if your population is defined as women in menopause, you will not find a list of names from any single source. Nor will you find complete lists of populations of heroin addicts, alcoholics, or persons with upper-respiratory infections. These populations have no central registry, no gathering place, and unless you redefine your population to include only those receiving some type of treatment, you will have no way to locate a list of the population. This is not to say that you cannot obtain samples of these populations but, rather, that the sample cannot be a probability sample and will have to be obtained by some more deliberate method. Keep in mind that the sample must fit the purpose of the study. Therefore, your goal must be to find the sample that best represents your population rather than one that uses the most sophisticated sampling technique. Nonprobability samples are particularly useful with patients when the total population is unknown or is not available.

Convenience Samples

A convenience sample (sometimes called an available sample) is a nonprobability sample that happens to be available at the time of the data collection. To obtain a convenience sample of patients, you could simply plan to include those patients who happened to come in to the clinic on data collection day, or choose the first 50 people who come into the emergency room on a particular Saturday night. There is no way of estimating the potential bias in this kind of sample, but it is possible to plan for objectivity so that subjects are not deliberately selected by the researcher.

Many samples in nursing studies are convenience samples because of the availability of patient groups through treatment centers. You will probably not know in advance who will come in for treatment, and you may have to wait for a sufficient number of new patients to arrive before the sample selection is complete. For example, if the target population is defined as new diabetics being treated for the first time in an outpatient clinic, it may take considerable time for a sufficient number of new diabetic patients to present themselves for diagnosis and treatment at the outpatient department. However, you can estimate approximately how long it will take to obtain your sample because you know from past information how many patients usually arrive at the clinic each month.

Other examples of convenience samples are all male Caucasian patients admitted to the coronary care unit for myocardial infarction during the month of February; all mothers whose premature infants are born during the study period; all children between the ages of two and four years who are admitted for tonsillectomy or herniorrhaphy during the study period.

Network Samples

A nonprobability sampling technique that is seldom discussed in the literature is network sampling.[2] This is a method that is useful in studies where it is difficult or impossible to locate the population. You may know that the population exists but have no idea where to look for a sample. Network sampling takes advantage of the fact that all human beings have social networks. Everyone has friends that have certain characteristics in common. For this technique, you need only locate one individual who has the desired characteristics and then ask that person to help you get in touch with friends who would also meet your sample criteria. Network sampling is extremely useful in finding socially devalued urban populations, such as addicts, alcoholics, child abusers, and criminals, because these people do not readily reveal themselves to strangers or outsiders. It is also useful for finding groups, such as successful dieters, widows, women experiencing menopause, and so on. These groups are hard to locate by the usual methods, but by finding a link in the social network, one subject will lead the researcher to others. Sometimes it is the only way to locate a difficult-to-find population.

Quota Samples

Like the convenience sample, the quota sample uses available subjects, but it takes additional steps to ensure inclusion of representatives from certain elements in the population. It can ensure that these elements are present in the same proportion in the sample as they appear in the population. This method is used when a convenience sample does not provide the desired balance of elements. For example, the postpartum unit in your hospital may have a patient population that is predominantly Hispanic; therefore, whites and blacks do not appear in sufficient numbers in this convenience sample. To counteract this problem, ethnic percentages are

---

[2]J. M. Saunders, personal communication, 1981.

specified so that the proportion of each group in the sample represents the ethnic breakdown of total population.

Like stratified random sampling, quota sampling allows you to control the numbers of sample subjects with desired characteristics. When you have several independent variables (for example, age, education, diagnosis, ethnic background), you will have to ensure that you have enough subjects in each category of independent variable so that you have enough data to analyze the relationships among your variables. For example, if you plan to categorize education according to levels so you can analyze the differences among them, you must have a sufficient number of subjects in each category for your analysis to be valid. In this instance, a quota sample would be appropriate, and it might be a good idea to have equal numbers of subjects in each group, instead of groups proportionate to the population distribution of educational level, to simplify the data analysis. Whether or not you decide to use a proportionate quota sample or an equal number depends on your research question. Whichever sampling technique best answers your question is the one to use.

Systematic Samples

You will find reference to systematic samples in published research reports and other research texts. Systematic sampling is the selection of every *nth* member of the available population, after beginning with a random start. If you used a telephone book or a list of students, you might select every fifth or every tenth person on the list. If you wanted to interview people on the street, you could decide to approach every third person. If you were interviewing inpatients you could select every other room or every room with an even number and interview every patient in the window bed. These are all predetermined methods of selecting a systematic sample that are obviously not probability samples but are not as subjective as convenience samples. The purpose here is to try to avoid the simple human biases that creep into nonprobability sampling techniques: interviewing people who make eye contact or smile at you, interviewing your friends, interviewing people who look good, and so on. The decision about who will be in the sample is predetermined rather than left up to the researcher at the time of selection. Systematic sampling is a type of nonprobability sampling technique that is intended to control investigator bias in sample selection but does not meet the criteria for probability sampling because it does not control for environmental bias and does not ensure random distribution of extraneous variables. In addition, a systematic sample can introduce bias into the sample if there is some bias to the order in which the population is listed. In using the telephone book, for example, the sample can omit entire ethnic groups and overrepresent others because of the alphabetical listing of the names. Choosing every other patient room in a hospital unit sounds objective, but there may be some bias of which you are unaware in the way patients are assigned to rooms. Therefore, you cannot know the distribution of the extraneous variables in your study, which is the important point in probability sampling.

Sample Size

The best advice for the novice researcher is to use as large a sample as possible. Large samples maximize the possibility that the means, percentages, and other statistics are true estimates of the population. They give the effects of randomness a chance to work. The chance of error goes down in direct proportion to the increased size of the sample. However, practical considerations are important, too—for example, how many people are available from your resources?

With random samples, it is possible to set the size of the sample according to how accurately you want to estimate the actual population parameters or how much sampling error you are willing to accept. The basic formula for computing the sampling error for a sample estimate of a population parameter is as follows:

$$\text{sampling error} = \frac{\text{variability of the measurement values among the sampling units}}{\sqrt{\text{size of sample}}}$$

It is possible to devise a number of sampling plans that will ensure that your estimates will not differ from the corresponding actual population figures by, say, more than 5% (sampling error) on more than 10% of the possible samples that you might draw from the population (level of confidence). You can also devise plans that will produce correct results within 2%, 99% of the time. In practice, of course, we do not repeat the same study on an infinite number of samples drawn from the same population, but it is possible to predict the probability that the sample will produce data within 5% of those resulting from a study of the whole population.

If you attempt to predict the necessary sample size for your study using the formula, you will see that the larger the percentage of possible error you are willing to accept, the smaller your sample can be. Therefore, the more accuracy you are trying to achieve, the larger the sample should be. However, this formula is applicable only to probability samples. When you do use it, you must know the variance of the measurement you plan to use with your population. This means that the measurement must be at least at an interval scale so that the variance can be calculated. The measurement must also have been used before with the same or a similar population so that the variance is known. You will find that if the variance is small, the sample size need not be as large as when the variance is large. When none of the measurements vary too far from the mean for the population, it takes only a small sample to obtain measurements that accurately reflect the population. But if there is a lot of variation in measurements, a larger group will be needed to incorporate the entire range of scores in the sample.

Another way to estimate the size of the sample you will need is to do a *power analysis*. A power analysis is a method of estimating that the sample is large enough to assume that your statistical analysis is meaningful and large enough to detect errors. A power analysis is itself a statistical analysis based on several factors: the amount of error you are willing to tolerate, the level of significance of the test (usually described as the p level), the size of the sample, the type of statistical test, and the effect size. A power analysis accounts for all these factors. If you know any three factors, the fourth can be calculated. There are books of tables and computer programs that estimate power based on these factors. (An excellent article on power analysis by Polit and Sherman is listed at the end of the chapter in the bibliography.)

If you know that you can obtain a probability sample and you know the variance of the measurement you plan to use, you can decide on your margin of error and select the optimal sample size to use. But, as mentioned before, there are practical factors that sometimes limit your ability to decide on sample size. If you have access to a group of women undergoing assertiveness training and they meet your criteria for inclusion in your sample, you will probably use the group for your study, no matter how large or small it may be. The practical factor influencing your decision is availability. If there is one such group available, take it. If there are many such groups available, you can plan for the best sample size.

When you have some choice in planning sample size but cannot use probability sampling, then the size of the sample will depend on the number and type of variables that you plan to measure—your goal, once again, is to ensure sufficient data for your analysis. If you plan to look at the relationships between variables, a handy rule of thumb is to plan for at least five observations for each category of each variable. If you plot your variables in a chart or table, you can see how many subjects you will need to have enough data. For example, Table 8-2 shows the relationship among gender, age, and postoperative anxiety level. With these variables

TABLE 8-2
Relationship among Age, Sex, and Postoperative Anxiety Level

	Males Age			Females Age		
Anxiety Level	**20–30**	**31–40**	**41–50**	**20–30**	**31–40**	**41–50**
Low	5	5	5	5	5	5
Medium	5	5	5	5	5	5
High	5	5	5	5	5	5

divided into three categories each, you would need at least 90 subjects. Each variable is then measured once for each subject.

If you plan to measure the same variable many times for the same subject over a period of time, then each measurement can be counted in the same way as you counted subjects in the last example. Look at the table again. If anxiety level is to be measured five times for each subject, you will need only one subject for each of the five observations. Therefore, the minimum sample size becomes 18. In exploratory studies, you will frequently make multiple, in-depth observations of the same subjects, which means that a small sample size will produce a large quantity of data.

Level of Study and Sample Selection

The type of sample you plan to select depends on the level of study you have chosen to do. Level I exploratory descriptive studies require non-probability samples for several reasons. First, there is usually an insufficient amount of information about the problem and the population to allow you to plan a probability sample. Second, because of the exploratory nature of the study and the flexibility of the data collection methods, it is rarely possible to generalize beyond the immediate sample. As is true with all sampling techniques, your major interest is to represent the population to the best of your ability. The reason for a representative sample at Level I, however, is to enhance your interpretation of the results and to give you a base on which to build further studies rather than to generalize to a broader population. Therefore, convenience, network, quota, and systematic samples are perfectly adequate techniques.

At the early stages of exploratory research, you begin with convenience sampling or network sampling to find subjects for the study. If you are studying patients on a ward or nurses in a hospital, you may use convenience sampling. But, if you are interested in people out in the community who are not easy to locate, you may have to advertise in newspapers for volunteers and ask people to refer their families and friends to you, using any network system to which you have access. Probability sampling is not possible in these studies.

At the exploratory level, the sample size is usually quite small because you are interested in doing an in-depth study. Sometimes you find that the entire population is very small and end up studying everyone. If, for example, you were interested in severe acute respiratory syndrome (SARS) and wanted to explore the characteristics of those who died from it, you would not wait for a large sample. Rather, you would begin to study all the victims. Five people may be a small sample, but at the time of your study, they might constitute the entire known population.

Another facet of sample selection in exploratory descriptive studies is the amount of time you have to spend collecting your sample. If your resources are limited, you must plan your study within a reasonable length of time. Your plan may call for a statement such as, "as many as possible from January to June who meet criteria, with a minimum of five." In this way, you have established a minimum sample size but will do your best to get a larger sample if you can. In a study of out-of-body experiences following cardiac or respiratory arrest, Joy (1979) found that only the pulmonary arrest patients recall these experiences 24 hours later. Although she interviewed 24 postarrest patients over a 6-month period (all that survived), her sample that reported out-of-body experiences was only three patients. At this point, the resources of the researcher determine whether to proceed with the study or whether to stop and analyze the experiences of three patients.

In using the multiple concurrent replication concept for exploratory studies, the sample size can be expanded considerably by having several investigators work at different locations, collecting data on different groups of people at the same time. In this way, also, the bias of the individual investigator can be described and accounted for because each one will be slightly different from the others.

Finally, the exploratory descriptive design is the most suitable for the case study approach using one subject or one small group (a total population) that the investigator studies in depth. This is the basis for biographical accounts and early studies of nursing interventions. Level I descriptive designs that look at the characteristics of a single population typically use either a total population or a simple random sample.

At Level II, the best approach to sample selection is the probability sample. Survey designs are based on the concept of generalizing to populations from samples. They also utilize nonprobability techniques when a probability sample cannot be obtained. At this level, any deviation from the probability sample must be explained as a limitation of the design because any such deviation diminishes the confidence you can have in the relationships you find.

Remember that at Level II you are looking for significant relationships between variables and that these relationships are meaningful only if you can apply them to populations (external validity). Level II studies utilize all three forms of probability sampling techniques, depending on the question asked.

Comparative designs are always found at Level II. The purpose of the comparative design is to compare groups to see if they are significantly different on some characteristic or trait. Usually the groups utilize a stratified random sample technique and are formed at the beginning of the study during sample selection. There are times, however, when the groups are not identifiable until the data have been collected using a simple random sample. In this case, during data analysis the groups will be separated on the variable and then compared. Thus, a Level II comparative survey can use either a stratified sample or a simple random sample with subsequent data analysis to form comparative groups.

Level III is similar to Level I in that nonprobability convenience sampling is the most usual. In experimental designs, the investigator must have full control of the variables. As far as the sample is concerned, this control is maintained through assignment to groups (see Chapter 7). The first concern in an experimental design is that the various experimental and control groups must be equivalent at the beginning of the study so that the effect of the independent variable can be measured. To ensure the equivalence of the groups, the members of the sample are randomly assigned to the various groups, thus producing groups that have equal distribution of the key variables (internal validity). This works well provided that the sample is large enough. If it is not, the researcher must ensure the distribution of key variables by some other method. Matching and selecting from a homogeneous population are two such methods. The use of random assignment at Level III provides control of sample variables essential to the experimental design. These samples are not, however, probability samples. In experimental designs, samples are obtained by asking people who meet the criteria to consent to be subjects—convenience samples. In clinical studies, the criteria for being in the sample usually involve being a patient with a particular problem at a given time. It is difficult, if not impossible, to obtain a random sample of patients who are in need of treatment at the time of the study. Frequently, the subjects are obtained sequentially, as they arrive for treatment. The population is unknown; therefore, probability sampling is impossible.

The main purpose of random sampling is to allow the results from the sample to be generalized to the population (external validity). Although it might seem advantageous to be able to do this at Level III, in reality it is usually impossible. Because of the researcher's concentration on control of variables, the sample is usually not representative of the population. The major emphasis is on identifying the effect of the independent variable on the dependent variable and on controlling all possible variables that might intervene in that relationship. Thus, because the sample is selected to hold many variables constant, many elements of the population are not included.

Bibliography

Beck, C. T. (1994). Achieving statistical power through research design sensitivity. *Journal of Advanced Nursing, 20*, 912–916.

Brink, P. J., & Wood, M. J. (1979). Multiple concurrent replication. *Western Journal of Nursing Research, 1*(2), 117–118.

Chein, I. (1976). An introduction to sampling. In C. Selltiz, L. S. Wrightsman & S. Cook (Eds.), *Research methods in social relations* (3rd ed., Appendix A). New York: Holt, Rinehart and Winston.

Cochran, W. G. (1963). *Sampling techniques* (2nd ed.). New York: Wiley.

Coyne, I. T. (1997). Sampling in qualitative research. Purposeful and theoretical sampling; merging or clear boundaries? *Journal of Advanced Nursing, 26*, 623–630.

Crosby, F., Ventura, M. R., Finnick, M., Lohr, G., & Feldman, M. J. (1991). Enhancing subject recruitment for nursing research. *Clinical Nurse Specialist, 5*(1), 25–30.

Fink, A. (1995). *How to sample in surveys.* Thousand Oaks, CA: Sage.

Ford, J. S., & Reutter, L. I. (1990). Ethical dilemmas associated with small samples. *Journal of Advanced Nursing, 15*(2), 187–191.

Hauck, W. W., Gilliss, C. L., Donner, A., & Gortner, S. (1991). Randomization by cluster. *Nursing Research, 40*(6), 356–358.

Ingram, R. (1998). Power analysis and sample size estimation. *NTResearch, 3*(2), 132–141.

Joy, F. (1979). *Patients' arrest experiences.* Unpublished master's thesis, University of California, Los Angeles.

Kachoyeanos, M. K. (1998). The significance of power in research design (Part I). *MCN, 23*(2), 105.

Kachoyeanos, M. K. (1998). The significance of power in research design (Part II). *MCN, 23*(3), 155.

Lentz, M. J. (1990). Time series—issues in sampling. *Western Journal of Nursing Research, 12*(1), 123–127.

Lipsey, M. W. (1990). *Design sensitivity: Statistical power for experimental research.* Newbury Park, CA: Sage.

LoBiondo-Wood, G., & Haber, J. (2002). *Nursing research: Methods, critical appraisal, and utilization* (5th ed.). St. Louis, MO: Mosby.

Morse, J. M. (1991). Strategies for sampling. In J. M. Morse (Ed.), *Qualitative nursing research: A contemporary dialogue* (Rev. ed., pp. 127–145). Newbury Park, CA: Sage.

Pavlovich, N. (Ed.). (1981). *Readings for nursing research.* St. Louis, MO: Mosby.

Polit, D. F., & Beck, C. T. (2004). *Nursing research: Principles and methods* (7th ed.). Philadelphia: Lippincott.

Polit, D. F., & Sherman, R. E. (1990). Statistical power in nursing research. *Nursing Research, 39*(6), 365–369.

Ruth, M. V., & White, C. M. (1981). Data collection: Sample. In S. D. Krampitz & N. Pavlovich (Eds.), *Readings for nursing research* (pp. 93–97). St. Louis, MO: Mosby.

Sharp, K. (1998). The case for case studies in nursing research: The problem of generalization. *Journal of Advanced Nursing, 27,* 785–789.

Sheldon, L. (1998). Grounded theory: Issues for research in nursing. *Nursing Standard, 12*(52), 47–50.

Waltz, C., & Bausell, R. B. (1981). *Nursing research: Design, statistics, and computer analysis.* Philadelphia: F. A. Davis.

Williamson, Y. M. (Ed.). (1981). *Research methodology and its application to nursing.* New York: Wiley.

Yarandi, H. N. (1991). Planning sample sizes: Comparison of factor level means. *Nursing Research, 40*(1), 57–58.

Zeller, R., Good, M., Anderson, G. C., & Zeller, D. L. (1997). Strengthening experimental design by balancing potentially confounding variables across treatment groups. *Nursing Research, 48*(6), 345–348.

CHAPTER NINE

Selecting a Method to Answer the Question

➤ **TOPICS**

Observation
Questionnaires and Interviews
Available Data
Physiological Measures
Bibliography

➤ **LEARNING OBJECTIVES**

- Discuss the relevance and utilization of observation in nursing studies.
- Outline the advantages of and basic considerations in designing a questionnaire.
- Describe the value of and operational considerations in using interviews in research.
- Explore the various sources of data in designing and conducting nursing research.
- Identify the value of physiological measures that may be used solely or in combination with other measures in nursing studies.

Choosing a method for data collection stems from the operational definitions of the variables in your study. At this point in your plan, it is time to examine these decisions in light of the overall design, and make sure that all the elements fit together. The method you choose to collect your data depends on several factors. First, it depends on the level of your question, or how much is known about your variables. For a Level I study, because there is little available information in the literature, you want to amass as much information as possible, and you are not sure what results to expect. In this case, the best methods are those that result in a lot of data being collected, as broadly as possible. These are methods such as unstructured observation, open-ended interviews and questionnaires, participant observation, and the use of written, available data. Data collection methods must be flexible because you may have to change the questions you ask or the situations you observe as you find out more about the variables. You cannot narrow down the topic too much because you do not know what data to expect, and trying to narrow down your focus could result in your missing valuable data.

For a Level II study, in which you are looking for relationships among variables, you must have accurate techniques for measuring your variables. Your data must be quantifiable because you are looking for statistical relationships among the variables. Here, structured observation, questionnaires, and interviews can be used, as well as physiological measures. Written, available data and projective tests may be considered. Questions and observations must be comparable from one subject to the next; even open-ended questions must be the same for each subject. The criterion here is accuracy rather than flexibility.

In Level III studies, you control the situation and the variables. Therefore, the method must be structured. Any method that produces structured, quantifiable data can be used. When there is a choice, you would use the most precise measure available. Conditions and measurements must be identical for all subjects because inferential statistics will be used to test the hypotheses.

Another consideration in selecting a method is which instruments are available and have already been tested and evaluated to measure your variables. During your search of the literature, some instruments may have come to light that other investigators have developed to measure the variables you are studying. If this is so, by all means use one of these instruments. Using an already tested instrument provides another link between your study and a growing body of knowledge about your variables. You will be adding to this body of knowledge with your data. But be sure that the instrument fits your definition of the variable. Does it measure exactly what you want to know? Only you can decide. Remember that it is possible to adapt an instrument to fit your question, provided you obtain permission from the person who developed it.

Developing your own instrument is not too difficult if you want to measure relatively concrete things like demographic characteristics, level of knowledge of a particular topic, or other factual reporting. If, however, you are attempting to measure an abstract concept, such as hope or grief, measurement becomes more complex. In this case, the development of measuring instruments is a science of its own, which is why beginning researchers should not attempt to develop their own instruments to measure complex concepts.

Instrument or tool development is a specialty area of research that requires advanced skill and experience. Where does it fit in the research paradigm? Exploratory studies can provide the basis for tool development by providing an in-depth description of the concept. For example, the concept of hope could be described as it is perceived by patients in a variety of settings and with various diagnoses and prognoses. From this exploratory work, the investigator might develop a theoretical perspective of the concept of hope. From this theoretical perspective, a tool might be developed to measure levels or types of hope. Using this approach, instrument development follows Level I studies and must be done prior to Level II or Level III studies in which the concept of hope is to be measured. Before the instrument is used, it must be tested extensively to establish its reliability and validity (see Chapter 10); this process becomes a study of its own.

If the literature review does not reveal any tools to measure a complex concept, the beginner should consider whether a Level I study would be more appropriate. If the study really belongs at Level II or III, there should be literature representing previous research on the concept, and a tool will be found that can be used or adapted for use in your study. This chapter focuses on some general guidelines for devising your own instrument or evaluating an existing one for your study.

Observation

Observation is a method of collecting descriptive behavioral data and is extremely useful in nursing studies because one can observe behavior as it occurs. Observation stops being a normal part of everyday life and becomes a research method if it is systematically planned and recorded and if both observations and recordings are checked for their validity and reliability. These factors make the difference between simply observing the world around you and collecting research data through observation.

Observation is the only way to gather some data. If the information you need cannot be obtained by asking questions, through available records, or by directly measuring some quality of the subject, you may have to observe the behavior of the subject and record what you see. Studying the behavior of infants, psychiatric patients, healthcare personnel inter-acting with dying patients; examining the verbal or nonverbal interaction between individuals or within groups; looking to see if people behave as they say they will—these are all well suited to observation.

In nursing studies, observation can provide a rich source of data that describe patient responses. Observation can be used alone or with other methods, and it will assist you in interpreting the results obtained through other methods.

For example, you can use observation in conjunction with interviews to validate self-report information. Many obesity studies are based on self-report (interviews about the individual's personal dieting and weight history) in conjunction with observation (observing the person's appearance and behavior during the interview), plus physiological measures (weighing the individual on a scale). Observations are frequently used when ques-tionnaires or interviews cannot be done because the subject is not able to respond to questions. Observation has produced excellent studies of infants, people who do not speak English, and brain-damaged individuals who have lost the ability to speak.

The act of observation itself is usually interactive. Unless you are be-hind a two-way mirror or viewing a videotape, you are a part of what you are observing. In addition, the act of observing is selective. It is impossi-ble to observe everything that is happening at one time. Finally, the act of recording observations is also selective—you can never record everything you observe.

Objects in the environment impinge on your consciousness as stimuli, some of which you select to observe and others which you do not. Some nurses, for example, have a tendency to observe interpersonal interac-tions and to neglect the physical environment in which they occur. Some nurses will observe nuances of facial expression but ignore room temper-ature, the passage of time, light sources, or weather. Another nurse might walk into a room, observe the equipment in great detail, and fail to notice the patient in the bed. So out of innumerable objects to observe, certain things are selected for observation. In addition, you will find that not all observations can possibly be recorded. Certain observations are selected to be recorded, and these then become the database. The way in which we select observations and record them is not random. Selectivity is highly patterned both by our culture and by our individual preferences.

All behavior can be observed from two points of view: (1) the insider's or actor's point of view or (2) the outsider's or observer's point of view. Both points of view are true. No two human observers observe the same thing or observe in exactly the same way. Observation is an expression of individuality, personality, preconceptions, and values. As an exercise, observe a social situation with two other people and then compare notes. You may be surprised at the results.

Human behaviors can be looked at as individual acts, unrelated to the setting, or they can be examined in the context in which they are occurring. For example, let us say you were observing the way in which people walk up and down a flight of stairs. The basic elements of the behavior are in the stepping procedures, either up or down. If you see a person alone, going up or down stairs, it is easy to examine the basic elements of how it is done. When you begin to observe the individual in relation to others, however, you begin to see patterns to the behavior that give you the idea that there are rules governing the behavior. You may notice that most people walk up on the right and walk down on the left side of the stairwell. You may also notice that if anyone walks up and down the stairs in a different pattern there are bodily collisions. You may begin to assume that there are rules governing on which side of the stairs one walks. You may also find that at certain times of the day, everyone is going up, and the stairs are treated as a one-way street. Someone attempting to go the other way will be trampled in the traffic. The people in the setting may not be aware of the rules. A stranger may not know the rules and always walk the wrong way until he or she becomes familiar with how things are done.

Recording observations provides a description of the behavior and the setting. The act of description (or recording) is in itself an analytical process that breaks down the observation into its most indivisible or basic parts and demonstrates how the parts fit together. Always record the behavior first, in the same way that you record behavioral data in the nursing process, and avoid labeling the behavior until you are ready for the analysis phase of your study. Labels represent a synthesis of your thinking or a conclusion that you have drawn from your observation. For example:

The patient was too weak to get out of bed.

The nurse was too tired to finish her work.

Both weak and tired are labels or concepts that stand for generalizations and value judgments. They are not descriptions of what was seen, heard, touched, tasted, or felt. After many subsequent observations, you will not remember when you go back and read your notes what those words meant. Was the nurse slumped in his chair? Did the patient look thin and pale? Did she try to get up slowly and without vigor?

The value of observation in research is that it provides the context in which social interactions occur. When you are observing a behavior, describe the setting from both the actor's and the observer's perception of the environment. Look for such things as the geographic setting, the time of day, the activity within the setting, the people present, and the relationships among them. Break up your observation into equal time periods. Try to discover the frequency with which situations are encountered in a typical setting. Develop an observational record chart with one observation per actor in every setting.

Notice the way the following recording of a Little League ball game is described. One activity or unit of behavior is listed per line. The focus is on the boy with the bat exclusively.

Boy hit ball.

Boy threw bat down.

Boy ran to the base.

Another form of recording is the paragraph summary, in which overall impressions of an event are listed. You might select one person or several persons to observe in the activity and summarize their activity in a paragraph. You might select a family observing a baseball game, or a player on the team, or even the concessionaire. This data will be quite different from the very focused recording of the baseball game itself. Using the paragraph summary, you will notice how much more detail you are able to rely on later when it comes to data analysis.

Check yourself as an observer. Try some of these observational exercises. Investigate the material objects in the setting, such as all the objects in the area where you brush your teeth. Observe other people's responses to you when you behave out of context (try walking up the down escalator). Watch a small group of your friends in a social situation and try to note what each person is doing.

The observational technique you use depends on the purpose of the study. If detail is not your interest, you need not have detailed observations and notes. But as in levels of measurement, detailed notes can be grouped into general statements, but general notes can never result in detailed analysis. Determining the appropriate observational technique ultimately depends on the research question being asked. Clinical studies that combine observation with another method of data collection make the most of the opportunity to study patient responses and will provide a depth of data not possible with only one method.

When you plan to use observation as a method of data collection, you need to make two decisions before you proceed. First, how involved do you intend to become with the subjects as participants? Second, how structured do you intend your observations to be?

Degree of Investigator Involvement

In participant observation studies, the observer is involved in the setting with the subjects. Examples include observations collected by nurses in the course of their patient care activities and studies where an investigator becomes part of the setting to collect data for research. In these studies, it is easy for bias to be introduced into the data collection process. Participant observers have unique opportunities to influence the behavior of their subjects; in fact, it is difficult to avoid doing so. If nurses are observing patient responses while they are giving patient care, it is easy to influence the patient's response through subtle changes in approach to the patient. As a matter of fact, the purpose of nursing care is to influence change in the patient. Participant observers frequently influence the subjects' behavior by communicating their expectations to the subject. These influences are difficult, if not impossible, to control because objectivity is influenced by interaction with subjects. There will always be some bias in participant observation studies even though the investigator may make every effort to remain objective and not influence the behavior of the subjects. Through detailed recording, however, the influence of the researcher will be described as part of the data.

When the observer is not a participant in the setting but is merely viewing the situation, there is less likelihood of undue influence on the participants by the observer. Frequently, there is some Hawthorne effect in the initial stages because the subjects are aware of being observed. This effect diminishes over time as subjects become accustomed to being observed. Nonparticipant observation studies can range from use of a one-way mirror for observing behavior to face-to-face observation of the subject. In any event, the observer must try to maintain the naturalness of the situation and be as unobtrusive as possible. The likelihood of subjects exhibiting normal behavior is directly related to the inconspicuousness of the researcher as observer. The goal in observational methods is always to maintain the normal environment of the subjects. This enables you to collect the type of data required by the study.

The advantage of nonparticipant observation is that the observed person will be less influenced by the researcher than will one who is actively involved with the researcher. Participant observation, on the other hand, has the advantage of providing a more normal environment for the subject because the observer either is a normal part of the environment or becomes so in the course of the study. In participant observation studies, the researcher begins the study as a stranger to the setting, so all subjects must teach the researcher how to behave properly. By the time the researcher becomes familiar with the people and the setting, the subjects simply forget the researcher is there.

In many observational studies, the subject is frequently a stranger to the setting (for example, rooms with one-way mirrors) and alters his or her behavior to meet the new and unfamiliar environment. If the researcher follows the subject around, a different dimension is added to the subject's life—namely, the researcher.

Determining the appropriate observational method ultimately depends on the research question being asked.

Degree of Structure

Observational methods vary greatly in the amount of structure provided for the observer. They range from very unstructured observations, which attempt to provide as complete and nonselective a description as possible, to very structured methods, which provide a complete list of expected behaviors and require only that the observer check which ones occurred.

An unstructured observation method might be used to describe the behavior of nurses immediately following the death of a patient. It would involve a complete description of everything the nurse says and does at this time. Remember that complete recording of an event is virtually impossible. Even with videotaping, exact replication will not be obtained because of biases introduced by camera angle and lighting. Selectivity is bound to occur. This fact should be recognized if you use unstructured observation. Even so, a rich depth of material can be gathered from unstructured observation—a depth that will never result from the use of structured methods. As long as the researcher accounts for possible bias in both data analysis and interpretation, this valuable method can be used to great advantage in nursing research. Of particular value is the combination of unstructured observation with structured methods, which gives the data more depth.

Structured observation can take one of several forms, but perhaps the most common is the checklist. A checklist allows the researcher to record whether or not a given behavior occurs. The desired behaviors must be explicitly defined so that there is no question in the mind of the observer as to whether or not they occur. For example, unhappy or sad are not suffi-cient descriptions. As it stands, the observer would have to interpret observations in light of a personal definition. A good checklist would spec-ify more operational definitions, such as visibly crying, refuses treatment, or turns back to nurse. These are all easily identifiable action definitions.

Structured observation requires a knowledge of the expected range of behaviors in a given situation. When developing a checklist, for example, the researcher must list all the expected behaviors related to the variable being measured so that the observer will be able to correctly identify all relevant behaviors in the subjects.

You can develop checklists for nursing studies when you know approxi-mately what behaviors to expect. Sometimes a pilot study can be done with a few subjects to give you an idea of the kinds of behaviors you can expect. A checklist will simplify data collection. A checklist makes it diffi-cult to record unexpected behaviors that are not included in the original list because the observer tends to watch for the expected behaviors on the checklist and can easily miss the unexpected.

An example of a checklist used in a nursing study is the following in-strument to measure nurses' monitor-watching activity in a cardiac care unit (CCU):

1. Looks at monitor only (at nurses' station).
2. Looks at monitor, goes to bedside, does not talk to patient.
3. Looks at monitor, goes to bedside, talks to patient.
4. Goes to bedside, talks to patient without checking desk monitor.

This instrument was developed to measure the number of instances in a given time period that CCU nurses behaved in one of the four listed ways. In this study, the researcher was interested only in those four activi-ties and, therefore, had no category for unexpected behaviors.

Structured observation, when appropriate, is an excellent method of collecting data. Many more subjects can be observed, in less time, than with unstructured observation, and the data analysis is much simpler. Taking results from a checklist merely involves counting how many times a particular behavior occurred. The results of unstructured observation, on the other hand, consist of quantities of descriptive data because the observer was trying to record everything that happened. These data must be sorted out to see if there are any patterns to the observed behavior—a very time-consuming process.

Timing of Observations

Because it is usually impossible to observe behaviors for extended periods because of fatigue and boredom, you must plan how and when you will make the observations. The two main methods are time sampling and event sampling.

In time sampling, it is customary to divide the day into units that are appropriate for your observation. For example, in the previous case of the CCU nurse activities, 15-minute periods make sense because they allow ample time for a nurse to exhibit any or all of the expected behaviors. One minute would not be sufficient time for one of the behaviors to occur. Several 15-minute periods during an 8-hour shift would provide a good sample of an individual nurse's behavior. The periods can be either randomly selected or predetermined according to the daily routine of the CCU.

Event sampling is used when you need to observe an entire event to give the subject the opportunity to perform all the expected behaviors. If your purpose is to record breaks in sterile technique during dressing changes by student nurses, the sensible approach would be to observe entire dressing change procedures. Time sampling would make no sense for this study. Describing nurse–patient interaction during admission to the hospital is another instance when event sampling might be used.

In all of these examples, observation is the best, if not the only, way to gather the required data. If you want to know about breaks in sterile technique by student nurses, your alternative research method is to ask the student or the patient. But neither of these approaches is likely to produce the data you need. Observation is the best method.

Type of Observation and Level of Study

The level of the study will affect the observational technique you choose to measure your variables. Unstructured observation is a method for use in Level I studies where flexible exploration is needed. This type of observation is not appropriate for Level II and III studies where precision in measurement of the variables is required. We have emphasized the concept that each level of research builds on the preceding level. To carry this idea through to choosing data collection methods, we look at the ability to provide structure in measurement as dependent on knowledge about the topic and/or variables. It is not possible to develop a structured tool to observe behavior unless you can base the tool on previous descriptions of behavior under the same circumstances. Therefore, developing a tool for a

Level II study requires the results of a Level I study on the same topic. For example, if you want to develop a structured tool to measure mothers' skills at managing the behavior of their toddlers, you would need detailed descriptive data from a Level I study. From the descriptive data, you could identify all the relevant behaviors that would be built into the structured tool.

In the same light, the tool used in a Level III study must be precise enough to differentiate between experimental and control groups. The tool, therefore, must be highly structured and based on considerable knowledge of the variable. Remember, the degree of structure increases with the level of the study and the extent of research and theory available to explain the action of the variables.

Questionnaires and Interviews

When your objective is to find out what people believe or think, the easiest and most effective method is to ask questions directly of the person. The purpose of asking questions is to find out what is going on in the minds of subjects—their perceptions, attitudes, beliefs, feelings, motives, plans, past events, and recall. In research, questionnaires and interviews are the methods designed to collect primary self-reported data.

Asking questions can provide measurement of many concepts and variables important to nursing research. Nurses ask questions frequently as part of assessment and evaluation of patient care. Although nurses are more accustomed to the interview technique, they quickly see the value of questionnaires and adapt easily to the idea that the patient's self-report is one of the most valuable data collection methods. The important thing to remember when choosing this method is that it must be the most appropriate one to measure the variables as you have defined them.

Whether or not you use the interview or questionnaire method (see Table 9-1), it must be because your operational definition calls for the subject's self-report. If it does not, or if there is reason to believe that the person cannot give a valid response (for example, if you are trying to measure an unconscious process), then these methods are not appropriate.

The major difference between questionnaires and interviews is the presence of an interviewer. In questionnaires, responses are limited to answers to predetermined questions. In interviews, because the interviewer is present with the subject, there is additional opportunity to collect nonverbal data as well and to clarify the meaning of questions if the subjects do not understand.

TABLE 9-1
Criteria for Selecting the Interview or Questionnaire

Advantages of the Interview	Advantages of the Questionnaire
1. The subject need not be able to read or write.	1. This approach is less expensive in terms of time and money.
2. The interviewer can observe the responses of the subject.	2. Subjects feel a greater sense of anonymity.
3. Questions may be clarified if they are misunderstood.	3. The format is standard for all subjects and is not dependent on mood of interviewer.
4. In-depth data may be obtained on any subject and are not dependent on predetermined questions.	4. Large samples, covering large geographic areas, compensate for the expected loss of subjects.
5. There is a higher response and retention rate.	5. A greater amount of data over a broad range of topics may be collected.

Advantages and Disadvantages of Interviews and Questionnaires

The written questionnaire has some advantages. For one thing, it is likely to be less expensive, particularly in time spent collecting the data. Questionnaires can be given to large numbers of people simultaneously; they can also be sent by mail, e-mail, or even posted on a Web site for participants to respond. Therefore, it is possible to cover wide geographic areas and to question large numbers of people relatively inexpensively.

Another advantage of questionnaires is that subjects are more likely to feel that they can remain anonymous and thus may be more likely to express controversial opinions. This is more difficult in an interview, where the opinion must be given directly to the interviewer. Also, the written question is standard from one subject to the next and is not susceptible to changes in emphasis, as can be the case in oral questioning. There is always the possibility, however, that the written question will be interpreted differently by different readers, which is one reason for carefully pretesting questionnaires to ensure that they are easily understandable. Otherwise the subject may come to a difficult question and just stop answering. Because there is no way to ask for clarification, the questionnaire may be discarded.

Interviews have many advantages, the most significant of which is questioning people who cannot write their responses (for example, patients with eye patches or in traction). This category also includes illiterate subjects or subjects who do not write as fluently as they speak. Oral responses from these individuals will contain much more information than would their written responses.

Another advantage of the interview method is that it usually results in a higher response rate than does the questionnaire. Many people who would ignore a questionnaire are willing to talk with an interviewer who is obviously interested in what they have to say. Hospitalized patients are a good example. Few patients refuse to be interviewed, but questionnaires left at the bedside or given to patients to take home have a much lower response rate.

When conducting an interview, you can be sensitive to misunderstandings by your subjects and provide further clarification if a subject misinterprets a question. In a questionnaire, on the other hand, you will not know whether the subject really misunderstood the question unless the response is quite bizarre. Even then, there is always some doubt as to what to do with such a response.

Another advantage of the interview technique is that you can plan to ask questions at several levels to get the most information from the subject. As an example, the sensory deprivation questionnaires developed by Jackson and O'Neil (1966) start by asking the patient some ambiguous questions, such as, How have you felt for the last three days? These are followed by more structured questions, such as, Did you experience anything out of the ordinary the last three days? If no reports of sensory disturbances are elicited by these two sets of questions, the interviewer goes on to the very structured questions: Sometimes people who are in the hospital with conditions like yours do have thoughts, feelings, and experiences that they wonder about. For example, they see things and wonder if they are real. If anything like this happened to you the last three days, would you describe it for me? This approach is unique to the interview. The combination of structured and unstructured questions can provide depth and richness to the data and, at the same time, elicit data that are comparable from one subject to the next.

Types of Questions

When looking for a questionnaire or interview schedule to use in your study or when developing your own tool, you will have to consider the various kinds of questions that you can ask to obtain a range of data, and then decide which method is best suited to your variables. The content of the questions must be considered first, then the amount of structure in the format.

Question content or the purpose of the question falls into two basic categories: those aimed at facts and those aimed at perceptions or feelings. Factual questions ask subjects for information about themselves or about events or people about which they know something. Questions asking for demographic data (for example, age, marital status, income, and education) fall into this category. So do questions asking the individual to recall an event or sequence of events (Tell me about the events leading to your coming to the hospital).

Nonfactual questions deal with the subjects' perceptions of what happened or their feelings about people, events, or things. They may also deal with the subjects' explanations for their behavior (Why did you call the doctor at that particular time?). In these kinds of questions, you are not interested in whether the subject's report is accurate but rather in the subject's perception, which may or may not accurately reflect the facts.

The format of interviews and questionnaires, just as that of observational methods, can range from very structured to very unstructured, depending on how much is known about the range of possible responses.

Degree of Structure in Questionnaires and Interviews

Structured questionnaires and interviews are those in which the questions are presented in exactly the same way, with the same wording, and in the same order to all subjects. The questions are standardized to ensure that the subjects' answers can be compared. The questions can be asked by an interviewer or can be given to the subject as a paper–pencil test; in either case, the questions are asked in the same order for all subjects so that the order of the questions cannot affect the subjects' responses.

The most structured questions are fixed alternative questions in which the subject is asked to choose one of the given alternatives. Some examples of fixed alternative questions are as follows:

A. Check the response that best describes how you feel about the statement, Alcoholism is basically a character disorder.

    ❑ Strongly agree   ❑ Agree   ❑ Neutral
    ❑ Disagree   ❑ Strongly disagree

B. Which of the following is your choice of specialty area? Choose only one:

    ❑ 1. Medical or medical intensive care

    ❑ 2. Surgical or surgical intensive care

    ❑ 3. Obstetrics: Labor and delivery, postpartum or newborn nursery, and area specialties

    ❑ 4. Pediatrics and area specialties

    ❑ 5. Psychiatry and area specialties

C. Which three of the following life events have been most difficult for you? Please rank your three choices in order from the most difficult (1) to the least difficult (3).

    ❑ 1. Childhood

    ❑ 2. Marriage

    ❑ 3. Retirement

    ❑ 4. Illness of self or spouse

    ❑ 5. Death of spouse or other close relative

    ❑ 6. Children leaving home

    ❑ 7. Parenthood

Questions such as these are the same whether used in a questionnaire or an interview. They are more commonly used in questionnaires but may be used in interviews, particularly if the subject is unable or unwilling to fill out a questionnaire.

In exploratory research, it may not be appropriate to structure the interview questions in advance, other than to decide on the opening statement or question. A flexible interview, properly used, can bring out much useful material because it allows the interviewer to pursue whatever seems to be important to the subjects and thus elicit the subjects' values, beliefs, and attitudes. Their responses will be completely spontaneous, self-revealing, and personal.

The flexibility of the interview is both an advantage and a disadvantage to the researcher. The results will not be comparable from one subject to the next because the interview format is never the same. However, the interview is invaluable in exploring the whole range of attitudes, thoughts, and feelings that exist for the topic.

Sometimes the interview has a focus, as in psychiatric evaluations, in which the interviewers have a list of topics to cover but can select their own method of eliciting the information. Also left up to the interviewer is whether to pursue an area of particular interest.

Another unstructured interview uses the nondirective technique. Here the initiative is almost completely in the hands of the subject. The interviewer's function is to encourage the subject to talk but with a minimum of guidance. The main function of the interviewer is to show interest in the subject and anything the subject cares to talk about, thus serving as a catalyst for the expression of the subject's feelings. This type of interview requires considerable skill on the part of the interviewer.

In a questionnaire, it is difficult to be unstructured. Some degree of structure is always required because you must set your questions in advance and cannot change them according to the subjects' responses. Questions that do not have fixed alternatives, however, are much less structured than those that do, because they require subjects to respond in their own words. The extent of the response that the subject must provide to answer the question will vary from a word to a sentence, a paragraph, or even an essay. The least structured questionnaires are those designed to elicit an extensive response from the subject. For example:

> Describe an event in your life that has had a significant impact on your present state of mind.

This questionnaire item is quite unstructured because it defines few parameters for the subject. The event described can be anything—a health problem, a social or cultural event, a positive or negative event. The choice is up to the subject.

Open-ended questions are less structured than the fixed-alternative kind and give subjects more leeway to provide their own answers. The question is designed to allow the subject a free response rather than a response limited to or guided by given alternatives. Some examples of open-ended questions are as follows:

- How do you feel about abortions?
- What do you think women should do to ensure equal rights?
- What do you like most about nursing school?

Setting Up Your Data Collection Instrument

In this age of computer literacy, you will find it helpful to design your questionnaire format so that your data can be easily entered into the computer.

When you are planning your format, remember that the computer reads only numbers and that it is set up to read across columns of numbers, either singly or by two or more numbers grouped together. Each variable that you want the computer to read can be set up on your questionnaire in numeric form. For example, rather than setting up your questionnaire to look like this:

What is your current age? _____

You might set up the same question to look like this:

What is your current age?   __ __

What you are doing is providing the correct number of spaces for marking a person's actual age. (If you are doing a study of children younger than age 10 years you will need only one space. If you are doing a study of the very old, three spaces will be needed.) The placement of the lines at the far right of the page facilitates entry into the computer because your eye will simply run down the right side of the page rather than searching all over for the input. Normally, the first few digits will be used for the subjects' identification number, after which you begin to enter the data from your questionnaire. Remember, also, that the computer cannot handle blank spaces, so if you have allowed two digits to record age, and one of your subjects is only six years old, the age must be recorded as 06 to not leave any blank columns. The same procedure would be done if you were asking for a person's weight. Rather than ask:

What is your current weight? _____

Format the question like this:

What is your current weight, in pounds?   __ __ __

As you can see, these are obviously numeric answers. What would you do if you had nominal or ordinal answers? Setting up the questionnaire for these answers is more complex but similar. For example:

Please circle your current marital status:

Never married   Married   Divorced   Separated   Widowed

If you were setting this up for a quick computer scan your answer sheet would look more like this:

Please indicate your current marital status: Never married 1. ___

Married 2. ___

Divorced 3. ___

Separated 4. ___

Widowed 5. ___

After you have set up your questions and answers for easy input into the computer, go through the questionnaire and number each space consecutively just as the computer does, leaving room at the beginning of your numbering system for the number you have given to each individual in the sample—two spaces if you plan scores lower than 100, three if higher. You may want to leave other spaces as well. Remember that your number system is zero to nine for any given space. If your number goes over nine, you will need two spaces. If it's over 99, you'll need three spaces, and so on. So plan ahead for data collection.

The most usual standardized or structured data you will plan to collect is the demographic data. Table 9-2 is an example of how to collect demographic data and how to set up the data collection sheet on each member of the sample.

Interviews

Although interviews and questionnaires can use the same questions, interviews are most effective when they are based on open-ended rather than yes–no or numeric answers. A major error that occurs with new researchers is to design an ordinal scale instrument and use it as the basis for an interview. Few people listening to an interviewer can remember the details necessary to answer the question. Likert scales were designed for questionnaires and are best limited to that method of data collection.

Projective Tests

There are times when the variables you are trying to measure are neither observable nor obtainable from the subject because they represent feelings or attitudes that the individual is unable or unwilling to report. Projective techniques are indirect methods of measuring these variables. They typically involve some type of imaginative activity on the part of the subject in response to an ambiguous stimulus. The use of these techniques requires intensive specialized training. Some nurses have this training, and others will have access to people who do; therefore, this discussion is appropriate.

TABLE 9-2

Demographic Data Sheet

Subject ID Number	___	___	___
	1	2	3

Age (in years)	___	___
	4	5

Gender

1. Male 2. Female	___
	6

Ethnic/Racial Identity

1. Native American   2. Latin   3. Caucasian

4. Black 5. Asian/Pacific 6. Other _____	___
	7

Marital Status

1. Never Married   2. Married   3. Separated

4. Divorced   5. Widowed

6. Other (Please describe.)	___
	8

Total Annual Income/Household	___	___	___	___	___	___
	9	10	11	12	13	14

Religion

1. Catholic

2. Protestant

3. Jewish

4. None

5. Other _____	___
	15

Education

(Circle highest degree.)

1. High School diploma

2. Certificate program (Please describe.)

3. Associate of Arts/Science

4. Baccalaureate (BA/BS/BEd, etc.)

5. Master's (MA/MS/MEd/MPH, etc.)

6. Academic doctorate (PhD, DSc, DNS, etc.)

7. Professional doctorate (MD, ND, DDS, etc.)

8. Other (Please describe.)	___
	16

The stimuli used in a projective test must be capable of arousing many different reactions; for example, an inkblot can appear to be many different things, a picture can elicit many different stories, and toys can be used to portray many people and events. The subject's perception of the stimulus, the feelings it arouses, and the way the subject organizes his or her responses provide the data for analysis by an expert. The responses are not taken at face value but, instead, are interpreted according to predetermined conceptualizations.

The Rorschach inkblot test consists of ten cards, each of which depicts an inkblot. The subject is shown each card and asked, What might this be? The thematic apperception test (TAT) provides a series of pictures about which the subject is asked to tell stories. Both of these frequently used techniques are designed to elicit a rich sample of responses from which a wide variety of inferences can be drawn. Other commonly used projective tests are word association, sentence completion, and figure drawing.

All projective tests rely on the fact that people often find it easier to be expressive when they are not talking specifically about themselves and their own feelings. Talking through the medium of the projective test allows the subjects to maintain a distance from their own thoughts and feelings, which enables them to talk impersonally about themselves. In addition, feelings of which the subject may not be consciously aware appear in the responses to the ambiguous stimulus.

If your operational definition calls for a projective measure, you will want to consider one of these approaches. Keep in mind, however, that most projective measures require the assistance of an expert to analyze the subjects' responses. If this help is not available, you may have to abandon this method of data collection even though it might be the most suitable.

Level of Question and Degree of Structure

With questionnaires, interviews, and observational methods, the level of the study is related to the degree of structure in the measurement tool. Unstructured interviews are appropriate for Level I studies but not for Levels II and III. Starting at Level II, questions must be standardized with fixed alternatives so that the responses of subjects can be compared. In addition, the responses at Level III must be sensitive enough to distinguish small differences between experimental and control groups; this task involves structured questions and answers. Therefore, only fixed-alternative questions may be used at Level III. You will find, when writing questions, that developing fixed-alternative answers requires a great deal of knowledge because you need to provide an alternative to fit every response. You can do it only if you know the whole range of possible responses. That means previous research has provided you with the necessary range of responses. If this knowledge is unavailable, the topic is not appropriate for a Level III study.

Designing the Questionnaire or Interview Guide

If you have decided to use a questionnaire or an interview guide, here are some suggestions on how to go about it.

1. List your questions in the same order to provide consistency and also to prevent the interviewers from forgetting something or from changing the order from one subject to the next. When determining the best sequence for the content of your questions, use the following guidelines:

   a. Order your questions from impersonal to personal topics.

   b. Order your questions from less sensitive to more sensitive (in this way the rapport with the investigator is established and trust is developed prior to asking personal or sensitive questions).

   c. In a list of options, alphabetize the order to minimize bias.

   d. Earlier questions may influence later questions, so begin from general questions first, and move to more specific questions later.

   e. Begin questioning with questions that arouse interest.

   f. Group questions by topic.

2. In exploratory studies, be as unstructured as possible while getting at what you want to know—the more you know, the more structured you can become. Examples of unstructured open-ended interview questions are:

   a. Think back to the most difficult experience you ever had. Tell me about it.

   b. In your opinion, why do people commit suicide?

   c. If you had it to do over again, what profession would you choose:

   Nursing?
   Medicine?
   Another health science?
   Liberal arts?
   Other?
   Why?

3. Base your questions on the literature as much as possible—if there is not enough literature, then ask logical questions—those derived from findings or unasked questions.

4. Start with topics you want covered. A handy rule is to follow the outline used in writing your problem. Give your initial questionnaire to others to critique prior to using it in your study (such as people who write questionnaires or people who know a lot about your topic). From their comments rewrite your questionnaire.

5. Pretest your questions on people similar to the sample you plan to study. Discuss the interview questions or questionnaire with the subject after the session is completed.

6. Remember, interviews take a long time.

Available Data

The health field offers a multitude of available data. Using this data is economical and has other advantages as well. Most official records have been collected over time, thus making it possible to follow trends. Time and money are saved by the availability of a large sample of records in one location.

An example of available data that comes to mind for nursing research is the medical record. Hospitals keep medical records on hand for at least five years and have records dating back much further that are retrievable for research purposes. Also available through hospital records departments are admission rates by age, gender, diagnosis, and other variables such as data on length of stay, types of surgery performed, and so on. Much information about work patterns of nurses can be found in personnel records and in the records of staffing patterns kept by nursing departments.

Data from entire communities can be found in census records and in records from public health departments. These can be used to look for trends within a community or to compare one community with another.

Less frequently, data from newspapers, magazines, professional journals, textbooks, and the like are used for research purposes. In historic studies, personal documents, such as autobiographies, letters, and diaries, can provide a wealth of data. Mass communication can also provide useful information. For example, consider the possibility of analyzing the image of the nurse as presented on television or in movies. Digital cameras, cell phone cameras, and similar technological advances present unique new methods to consider for data collection, assuming that ethical considerations can be resolved.

Unwritten sources of available data include television, motion pictures, tape recordings, photographs, and, in rare cases, a historian studying a culture without written records. The use of historic artifacts, buildings, architecture, clothing, and the like are examples of unwritten available data and are possible sources of data for nursing studies.

If your study requires a large sample, consider using available data collected for another study or by a government agency, perhaps for policy research. If such data is available, it can make it possible for you to utilize a large database without the expense of collecting the data yourself. Secondary analysis of data is an excellent way to maximize resources.

The major drawback in using available data, no matter how they were collected, is that they were not compiled primarily for your study and, therefore, may not quite fit your definition of terms. For example, if you were collecting data on the number of times patients are transferred from room to room during their hospital stay, you might go to the hospital daily census as a source only to discover that this document lists only transfers from one nursing unit to another and not those made from room to room within the same unit. Hopefully, this is something you would find out before you began to collect data, but sometimes there is no way of knowing how the data were collected and how the recorders defined the categories of data. You can, therefore, obtain misleading results from available data.

For example, suppose you wanted to compare the nurse–patient ratio among several hospitals in your area. Each hospital has data available that can be translated into a nurse–patient ratio. However, you might find that one hospital that appears to have fewer patients per nurse actually includes head nurses and unit secretaries in its staffing figures, whereas other hospitals do not. If you are not aware of how the data are reported, you may be misled by your findings.

When using nurses' notes as a source of data, you must take into account the fact that the nurses doing the recording had no common operational definitions for the terms used. Even simple terms like slept well have different meanings for different nurses. An operational definition established for research purposes has to specify exactly what is meant by slept well and how it is to be differentiated from slept poorly or other categories. Thus, slept well might become, when checked every half hour during the hours of midnight to 6 a.m., the patient was asleep. When operational definitions are not available, the individual data collectors use their own definitions. As long as this fact is taken into account, much valuable information can be found in nurses' notes and other such records.

The amount of structure used to collect available data can usually be determined from the method of data recording. If predetermined categories were used, such as checklists or fixed-alternative responses, the data will be more structured than if the recorder used a personal diary or journal to record the data. Looking at a medical record, you will find many examples of unstructured data. Progress notes and daily nurses' notes are usually written in the individual's own words. A physical examination, on the other hand, may be recorded on a checklist, with few statements by the individual. Vital signs, medication dosages, and surgical checklists are other examples of structured available data.

Many Level I and Level II studies can utilize available data; unstructured data will be appropriate only at Level I. Available data can never be used in experimental designs exclusively because they have, by definition, already been collected and therefore cannot be manipulated to measure the effect of an experimental independent variable. In Level III studies, however, available data may be used to provide background information about the sample but not to provide measurements of the independent and dependent variables.

Physiological Measures

As a method of data collection, nurses have the opportunity to utilize a wealth of physiological measures. These provide objective data relating to patients' responses to nursing care and should not be overlooked as sources of valuable data. Physiological methods can be used alone or with other methods. They can be used as the data collection method for your study, or the results of physiological measures can be obtained from available records, such as patients' charts.

Physiological measures available to nurses range from simple (such as weight, blood pressure, pulse, and temperature) to more complex (measurement of blood and urine chemistries, neuroendocrine measures, etc.). Nurses can use measurements, such as tidal volume and blood gasses, to measure the response to treatment of respiratory patients. Woods et al. (2008) tested the feasibility of saliva collection for cortisol measurement in nursing home residents with advanced dementia. They were able to demonstrate that this simple technique could provide a valid and reliable measure of stress. With the complex monitoring equipment available in critical care units, nurses have the opportunity to study many variables that formerly could not be accurately measured. Instant and continuous measures of physiological response can be obtained for patients in critical care units. In addition, nurses engaged in physiological research can receive funding to set up laboratories to handle biological specimens and can do the analysis themselves.

Bibliography

Bonmi, A. E., Kernic, M. A., Anderson, M. L., Cannon, E. A., & Slesnick, N. (2008). Use of brief tools to measure depressive symptoms in women with a history of intimate partner violence. *Nursing Research, 57*(3), 150–156.

Cassiani, S. H. B., Zanetti, M. L., & Pela, N. T. R. (1992). The telephone survey: A methodological strategy for obtaining information. *Journal of Advanced Nursing, 17*(5), 576–581.

Creswell, J. W. (2007). *Designing and conducting mixed methods research.* Thousand Oaks, CA: Sage.

Denny, E. (1991). Feminist research methods in nursing. *Senior Nurse, 11*(6), 38–40.

Dillman, D. A. (2009). *Internet, mail, and mixed-mode surveys: The tailored design method* (3rd ed.). Hoboken, NJ: Wiley.

Doll, M., Ball, G. D. C., & Willows, N. D. (2004). Rating of figures use for body image assessment varies depending on the method of figure presentation. *International Journal of Eating Disorders, 35*(1), 109–114.

Drahota, A., & Dewey, A. (2008). The sociogram: A useful tool in the analysis of focus groups. *Nursing Research, 57*(4), 293–297.

Fink, A. (2009). *How to conduct surveys: A step-by-step guide.* Beverly Hills, CA: Sage.

Jackson, C. W. & O'Neil, M. (1966). Experiences associated with sensory deprivation reported for patients having eye surgery. In J. E. Jeffries & J. C. Rundels (Eds.), *Ross Roundtable on Maternal and Child Nursing* (pp. 54-69). Columbus: Ross Laboratories.

May, K. (1991). Interview techniques in qualitative research: Concerns and challenges. In J. M. Morse (Ed.), *Qualitative nursing research: A contemporary dialogue* (Rev. ed.). Newbury Park, CA: Sage.

McNees, P., Meneses, K., & Su, X. (2008). Live item index technique: An intervention research tool. *Nursing Research, 57*(2), 69–74.

Moser, D. K., Riegel, B. H., McKinley, S., Doering, L. V., Meischke, H., Heo, S., et al. (2009). The control attitudes scale—revised: Psychometric evaluation in three groups of patients with cardiac illness. *Nursing Research, 58*(1), 42–51.

Patton, M. Q. (2002). *Qualitative evaluation and research methods* (3rd ed.). Newbury Park, CA: Sage.

Payne, S. L. (1951). *The art of asking questions.* Princeton, NJ: Princeton University Press.

Roberts, B. L., Srour, M. I., & Winkelman, C. (1996). Videotaping: An important research strategy. *Nursing Research, 45*(6), 334–335, 338.

Spradly, J. P. (1979). *The ethnographic interview*. New York: Holt, Rinehart and Winston.

Spradly, J. P. (1980). *Participant observation*. New York: Holt, Rinehart and Winston.

Sue, V. M., & Ritter, L. A. (2007). *Conducting online surveys*. Los Angeles: Sage.

Tappen, R. M., & Williams, C. I. (2008). Development and testing of the Alzheimer's disease and related dementias mood scale. *Nursing Research, 57*(6), 426–435.

Vincent, D., McEwen, M. M., & Pasvogel, A. (2008). The validity and reliability of a Spanish version of the Summary of Diabetes Self-Care Activities Questionnaire. *Nursing Research, 57*(2), 101–106.

Waltz, C. F., Strickland, O. L., & Lenz, E. R. (1991). *Measurement in nursing research*. Philadelphia: F. A. Davis.

Webb, C., & Kevern, J. (2001). Focus groups as a research method: A critique of some aspects of their use in nursing research. *Journal of Advanced Nursing, 33*(6), 798–805.

Woods, D. L., Kovach, C. R., Raff, H., Joosse, L., Basmadjian, A., & Hegadoren, K. (2008). Using saliva to measure endogenous cortisol in nursing home residents with advanced dementia. *Research in Nursing and Health, 31*(3), 283–294.

CHAPTER TEN

Reliability and Validity of Measurement

➤ **TOPICS**

Errors in Data Collection Procedures
Validity
Reliability
Reliability and Validity Issues in Field Research Using
    Participant Observation
Reliability and Validity in the Research Plan
Self-Test
Bibliography

➤ **LEARNING OBJECTIVES**

- Define the types of error in data collection.
- Understand the concept of validity in research.
- Describe the various methods of establishing validity.
- Understand the concept of reliability in research.
- Describe the various ways in which reliability is established.
- Discuss appropriate ways of establishing reliability and validity for research designs.

Each step of the research process depends on the preceding steps. If a step is missing or inaccurate, then the succeeding steps will fail. When developing your research plan, be aware that this principle critically affects your progress. For example, if you asked your question correctly, you can perform an adequate literature review. A good literature review is basic to the purpose of the study. The purpose of the study is basic to the operational definitions. After you have operationalized your terms, you can proceed with the design, sample selection, and method of data collection. The concepts of reliability and validity will be discussed now because they ultimately will influence the data analysis and the outcome of the final report.

Reliability and validity, in research, refer specifically to the measurement of data as they will be used to answer the research question. The data you collect will only be as good as the instrument you use to collect it, and your goal is to have accurate data that represents exactly how your study participants rate on the variables you are measuring. In other words, the instrument that measures your variables is the central issue in determining the reliability and validity of the data.

Whatever data collection method is used, the intent must be accuracy. How much you can rely on the results depends on the consistency, stability, and repeatability of your data collection instrument—in other words, its reliability. If you were to measure the same variable in the same person again, under the same circumstances, would your result be the same?

In addition to reliability, you need to know if the measurement technique used to collect data actually measures what it is supposed to measure; in other words, is it a valid technique? If you use a questionnaire to measure an individual's moral values, did the questionnaire, in fact, measure that concept or something entirely different, such as religious beliefs? The degree to which answers actually reflect the individual's moral values represents the validity of the questionnaire.

Data collection in nursing research is not a precise science, and there are many factors that can affect the reliability and validity of the results. Estimating the degree to which an instrument is valid and reliable is a critical step in the research process because this determines how much weight can be placed on the results. This is a crucial part of evaluating research for application in practice as well and will frequently make the difference in a decision relating to evidence-informed practice.

This chapter deals with the concepts of reliability and validity of the instruments used to measure variables. The issues related to the validity of the research result are covered under the discussion of internal and external validity in Chapter 7 (Selltiz, Wrightsman, & Cook, 1976).

Errors in Data Collection Procedures

The whole point of doing research is to measure differences among the subjects in the sample. When you are evaluating nursing interventions, you want to know whether the intervention really made a difference to the outcome for the patient or whether the result reflects an error in the data collection process. What you are looking for are the true differences that occur among patients as a result of the nursing intervention. These true differences are the research objective. Any other differences are errors in the measurement process. Some errors may be due to the way data were collected, others to the characteristics of the subjects.

When you are measuring or testing a variable, you want to be sure that what you are measuring reflects the true differences in the subjects and not an error either in relation to the characteristic you are measuring or to the measurement process itself. The process of measurement, however, is easily affected by error, particularly when we are measuring abstract concepts that may not be fully understood at the present time.

Errors in the measurement process can be either constant or random. A constant error will consistently affect the measurement of the variable in the same way each time measurement is done.[1] It will provide an incorrect measure of the variable, and the error will be the same for all subjects. An example is a weight scale that consistently weighs 2 grams over the actual weight. The measurement will appear to be reliable because repeated measures of the same item will result in the same weight. The measurement, however, will not be a valid weight because it is always 2 grams over the actual weight of any item.

The two most stable and problematic constant errors in social science research are social desirability (where the research subjects respond with what they believe is the positive social response whether or not it is true) and acquiescent response set (consistently agreeing or disagreeing with the questions). These two sources of error are examples of constant error in that they are always present in some people, and those people will consistently bias their responses to any questionnaire or interview. For this reason, in any personal interaction with human subjects for the purpose of obtaining information, the researcher must be very careful to present questions in such a way as to avoid either of these sources of error. Constant error affects the validity of the measurement or its ability to arrive at true differences among subjects. Other traits of individuals can also produce constant error in measurement. Intelligence and test-taking skill are two examples. Both characteristics can influence a subject's performance on a paper-and-pencil test and thereby contaminate the true differences that the

---

[1]The basic concepts used here in reliability and validity were adapted from Selltiz, C., Wrightsman, L., & Cook, S. W. (1976). *Research methods in social relations*, (3rd ed., chap. 6). New York: Holt, Rinehart and Winston

researcher is looking for on the trait actually being measured. When developing questionnaires, it is up to the researcher to demonstrate that the tool is not being affected by traits such as these, and because we are unable to know directly an individual's true position on many of the variables that we measure, we judge the validity of the instrument by the extent to which its results are comparable with other evidence. Because there are differences in the types of evidence that are available to establish the validity of various instruments, there are different levels and types of validation.

Constant error can be introduced with the independent variable in a Level III study. This problem is a result of the two-group design, in which one group receives the nursing intervention and the other group does not. The validity of the independent variable can be questioned any time there are only two groups, one of which receives no treatment, because we know that some improvement will be noted in any study simply from the extra attention provided to the intervention group, regardless of the efficacy of the intervention. For example, suppose a special technique of crisis intervention is being tested for its ability to decrease anxiety. In this study, the experimental group receives 1 hour of intensive crisis intervention, and the control group receives no special intervention. This design sets up a special case of constant error because it does not separate out the attention paid to subjects from the actual intervention. It therefore does not achieve a valid measurement of crisis intervention. What is really being tested is something versus nothing. There is no way of truly isolating the effect of the crisis intervention. This creates a constant error in applying the independent variable and affects the outcome of the study. In this case the error is built into the design and will be a factor with each and every subject in the study. The design can be corrected easily by including more variation in the independent variable. For example, adding one other form of counseling in the form of a second experimental group will improve the validity of the measurement of crisis intervention in the original group.

Random error, in contrast, is unpredictable error that varies from one measurement to the next even though the characteristic being measured has not changed. Random errors are transient in nature and result in inconsistent data. If measurements are repeated on the same subjects, the results will not be the same. Random errors directly affect reliability, but because valid measures must also be reliable, random errors also indirectly affect the validity of the measurement technique.

Random errors can result from many factors related to the research situation. The subject's mood, attention span, state of health, and level of pain are all examples of transient personal factors that can cause unreliable responses to measurement and can result in different measurement scores from one time to another. The researcher's general state of well-being may also contribute to random error, in that situations where the data collector is feeling fatigued, impatient, bored, ill, or distracted can affect the subjects' responses to measurement. These possibilities for random error need to be considered in planning the process of measurement in any study because the goal is to maximize the reliability of the results.

Other transient factors that cause random error in measurement can stem from the physical environment in which the research occurs, such as weather, temperature, lighting, noise, and interruptions. Privacy may be a factor in some studies when subjects may hesitate to answer accurately if they fear they may be overheard by family members or others in the environment. Care must be taken in planning the procedures for data collection so that random error is kept to a minimum.

The wording of the questions can affect both the reliability and the validity of the tool used for an interview or questionnaire. Unclear questions can affect reliability if they lead some subjects to misinterpret the question. They can affect validity if they lead to systematic misinterpretation by all subjects. Either way, they produce both constant and random errors in measurement.

When you develop a research instrument, there is no way you can possibly ask every conceivable question about the concept you are trying to measure. You must include some questions and exclude others. In effect, you are sampling the universe of possible data about your variable, thus choosing to collect some data and not others. The sample you select must be representative of the universe of what is known about your variable. Ensuring this representativeness is a difficult process. You can never be completely sure that you have selected a truly representative sample of content for your tool. If you underrepresent the content needed to measure a concept, the error affects the validity of your instrument because it will provide a source of constant error for all your subjects. If you ask many more questions than you need to estimate the concept you are measuring, you could create boredom or fatigue in your subjects, which may affect reliability.

A final source of error comes not from the process of data collection, but rather from the process of data analysis. Here, you may introduce error in coding answers when you transpose from one page to another. Or, you might make a mathematical error in calculating the results of the answers. These are random errors and will affect the reliability of the final data.

Error can be permanently damaging to the research project and very serious or it can be superficial and easily corrected. Error can be obvious to any external reader or it can be hidden from everyone. Error can be a problem or a minor irritant. In any case, every researcher attempts to remove as much error as possible from the research study during the planning phase to increase the credibility of the results.

Bailey presents a table showing the type of error that is likely to occur during different phases of the research process. The serious researcher looks for sources of error during the planning phase, accepting critique from peers and supervisors early in the process to produce as valid and reliable a study as is possible under the circumstances (see Table 10-1).

The concepts of reliability and validity presented here are the basic concepts as they apply to measurement. This chapter is not intended to

TABLE 10-1
Error in the Research Process

Phase of the Research Process	Type of Error

1. The research question
   The research problem
   Operational definitions
	1. Lack of face validity

2. Construction of measurement
   instrument (questionnaire)
	2. Faulty or ambiguous wording
	   of questions
	   Categories not mutually exclusive
	   Not representative of content

3. Sampling	3. Lack of external validity
	   a. Sampling error
	   b. Not representative

4. Data collection (failure to control)	4. Reliability issues:
	   a. Environment (lighting, heat)
	   b. Personal characteristics of respondent (fatigue)
	   c. Relationship between researcher and respondent
	   d Mechanical defects (faulty recording,
	      equipment failure)

5. Coding	5. Coding errors such as missing data, incorrect recording, illegible coding
6. Data analysis	6. Incorrect statistics Faulty interpretation of data

Source: Adapted from Bailey, K. D. (1978). *Methods of social research.* New York: Free Press.

provide the mechanisms for testing reliability and validity above the basic level, but it will give you a good idea of what to look for when you are choosing a tool to measure your variables and how to decide if the reliability and validity of your measures are adequate for your study. This chapter will not enable you to develop a reliable and valid measure if one does not presently exist.

Validity

There are three major methods of estimating the validity of a data collection instrument or the investigator as a valid participant observer. The greater the degree of validity of the data collection device, the more confident you will be that the results you achieve reflect true differences in the scores of your subjects and not some random or constant error. Because our concern with validity is primarily one of constant error, the degree of validity will reflect the degree to which we are controlling or accounting for constant error.

The degree to which valid measurements can be achieved is directly related to the level of the study design. Exploratory descriptive designs, by nature, have a low level of validation and must rely heavily on estimates of reliability. Level II descriptive survey designs can achieve a greater degree of validity but still rely heavily on reliability estimates. Level III demands the highest degree of validity and reliability testing. Just as control over the independent variable must increase with the level of design, so must control for error in data collection. Methods of establishing validity of the measurement technique fall into one of three categories: self-evident measures, pragmatic measures, and construct validity.

Self-Evident Measures

These methods of establishing validity deal with basic levels of knowledge about the variable and look at an instrument's apparent value as a measurement technique rather than its actual value. In other words, self-evident measures refer to the fact that the instrument appears to measure what it is supposed to measure.

Face Validity

At the most basic level, when little or nothing is known about the variable being measured, the level of validity obtainable is called face validity. "On the face of it" merely establishes that the tool seems to be an appropriate way to find out what you want to know. Looking at the questions you have developed to ask your subjects, you can say, I think I will find out what I want to know by asking these questions. It looks all right to me. This is the extent of face validity. It is the lowest level of validation and is used only when you are beginning to study a particular idea and have no prior research literature to provide more information. If there is literature on the variable, either theory or research, then face validity is not sufficient. If you have chosen to study a variable that has not been studied before, you usually will start with face validity because it is the beginning step of the validation process.

Let's say that you are interested in discovering patients' attitudes toward the labels they are given by nursing staff, and you want to know what patients would like to be called. You may have found no previous studies that relate to this area and no questionnaires previously developed, and therefore you plan to develop your own tool—a questionnaire or interview schedule. The first step is to write down some questions. For example, you might decide to ask these questions:

What are the different ways that nurses address patients?

Which of these have been used by nurses who have addressed you?

How do you prefer to be addressed by nurses?

After writing your questions, you look them over and you think they make sense. Next, you give the questions to your family and friends, and they agree that the questions make sense. You now have established face validity. You might also give the questions to some staff nurses and some patients. You are developing more confidence in your questions because these groups also agree that they make sense, and you can now say that your questions have face validity.

Content Validity

Content validity is also a self-evident measure but involves comparing the content of the measurement technique to the known literature on the topic and validating the fact that the tool does represent the literature accurately. You want to obtain an adequate sampling of the content area being studied. Content validity is frequently estimated from the review of the literature on the topic or through consultation with experts in the field who have become experts by having done unpublished research in the area. After you have critically reviewed the literature, you construct your questions or instruments to cover the known content represented in the literature.

Content validity is a self-evident measure because it relies on the assurance that you can demonstrate an adequate coverage of the known field. An expert should be able to judge whether or not the tool adequately samples the known content. Researchers, therefore, frequently call on experts in the field to verify content validity for newly developed tools.

In exploratory descriptive studies using participant observation, you may be in situations where you do not know either the setting or the population. You assume that the persons you select to represent the population are knowledgeable about the content you are trying to elicit. In this case, you assume that the members of a group or population have face validity as experts in their culture or social roles, and you try to further validate each person's report by talking with as many experts as possible. The more people you question, the more content you will gain and the more depth of data you will have at your disposal. On the face of it means your informants appear to have face validity; you establish content validity of the data by cross-checking the answers with several informants until you are satisfied that the content is accurate.

Use of Judge Panels

There are times when you want validation from others that, on the face of it, your data collection instrument is collecting what it is supposed to or that your categories for discriminating data in content analysis seem appropriate. In this case, you put together a group of people who you believe are knowledgeable about the content you are testing or the process of developing questions. This panel of experts is asked to judge whether or not, on the face of it, your work appears to be sound, that it will do what you want it to do. This is your judge panel.

Students can use classmates, a thesis committee, clinical staff (if it is a clinical study), and so on. Faculty use one another, students in their courses, as well as clinical and administrative staff where appropriate. Clinical agency personnel use one another, visiting faculty, and students. The point is to get opinions other than your own. We become so close to our own studies we tend to lose sight of alternative responses. The use of a judge panel, and taking its advice if it is asked for, is a first step in the development of the validity of your data collection instrument(s). Even if you are using someone else's instrument, the use of the judge panel will assist you in determining its appropriateness to your study.

One use of a judge panel is more closely allied with content validity than face validity. In this instance, the panel of experts is drawn together because it is familiar with the content area or theoretical formulation of your study. The judges are usually researchers in the field. You ask them to look over your questionnaire, interview schedule, or observational tool to judge whether or not your instrument adequately represents the known universe of content you want to cover. Their responses are reported in your proposal according to the percentage of agreement among the judge panel members with the items you have developed.

Pragmatic Measures

Pragmatic measures of validity essentially test the practical value of a particular research instrument or tool and focus on the questions, Does it work? Does it do what it is supposed to do? Pragmatic validation procedures attempt to answer these questions. The two types of pragmatic measures are called concurrent validity and predictive validity.

Concurrent Validity

Instruments that attempt to test a research subject on some current characteristic have concurrent validity if the results are compared and have a high correlation with an established (tested) measurement. Suppose you had developed a behavioral checklist to measure nurses' job satisfaction. To validate this test, you would need to compare it with the results of an established job satisfaction instrument shown to be valid for nurses. A high correlation between the results of the two dissimilar tests would indicate concurrent validity for your checklist.

A classic study by Walbek and Gordon (1980) assessed the concurrent validity of three self-report measures of assertiveness by comparing them with trait ratings of experts in assertiveness behavior. They found that although the three self-reports correlated highly with one another, there was not a high correlation between any of them and the trait ratings. Therefore, concurrent validity was not established for the self-report measures. This example points out the necessity of requiring either a test for which validity has been established or a measure that approaches the concept differently as a criterion for concurrent validity.

Predictive Validity

Instruments that accurately predict some future occurrence have predictive validity. Measures designed to predict success in educational programs fall into this category, as do aptitude tests. They are designed to measure some current characteristic that is expected to predict something that will occur sometime in the future. Predictive validity is established by measuring the trait now and waiting to see if the event occurs as predicted. Once predictive validity has been established, the instrument can be used with confidence to discriminate between people on the basis of expected outcome.

Both concurrent and predictive validity can be used for the same instrument, as in the following example by Selltiz and Kidder (1981). A test was designed for insurance salespeople that attempted to predict their ability to sell insurance. To be validated, the test was first given to a sales force currently selling insurance. Scores were compared with the amount of insurance each person sold in the prior year. This established the concurrent validity of the test. The next step was to follow a new sales force for five years, giving them the test initially and then keeping track of their sales records and noting those who stopped selling insurance. The extent to which the test was able to predict the ability to sell insurance was determined by the accuracy with which it differentiated between successful and unsuccessful salespeople at the end of a five-year period.

This two-step process can be used to develop many instruments intended to predict success. First, concurrent validity is tested by giving the test to groups who are currently demonstrating the characteristic being measured: selling insurance, practicing nursing, and recovering from surgery. If it discriminates between degree of success and failure in a population currently demonstrating the characteristic, then it has some concurrent validity and can be tested further on other groups to determine its value as a predictor. The second step, predictive validation, involves a longitudinal approach, following a sample of people over time to validate the prediction.

In exploratory descriptive studies with no structured tests available and little knowledge of the characteristics held by people in the sample, you must depend on others in the society to point out this information. As a participant observer in a new setting, you often do not know who is a good nurse or who does the best nursing care plans, so you must ask other people in the setting to point out the person to whom you should speak. This is the most fundamental step in concurrent validation of the source of your data—the discovery of who possesses the particular trait or characteristic that you want to find. When you are in an unfamiliar setting and you don't know the rules of the social system, you must rely on pragmatic validation procedures, such as asking other people.

In participant observation you can use predictive validity also. Here, you ask your informants to predict what will occur in a given situation and then actually observe the event with the informant. Then, if something happens that was not predicted or happens differently from prediction, you can ask for clarification at that time. This is a beginning level of predictive validation prior to the development of a standardized and structured test or measuring instrument.

Construct Validity

Construct validity is useful mainly for measures of traits or feelings, such as generosity, grief, or satisfaction. The theoretical base for the concept is tested by determining the extent to which the instrument actually measures that concept. Construct validity can be determined using one of three approaches:

- Contrasted groups
- Experimental manipulation
- The multitrait–multimethod approach (Waltz, Strickland, & Lenz, 1991)

The contrasted groups approach is carried out by comparing two groups, one of which is known to score very high on the concept being measured by the tool and the other very low on that concept. For example, a group of recently bereaved individuals would be expected to score very high on a measure of grief, whereas a group of people who have not suffered any losses should score very low. The tool can be given to both groups and the scores compared. If the tool is valid, the mean scores of these two groups will be significantly different.

Experimental manipulation requires that an experiment be designed to test the theory or conceptual framework underlying the instrument. Such an experiment would have hypotheses that predict the behavior of people who score at various levels on the tool. Data will then be collected, testing the hypotheses to determine whether the theory underlying the tool is adequate to explain the data collected (Waltz, et al., 1991).

The third method, the multitrait–multimethod approach, was proposed by Campbell and Fiske in 1956 to evaluate of the validity of measurement tools. This is the preferred method of establishing construct validity whenever it is possible to use it. The multimethod approach is based on the premise that different measures of the same construct should produce very similar results and that measures of different constructs should produce very different results. To perform this type of validity, you must have access to more than one method of measuring the construct under study, and you must be able to measure another construct at the same time. Thus, you have data from two or more tools designed to measure the construct you are studying and one or more measures of a different construct. If there is good construct validity, you will see a high correlation between the tools that are measuring the same construct. In addition, the measurement of the different construct will allow you to discriminate between the two constructs, and it will be clear that the tools are measuring different traits (Galassi, Delo, Galassi, & Bastien, 1979).

For example, Galassi and others (Gough & Heilbrun, 1979) have reported extensive construct validity testing on a College Self-Expression Scale (CSES). This scale measures general assertiveness. The key concepts were determined to be assertiveness, self-expression, and self-denial. The authors correlated the scores of their CSES with the 24 scales of Gough and Heilbrun's adjective checklist (1979). The two scales were found to correlate highly on defensiveness, self-confidence, achievement, dominance, exhibition, and autonomy. The new scale was shown to correlate highly with an existing measure on some of the concepts falling within the construct of assertiveness. Next, the CSES scale was determined to be different from similar constructs, such as aggressiveness. Each step increased the construct validity of the instrument. Each step actually tested the theoretical construct of assertiveness, as defined by the authors.

Reliability

Reliability refers to the consistency, stability, and repeatability of a data collection instrument. A reliable instrument does not respond to chance factors or environmental conditions; it will have consistent results if repeated over time on the same person or if used by two different investigators. The reliability of an instrument says nothing about its validity. It can be measuring the wrong concept in a consistent, stable fashion. Reliability only means that the instrument provides consistent, stable, and repeatable results.

Even if you plan to carry out construct validation procedures on your measuring instrument, you still need to be concerned about its reliability. If an instrument could be proven to have absolute validity, there would be no need to test for reliability because the instrument would automatically have perfect reliability. But because no measurement instrument can have absolute validity, we test for reliability of all instruments, and you will need to include reliability testing in your research design.

There are three methods of testing the reliability of research instruments: tests for the stability of the instrument (how stable it is over time), tests for equivalence (consistency of the results by different investigators or similar tests at the same time), and internal consistency (the measurement of the concept is consistent in all parts of the test). Each test of reliability looks at a different aspect of the instrument. When developing, adapting, or utilizing someone else's research instrument, you need to use one or more of these tests to establish the level of reliability of the instrument for your own use.

Tests of Stability

Stability is undoubtedly the best indicator of an instrument's reliability. A stable research instrument is one that can be repeated over and over on the same research subject and will produce the same results. Testing for stability, however, has one major limitation: it can be done only when you can assume that the trait being measured will remain constant over time. An example of a stable concept is intelligence. It should be possible to measure intelligence repeatedly, at regular intervals, and to obtain the same score. An unstable concept such as pain, on the other hand, is changeable and subject to frequent fluctuations even in persons with chronic pain. Repeated measures of pain in a subject would result in widely different scores. These differences would not mean that the instrument was unstable, but rather that the individual's pain was changing. This reflects expected differences due to changes in the variable being measured. Tests of stability will not be able to make this distinction. Thus, although stability is a good indicator of reliability when the variable being measured remains constant, it is not useful in the measurement of changeable or transient states. Tests of stability are in two categories: test–retest and repeated observations.

Test–Retest

The classic test of stability is test–retest. Repeated measurements over time using the same instrument on the same subjects is expected to produce the same results. It is easiest to visualize in the field of education for the development of reliable tests of knowledge. For example, a test is developed to measure knowledge of mathematics. The test is given to a group of students and repeated two weeks later. Assuming that the students have had no additional instruction in mathematics during the two-week period between tests, their scores will be very similar at both testings if the test measures reliably. Knowledge of mathematics is not a trait that is expected to change significantly according to the day of the week or the weather. Results from the first testing can be correlated with results of the second testing, and a high correlation should result (+0.8 or higher). Any time you are measuring a relatively stable trait or characteristic, you should be able to ask the same questions and get the same answers every time, regardless of the individual's mood or frame of mind. A reliable questionnaire will give you consistent results over time. If the results are not consistent, the test is not considered to be reliable and will need to be revised until it does measure consistently. Test–retest is used primarily with questionnaires, but the concept of repeated measurement to establish stability can also be used with such tools as thermometers and hemodynamic monitors and in instances where the variable being measured is not expected to fluctuate.

Test–retest is used in interviewing as well as in examinations and questionnaires. Here the investigator interviews the research subject over time on the same topic. Assuming that the topic of the interview is a stable one, the answers to the same questions should be the same. The only allowable differentiation is that frequently subjects will remember more about a topic when interviewed and will expand on all subsequent interviews. Subsequent interviews will incorporate questions on the new material and be asked about as a test–retest. Test–retest would be an inappropriate test of reliability if you were interviewing subjects on, What did you have for dinner last night? Dinner menus are expected to change. But if the question was, What did you have for dinner last Thanksgiving? the answers should be consistent from interview to interview with the addition of recalled food items between interviews. Then, these added items also should be recalled over time.

Repeated Observations

When using observational methods of data collection, the test of stability of the instrument is called repeated observations. This method has the same basic elements as test–retest. The measurement of the variable or trait is repeated over time, and the results at each measurement time are expected to be very similar. If you have developed an observational scale to rate nurses' behavior during the process of counting narcotics, you would expect that the same nurse who counted narcotics three days in a row would have a similar rating each day. If you get different ratings each day, you will question: (1) whether or not you have a reliable rating, (2) whether or not you are measuring a stable trait or characteristic, or (3) whether or not you are observing the same way each day (that is, whether you are a consistent observer). This last point is not a problem when your instrument is a questionnaire, but when you are using observation as your method of collecting data, an evaluation of your reliability as a data collector is part of the testing of the instrument.

Tests of Equivalence

When the concept or trait being measured is not a stable one, the reliability of an instrument cannot be tested by repeated measures. When a group of subjects is collected to test an instrument's reliability on a trait that is known to fluctuate over time, any testing will have to be done within a short enough time so that the trait will not have changed and an estimate of the consistency of the instrument to measure the trait can be obtained. Tests of equivalence attempt to determine if similar tests given at the same time yield the same results, or if the same results can be obtained using different observers at the same time. Equivalence is based on the idea of using alternate forms of measurement of the same trait at the same time and comparing the results.

Alternate Form

A test of equivalence using alternate forms of paper and pencil tests consisting of two sets of similar questions designed to measure the same trait is called alternate form testing. The two tests are based on the same content, but the individual items are different. When these two tests are administered to subjects at the same time, the results can be compared just as with the test–retest method, only this time it is the equivalence of the two measures that is tested rather than the stability of one instrument. Obtaining similar results on the two alternate forms of the instrument gives support for the reliability of both forms of the instrument.

A number of alternative forms of objective tests are used in education. For example, an instructor in the public school system might use this concept for examinations of students in high school courses. Here the instructor, using the same content but different questions, develops two tests for use in the same course. Sometimes the instructor will pass out two sets of examinations alternately to the class at the same time. In this way, if a student looked over another student's shoulder, he or she would see a different test. In this case, the alternate form of the test is to prevent dishonesty among the students rather than to measure the reliability of the test. At other times the alternate test is used for makeup examinations for students who missed the examination due to illness. The idea of alternate tests is that the tests will be equivalent. If one student were to take two forms of the test, the results should reflect the same level of knowledge, if the tests are reliable.

Alternate form is used in interview situations in very much the same way as it is used in questionnaires. Because interviews generally take much longer to complete than questionnaires, the interviewer will not repeat all of the content in an alternate form, but rather will incorporate into the interview schedule a few questions that ask for the same content in a different way. The way in which the subject answers the questions provides a measure of the consistency or reliability of the questions.

The major problem with alternate form questions is that they tend to be boring for the subject. When the questionnaire or interview is already very long, the addition of another questionnaire of the same length or even the addition of a few extra interview questions may be too tiring for the subjects, and you may actually be introducing new sources of error through subject fatigue and boredom. This is the major factor to consider when deciding whether you can use the alternate form method to test for reliability.

Interrater Reliability

This is the method of testing for equivalence when the design calls for observation. It is used to determine whether two observers using the same instrument at the same time will obtain similar results. A reliable instrument should produce the same results if both observers are using it the same way. An observational tool designed to measure assertiveness in social interactions is an example of an appropriate use of interrater reliability. Two researchers observe an interaction together, and each one separately rates the assertiveness of the participants using the same scale. These ratings are then compared for equivalence. The extent to which they agree serves as a measure of the reliability of the tool.

Interrater reliability is the most common method of testing observational tools for reliability because it can be used with situations that are changeable. Most social interaction situations are not repeated, and so you will rarely get to do repeated observations to test the reliability of your observational tool. However, you can usually find another observer to work with you in testing the tool.

This method is also very useful to test the reliability of interpreting physiological tools. For example, you might expect that every nurse who reads a glass thermometer will read it in the same way and come up with the same results. Nothing could be further from the truth. In actuality, thermometer reading can be quite unreliable unless the data collectors are all trained to read the thermometer exactly the same way specifically for the research project. Although the thermometer being used for the research may have been shown to be reliable on test–retest when read by one individual, when two different individuals read the same thermometer they may not arrive at the same numeric score. To test for the equivalence of their thermometer readings, interrater reliability testing is used prior to the onset of the actual data collection.

Manual blood pressure readings using a stethoscope and sphygmomanometer will also appear to provide unreliable data on test–retest when the reading is done with less than ten minutes between tests. This is because blood pressure readings change before and after the use of a tourniquet—a blood pressure cuff—so sphygmomanometers are known to result in different readings on a test–retest procedure. To test the interrater reliability of a blood pressure reading, a double stethoscope is used, which enables two people to listen and agree on blood pressure readings at the same time.

The concepts basic to equivalence are the use of two measures using alternate form questions or two observers comparing their ratings of the same event using the same data collection tool. Equivalence is used in situations where the characteristic being measured is changeable and is not expected to remain stable over time.

Tests of Internal Consistency

Internal consistency refers to the extent to which all parts of the measurement technique are measuring the same concept. For example, when developing a questionnaire to measure depression, each question should provide a measure of depression consistent with the overall results of the test. In laboratory tests, this concept includes the idea that the results obtained from counting the red blood cells in one drop of blood from a specimen should be the same as those obtained from another drop of blood from the same specimen. Hospital laboratories commonly check their own reliability by reserving parts of blood and tissue samples to be separately run through the appropriate testing procedures. Comparison of the results gives a measure of the reliability of the procedures.

All structured questionnaires designed to measure single concepts, traits, or phenomena on a quantitative scale are tested for internal consistency to ensure that all items on the questionnaire are contributing consistently to the overall measure of the concept. Internal consistency is usually established in addition to tests of stability or equivalence that may be used as measures of reliability. Sometimes, however, internal consistency may be the only measure of reliability that can used with a particular instrument. If the trait being measured is a changeable one, test–retest cannot be used. If alternate form questions are not possible because the length of the questionnaires would prohibit asking subjects to complete two at the same time, then equivalence is not an option. Internal consistency will provide a useful measure of reliability in these cases.

Tests of internal consistency are based on the idea of split-half correlations in which scores on one half of a subject's responses are compared to scores on the other half. If all items are consistently measuring the overall concept, then the scores on the two halves of the test should be highly correlated. To provide a good measure of reliability, the division of the test into halves must be done in an unbiased manner. Random division is best because all choice will be removed from the researcher. Special statistical tests have been developed to provide measures of internal consistency for questionnaires. Cronbach's alpha coefficient is the test most frequently used to establish internal consistency (1990). The alpha coefficient correlates each individual item with each other item and the overall score, thus giving an overall measure of the consistency with which the score on an item can be used to predict the overall attribute being measured. In addition to providing a measure of reliability, it also assists the researcher in identifying individual problem questions. Internal consistency must be established before an instrument can be used for research purposes. Any new instrument that you might develop will require pilot testing before you use it in your research project. If you revise an existing tool, you should treat it as a new tool for purposes of reliability testing, and even an established instrument should be tested for internal consistency each time it is used with a new population.

Internal consistency is a useful device for establishing reliability in a highly structured quantitative data collection instrument. It is not useful in open-ended questionnaires or interviews, unstructured observations, projective tests, available data, or other qualitative data collection methods and instruments.

Reliability and Validity Issues in Field Research Using Participant Observation

When research is conducted in naturalistic or field settings using qualitative or predominantly unstructured data collection instruments, repeatability of the research procedures and reliability of outcomes is difficult to achieve. The reasons are inherent in the setting itself. Field settings are in the process of change all the time. Social interactions among the same participants will differ from one hour to the next. What was studied one year will probably not be the same the next year in the same setting. The people have changed, the setting has changed, and possibly even the problem has changed—sometimes perceptibly, sometimes imperceptibly. For this reason, a second researcher entering the field to study the same phenomena using the same data-collection procedures will be unlikely to replicate the original study and produce the same results.[2] Many quantitative researchers question the validity of qualitative field research, particularly when participant observation is the major method of data collection. In nursing, however, these types of studies are gaining more acceptance as we are able to see the wealth of data they produce about the behavior of people and to gain an appreciation for the value of this research.

Due to the problem with replication and control over the field situation, field researchers, of necessity, have developed strategies for ascertaining the validity and reliability of their research using slight modifications of the concepts discussed previously.

A significant difference between field and laboratory research is that in field research it is the researcher, particularly as a participant observer, that is the primary research instrument. It is the researcher, not a mechanical research instrument or measurement device, that collects and measures the data through observations and talking to people. The researcher, using participant observation as the major data collection method, is the principal research instrument.

Field research was developed by anthropologists and sociologists to study human behavior over time in natural settings. The researcher, as participant observer, either lives with the subjects, as anthropologists do, or spends time collecting data by visiting the research site regularly over a long period of time. Fieldwork consists of a combination of the following data collection methods: participant observation, in-depth interviewing of key informants, life histories, census taking, kinship charts (genealogies or genograms), collection of written and unwritten available data, photography (stills, movies, and videos), audio recording of events and interviews, observation of special and repetitive events, and participation with informants in all social events. The purpose of the researcher is to live the life of the subjects as much as possible, to learn the rules of behavior as well as

---

[2]This was the famous case of Tepotzlan, where Oscar Lewis and Robert Redfield arrived at totally different ethnographic accounts of the same Mexican town. The fact that they talked to different people during different time periods and asked different questions yielded different pictures of the same place.

possible by living them, and eventually to describe the social life of the people being studied from their perspective. Because data are collected using many instruments or data collection devices; because data collection occurs over long periods of time; because the researcher's training in field methods, objectivity as an observer, ability to record with clarity and precision, sensitivity to the nuances of behavior, and ability to ask relevant and clear questions are critical to the outcome of the research, the issues of reliability and validity and sources of error become very complex.

Issues of reliability are concerned with the consistency, stability, and repeatability of the informant's accounts and the investigator's ability to collect and record information accurately. When key informants are interviewed over time, their responses to the same questions on the same topic should be answered with essentially the same information. This is a type of test–retest of the same informants on the same material. To further test the reliability of the informants, the researcher tape records interviews, transcribes them, then presents the informants with literal transcriptions of the interviews for verification of what was said. Frequently these verification sessions will clarify the content as well as the verbatim terminology, expand on the information by clarifying unclear or incomplete materials, and essentially validate that this material is correct. Over time, this procedure is repeated with the same informants, until by the end of the fieldwork period, the material is considered to be both valid and reliable.

When the field researcher is interviewing an informant for a single time only, the use of alternate form questions within the interview itself is a standard test of the reliability of that particular informant. The same question will be asked in the same way two to three times during the interview as a measure of stability. In addition, the subject will be asked two to three different types of questions on the same topic for alternate form reliability.

Several methods are used in the field situation to establish the reliability of the investigator. Because participant observers are often alone in the field and cannot use equivalence with another researcher, equivalence is developed by working with informants. Early in the fieldwork situation when the investigator is a stranger and unfamiliar with the rules of behavior and the setting, establishing equivalence of observation of events is critical. In the traditional anthropology situation, the investigator usually hires an informant, who observes the occasion also. The investigator then records the activity on the spot, either taking field notes, taping a running documentary of the events, or photographing events in still photographs or on film. (A written record along with photographic evidence has greater validity than either one alone.) The written record is then reviewed with the informant for completeness and comprehensiveness of the coverage. Any conclusions or inferences drawn are also verified with the informant. This is also an excellent time for the informant to explain what has occurred and why (this discussion–interview is, of course, tape recorded). Taking along an informant during these observations is critical to the field-work because questions about the event can be asked and answered at the time it is being observed so that discrepancies between what is observed and what is explained can be clarified. Also, the informant is more inter-ested and involved at the time of the activity and so is more willing to dis-cuss it. The researcher does not have to rely on anyone's memory of the event and thus avoids distortion caused by selective memory.

Validity issues are of greatest concern in field studies. Social desirability and acquiescent response set are as much a factor in field studies as in other questionnaires or interviews, thus the fieldworker needs to try to minimize these sources of error. Although all field researchers usually give their final reports to their informants for verification, many informants will not critique the material. They may not want to contradict the investigator, whom they see as a high-status individual; or they may deliberately want to keep their world a secret and want falsehoods to be published. Final reports are often shared with other researchers in the area as well as with several key informants, not just one. All comments are recorded to find dis-crepancies between comments and the final report.

A major method of verification of the truth of the data is by the use of multiple methods. Here we are relying on pragmatic validation proce-dures. Interview materials are always verified by direct observation of the event, interaction, or person. Any discrepancy can be examined more closely. If you are studying mother–infant interaction, it is not sufficient to ask mothers what they do in particular situations; the field researcher knows that what one says is not always what one does. Therefore, obser-vations of mother–infant interactions are critical validation procedures. It is insufficient to interview informants about birth customs without also validating those reports by observing birthing. Both the observation and the interview (verbatim to the degree possible) are reported. This estab-lishes the reporter's verification procedures and assures the reader that the results are reliable.

The fieldworker always looks for written reports on the groups being studied, whether they are reports of colonial officers, prior research reports, letters, diaries, newspapers, or historic documents; all are sought for verification purposes. The use of videotaping and photography vali-dates observational notes (concurrent validity) and also provides a means for repeated observations of the same event (stability). Tape recordings of interviews and social events not only allow for repeated replay (stability) but also can be used as the basis for further interviewing, for clarification of previous interviews, or to elicit new material.

These methods are all critical for an anthropologist working in a field setting, such as an African village, particularly when the researcher is not facile with the language and the customs. When the researcher enters the field as a stranger, everything is new and unfamiliar. Validation of learning is essential while you are becoming familiar with the setting. For the participant observer, fortunately, many social events and interactions are patterned and repetitive; through repeated observations many social rules of behavior are learned early. The observer then uses this knowledge (content validity) and through trial and error discovers what is being done correctly and what is being done incorrectly and why (pragmatic validation). Over time and with greater familiarity with the culture, more and more observations and interview data (both formal and informal) are collected and verified, proving—simply by weight of evidence—that the material is correct. Intensive interpersonal contact with research subjects over long periods of time provides repetitive, and sometimes overwhelming, amounts of data on the topic. The degree to which the field researcher has collected and transcribed data verbatim (in the subject's own words), has verified each transcription with the original informant, and has cross-checked all data against all forms of data collection establishes the validity of the collected data.

Reliability and Validity in the Research Plan

In exploratory descriptive studies, validation procedures frequently reflect self-evident measures or, at most, pragmatic measures; they rely heavily on reliability tests. If you were interested in developing a research program designed to describe and eventually test certain types of nursing interventions, you might begin your program at the exploratory descriptive level by observing nurses intervening with patients in particular settings. You might be interested in specific nursing diagnoses found in the nursing care plans and observe each nurse at planned intervals as care relative to those diagnoses is given. You then interview these nurses to see what nursing interventions they said were used. Your observations are repeated over time as you observe the same nurse with the same patient. In addition, you observe different nurses with the same patient and the same nurse with different patients. To test for equivalence, you would need another person observing with you in certain selected situations, thus determining your reliability as an observer. By virtue of the in-depth study, you have utilized both self-evident and pragmatic measures of validity, as well as stability and equivalence as measures of reliability.

At the descriptive survey level of design, you need to be concerned with the reliability of your measurements because accuracy in measurement is the key to a reliable Level II study. Instruments must be tested for reliability and validity, and frequently this is done in a pilot study. Even if the instrument has been previously tested in another study, it should be retested as part of your study because it has been shown that both reliability and validity can change over time. Neither is constant.

Level III experimental designs ideally require instruments that have construct validity. Only in this way can there be true confidence in the results of experiments. So few instruments in nursing research have reached the construct validity level of sophistication that studies often are carried out without the validation. This factor must be considered in interpreting the results of these studies.

Each level of research requires some facet of reliability and validity testing of the measurements, whether the research tool is you, the observer, a questionnaire, or a mechanical device. The point is that the results obtained from your measurement should be true results and not due to errors in your instrument. These critical concepts of reliability and validity can make the difference between good research and poor research.

Self-Test

The following is a series of examples of research measures commonly used in nursing studies. We first give you the item and ask you what kind of reliability or validity test you would want to use to detect either constant or random errors, then we give you some answers. You may find other answers just as appropriate.

Test Measures

1. A 40-item questionnaire to measure knowledge of diabetes to be used in a before–after experimental design.

2. An observational scale to measure a nurse's assertiveness in role-playing situations. Responses to be rated as passive, assertive, or aggressive.

3. Blood pressure readings using a sphygmomanometer and stethoscope.

4. Twenty-four-hour urinalysis for sodium, potassium, and catecholamines as a measure of stress.

5. Unstructured interview designed to elicit patients' understanding of their diagnoses or surgery, to be subjected to content analysis.

Answers

1. You can use a test of internal consistency, such as Cronbach's alpha, and you can use a test–retest procedure on the control group as part of your before–after design. In addition, you may build in alternate-form questions as a test of equivalence. If the test was based on the literature on diabetes, and you have subjected it to a panel of expert judges who confirmed that it covered the material necessary for diabetics to know, then you have self-evident validity. You may use a different test in conjunction with this one as a test of concurrent validity. You also may use a test with construct validity.

2. If the observational scale is being used for the first time, ask two observers to use it and compare their results—a test of equivalence. If their results are discrepant, train them to use the scale, then give them another assignment and compare those results. If their results continue to be discrepant, either the tool needs revision or you need two new observers. The validity of the tool should reflect content validity—the items have been developed from the literature. Document the source of each item and write a rationale for inclusion.

3. The test of blood pressure has a physiological explanatory base, so the use of the instrument has construct validity. We must, however, check to be sure that the particular instrument we are using in our research is both valid (measures accurately) and reliable (is consistent). We can check its accuracy by comparing the results of our blood pressure equipment to another means of measuring blood pressure, such as a cardiac monitor. We can check the reliability of our observers by training two observers to use the equipment (equivalence) and providing a stethoscope with two sets of earphones so they can listen simultaneously and compare readings. We can check the reliability of the cuff by using it on a subject in a test–retest situation, allowing enough time to elapse for the pressure in the arm to return to baseline.

4. These measures of stress must be validated and justified by the literature. If you are looking at stress as a short-term phenomenon (ten-minute stress), is a 24-hour urine specimen appropriate to test the theory? To test your assumption, use a different measure of stress while collecting the 24-hour urine specimen. Compare the results (concurrent validity). Urine is easily tested for internal consistency by sending two specimens from the same collection to the same laboratory and the same technician. If the results are identical, both the technician and the equipment used are reliable on test–retest. Two samples of urine can be sent to two different technicians for a test of equivalence of the technicians.

5. In unstructured interviews the subject has face validity—you assume the subject is telling the truth. You can build in a few alternate form questions for equivalence to see if the subject answers with the same information. The questions also may have face validity if the subject gleans what the researcher wants to know. The questions also may have content validity if they are based on relevant literature. The interview can be pretested prior to the study to determine whether the subject understands the question and if the interviewer asks questions consistently. Using a tape recorder to review interviewing techniques is a useful test of both reliability and validity.

Bibliography

Barnason, S., Zimmerman, L., Atwood, J., Nieveen, J., & Schmaderer, M. (2002). Development of a self-efficacy instrument for coronary artery bypass graft patients. *Journal of Nursing Measurement, 10*(2), 123–133.

Beck, C. T., & Gable, R. K. (2001). Ensuring content validity: An illustration of the process. *Journal of Nursing Measurement, 9*(2), 201–215.

Brink, P. J. (1991). Issues of reliability and validity. In J. M. Morse (Ed.), *Qualitative nursing research: A contemporary dialogue* (Rev. ed., pp. 164–186). Newbury Park, CA: Sage.

Campbell, D. T., & Fiske, D. W. (1959). Convergent and discriminant validation by the multitrait–multimethod matrix. *Psychological Bulletin, 56*(2), 81–104.

Considine, J., Botti, M., & Thomas, S. (2005). Design, format, validity and reliability of multiple choice questions for use in nursing research and education. *Collegian, 12*(1), 19–24.

Cronbach, L. J. (1990). *Essentials of psychological testing* (5th ed.). New York: Harper & Row.

DeVon, H. A., Block, M. E., Moyle-Wright, P., Ernst, D. M., Hayden, S. J., Lazzara, D. J., et al. (2007). A psychometric toolbox for testing validity and reliability. *Journal of Nursing Scholarship, 39*(2), 155–164.

Galassi, J., Delo, J., Galassi, M., & Bastien, S. (1979). College self-expression scale (CSES). In M. J. Ward & M. E. Felter (Eds.), *Instruments for use in nursing education research* (pp. 108–111). Boulder, CO: WICHE.

Gough, G. H., & Heilbrun, A. B. (1979). *The adjective checklist: Manual.* Boulder, CO: WICHE.

Higgins, P. A., & Straub, A. (2006). Understanding the error of our ways: Mapping the concepts of validity and reliability. *Nursing Outlook, 54*(1), 23–29.

Houser, J. (2008). Scientific inquiry. Precision, reliability and validity: Essential elements of measurement in nursing research. *Journal for Specialists in Pediatric Nursing, 13*(4), 297–299.

Irvine, D., O'Brien-Pallas, L. L., Murray, M., Cockeri, R., Idani, S., Saurie-Shaw, B., et al. (2000). The reliability and validity of two health status measures for evaluating outcomes of home care nursing. *Research in Nursing and Health, 23*(1), 434–454.

Mishel, M. H. (1998). Methodological studies: Instrument development. In P. J. Brink & M. J. Wood (Eds.), *Advanced design nursing research* (2nd ed., pp. 235–282). Newbury Park, CA: Sage.

Nolan, M., & Ruhi, B. (1995). Alternative approaches to establishing reliability and validity. *British Journal of Nursing, 4*(1), 587–590.

Nolan, M., & Ruhi, B. (1995). Validity: A concept at the heart of research. *British Journal of Nursing, 4*(9), 530–533.

Polit, D. F., Beck, C. T., & Owen, S. V. (2007). Is the CVI an acceptable indicator of content validity? *Research in Nursing and Health, 30*(4), 459–467.

Selltiz, C., & Kidder, L. H. (1981). *Research methods in the social relations.* New York: Holt, Rinehart and Winston.

Selltiz, C., Wrightsman, L. S., & Cook, S. W. (1976). *Research methods in social relations* (3rd ed.). New York: Holt, Rinehart and Winston.

Thomas, S. D., Hathaway, D. K., & Arheart, K. L. (1992). Face validity. *Western Journal of Nursing Research, 14*(1), 109–112.

Van Ness, P. H., Towle, V. R., & Juthani-Mehta, M. (2008). Testing measurement reliability in older populations: Methods for informed discrimination in instrument selection and application. *Journal of Aging and Health, 20*(2), 183–197.

Walbek, N. H., & Gordon, V. C. (1980). Concurrent validity of three self-report measures of assertiveness. *Research in Nursing and Health, 3,* 159–162.

Waltz, C. F., Strickland, O. L., & Lenz, E. R. (1991). *Measurement in nursing research* (2nd ed.). Philadelphia: F. A. Davis.

Windle, P. E., & Throckmorton, T. (2008). Finding, selecting, and evaluating instruments to support decision making: Reliability and validity. *Journal of Perianesthesa Nursing, 23*(1), 60–62.

CHAPTER ELEVEN

Ethics in Nursing Research

➤ TOPICS

Problems Involving Ethics
Informed Consent
Balancing Potential Benefit Against Actual Cost
Maintaining Anonymity and Confidentiality
Federal Guidelines on the Submission of Proposals for Review
Ethical Principles Underlying Protection of Human Subjects
Bibliography

➤ LEARNING OBJECTIVES

- Outline why it is necessary to protect the rights of human subjects in research.
- Identify some of the problems that have arisen as a result of violations of the rights of individuals participating in research projects.
- Describe the meaning of informed consent and identify issues relating to it in research on human subjects.
- Determine the considerations that must be weighed when balancing potential benefits and costs in research with particular reference to maintaining subjects' anonymity and confidentiality of information.
- Outline the nature of federal guidelines for the review of research proposals involving human subjects.
- Discuss the major ethical principles that guide researchers in their work.

What happens to people who take part in research? Who is concerned with their welfare? Until recently, these questions received little attention. In the past, some researchers involved their subjects in research without obtaining their permission, gave false information about the subjects' role in the study, or involved people in physically and psychologically harmful experiments. Little attention was paid to the rights of subjects. The scientific contribution of the research was all-important.

Today, the rights of research subjects in all disciplines must be protected to the fullest possible extent. When subjects are vulnerable (as is true of clients of the healthcare system), the research proposal must explain how subjects' rights will be protected.

The movement to protect human rights in research began after the Nuremberg trials that followed World War II. The world was so appalled by the biomedical experiments conducted on concentration camp prisoners that a code of behavior for researchers was drafted. The Nuremberg Code, drawn up and accepted by the United Nations in 1948, was the first set of guidelines protecting the rights of research subjects. It was an excellent beginning but left out two major classes of research subjects: children and the mentally incompetent. The Declaration of Helsinki, originally written in 1965 by the World Medical Association and updated through 2009, remedied that omission by including children if parental permission was obtained and the mentally incompetent if proxy consents were obtained. Between 1945 and 1966, 2000 research projects were approved by the National Institutes of Health (NIH) where informed consents were not required of participants. During this time the drug thalidomide was being developed. Even though the drug had not received US Food and Drug Administration (FDA) approval because there were concerns about its safety, it was prescribed for thousands of women in the United States and Canada who were not informed of the risks of the drug. They essentially took part in a drug trial without their knowledge or consent. The scandal that erupted following the birth of the babies with severe birth defects born to women who took thalidomide led to amendments to the Federal Food, Drug, and Cosmetic Act. As a result, physicians were required to inform individuals if they were taking a drug that had not received FDA approval.

In 1966, the surgeon general of the United States issued guidelines to protect the rights and welfare of research subjects. These guidelines initiated a system of review of research proposals at the local level (institutional review boards) and accepted the notion of proxy consents. The guidelines also established rules that researchers must follow to obtain informed consent for drug trials.

Problems resulting from biomedical research were the subject of Senate hearings in 1973. Two of the most famous were the Tuskegee case and the Willowbrook case (Veatch, 1977). The Willowbrook case concerned an experimental design in which children living in an institution for the mentally retarded were injected with hepatitis virus. In the Tuskegee case, black male prisoners were used for a classic experimental design for treatment of syphilis. One group of infected men received no treatment, and their disease progressed to third-stage syphilis. These cases, among others, raised several ethical issues requiring a set of guidelines and principles on which to judge the ethical nature of research.

In 1974, Congress established the National Commission for the Protection of Human Subjects of Biomedical and Behavioral Research. This commission explored basic ethical issues of human subjects in research and identified principles to assist with the planning and conducting of ethical research. The 1979 Belmont Report summarized the basic ethical principles developed by the commission and addressed informed consent. Recommendations specified that researchers have a duty to keep subjects informed throughout a research project and explain the risks and benefits fully to ensure subjects' understanding. These recommendations applied to all health-related research, including nursing studies.

In Canada, the Tri-Council Policy Statement: Ethical Conduct for Research Involving Humans has been widely adopted as the definitive policy statement for health research. Research conducted in a wide variety of Canadian agencies is governed by the principles and standards specified in this document. The principles discussed in the report are based on guidelines of the federal research councils over a period of some years and on standards widely accepted in the international community.

As nurses become more involved in research, the issue of protection of human subjects becomes critical. The profession is responsible for establishing guidelines for ethical practices in nursing research. The International Council of Nurses developed the Code for Nurses: Ethical Concepts Applied to Nursing in 1953. Although no reference was made to research at that time, the most recent update (2000) of the code specifies that ethical principles outlined shall apply to research.

But you may ask, Why do we need to bother about ethical guidelines for research? Aren't people protected by law? The law is a written mandate for behavior, based on what people believe is good and bad behavior—their ethics. Before writing down laws, people must decide what they believe in. Frequently, laws are a set of instructions on what you are not allowed to do rather than a set of instructions on what you should do. Ethics outlines a set of principles that can be used to determine which actions are right and which are wrong. Ethical judgments are the decisions a person makes on whether a particular act is right or wrong. Finally, ethical theory provides a means of understanding ethical principles, and bioethics is the application of general moral principles to the area of health–illness action and events (Beauchamp & Childress, 1979). When an action deriving from an ethical principle becomes law, people can be punished for immoral behavior. The law is normally in a catch-up position in relation to ethical values and practices. Ethical values and practices change over time, and there may be a need to enact laws to ensure that they are observed. The question of do-not-resuscitate (DNR) protocols is a good example of a change in practice based on ethics. The development of laws to ensure that DNR protocols are allowed in particular circumstances is occurring throughout the Western world. The problem arose because the development of lifesaving technologies led to the possibility of maintaining or restoring life following adverse health events. Many people had difficulty with the idea of themselves or their loved ones being kept alive through artificial means. Health professionals also had difficulty in such circumstances. After many court challenges over cases where people were being kept alive by artificial means, laws are gradually being enacted to allow the use of DNR protocols under particular circumstances. Because the law is frequently many years behind ethical–moral conduct, it cannot be relied upon to set guidelines for ethical behavior in nursing practice or research. Therefore, you need to think through the situations you will face in your research and make decisions based on what is reasonable and ethical in each particular situation.

Problems Involving Ethics

Anything that violates an individual's basic rights becomes an ethical issue. There are many such occurrences in research. Most violations arise from the difficulty of obtaining truly informed consent, whether this stems from the subject's lack of understanding or the researcher's failure to inform the subject adequately. Expert views on the topic of informed consent vary widely, from those who believe that everyone has a moral obligation to participate in biomedical research for the good of humanity (Visscher, 1981) to those who think that no one but another researcher in the same field can truly give informed consent (Ingelfinger, 1981). The chances that the subject has complete understanding of the research and feels totally free to make a choice are perhaps unlikely. If the subject is a patient in the health-care system, there are additional constraints to free choice. The patient may feel it is necessary to please those on whom he or she is dependent, such as the physician or nurse. In nursing, as in other professions, the state of the art cannot move forward without research. Therefore, human subjects must be solicited to test ideas and answer questions. The protection of the subject is the obligation of every nurse researcher.

If the subject is not aware of the true nature of the research and the subject gives consent willingly to participate in a research project, the consent is not informed. The researcher has not obtained an informed consent if only partial information is given about the study in general terms or if false information about the purpose of the study or the procedures to be followed is provided. Both methods of obtaining consent are questionable in that both inhibit the right of free choice. The use of deception is considered more unethical than the withholding of information, although the line separating the two may be undistinguishable. Withholding of information is widely used in studies where it is believed that complete information about the purpose of the study will influence the subject's response. Thus, subjects might be told they will be participating in a study to improve nursing care, when the actual question could be, What are patients' attitudes toward male nurses? or What is the relationship between ethnic background and perception of pain?

Another instance of withholding information is found in the use of placebos to compare the effect of the real treatment. Participants are not informed whether they are receiving the placebo or the real treatment. For example, when testing the effect of a new teaching method on the abilities of diabetic individuals to control blood sugar, study participants might not be told whether they are receiving the new or the old teaching method in an attempt to prevent this knowledge from influencing the results. These practices are so widely accepted that the participant's right to complete knowledge before consenting is rarely considered.

The National Commission for the Protection of Human Subjects of Biomedical and Behavioral Research has considered the problem of withholding information from subjects. A commission report states strongly that such research can be justified only if the researcher can demonstrate that informing the subjects would truly invalidate the research and not just cause the researcher inconvenience. In addition, there can be no undisclosed risks to the subjects. If these criteria are met, the research might be approved, but there must also be a plan for giving the subjects complete information after the study is over. Under no circumstances may the investigator lie to the subject, even though a direct answer may make that particular subject ineligible for the study.

Professionals use a number of rationalizations for withholding information from participants. One is that informed consent is necessary only when there is some risk for the participant. If the researcher determines that no risk factor exists, that individual may reach the conclusion that subjects do not need complete information about the study. Another rationalization is that researchers are obligated to give only the information that the subject requests about the study and that the responsibility for ensuring informed consent, therefore, belongs to the subjects. An assumption that often underlies this rationalization is that people are not really interested in the research question, only in what will happen to them as subjects. None of these positions can override the subject's basic right to autonomy and respect, and, therefore, none are acceptable practices.

Deliberate deception of human subjects was a common practice among researchers at one time. A number of outstanding studies based on deception produced far-reaching results and provided previously unavailable information about human behavior. This practice was based on the belief that the data would not have been obtainable if the subject knew the true nature of the research. For that reason, subjects were deliberately misled about the study or the experiment. In some cases, subjects received the results of the study after it was completed. In others, the subjects never knew.

Examples of deceiving research subjects include telling subjects that they are being tested for one thing when they are being tested for something else, not telling control subjects that they have received a placebo when they have come for the experimental item (such as birth control methods), telling subjects that someone else is being observed instead of them, and not telling subjects that they are involved in a research project even when they ask. Deception of research subjects is unethical.

Coercion of Subjects to Participate

The assumption behind the concept of informed consent is that, given sufficient information on which to base a decision, the subject's consent to participate is made freely. However, there are various ways in which consent may be partly, or even wholly, coerced by the circumstances under which it is obtained.

Many times, the researcher is in a position to influence subjects' participation in the study. For example, the researcher may be the subject's employer or teacher and thus may exert considerable control. An employer or a teacher may require that individuals participate as a condition of remaining employed or passing a course. Without question, this is coercion.

Another type of coercion occurs when individuals are required to give consent to participate in research to be accepted for treatment at a particular healthcare facility. This might happen in medical centers and specialty hospitals, such as those specializing in the treatment of catastrophic illnesses. The individual is likely to feel that the last chance of being accepted rests with that institution and, therefore, feels compelled to consent to anything.

Coercion also occurs when people are given the option to refuse but with the sense that refusal will not go unpunished. For example, when a nursing supervisor brings questionnaires to a nursing unit, distributes them, and says she will be back to pick them up in an hour, at least some of the nurses are likely to feel that a refusal will offend their supervisor, even though they are given the option, perhaps thinking it will have an effect on their days off or their shift rotation.

Healthcare clients are particularly vulnerable to requests to participate in research when the person making the request is someone on whom the individual must depend for critical needs. The physician and the primary nurse can easily take advantage of an individual's vulnerability.

The ethical position is to recognize that people are never obligated to assist with research. Many times it may seem obvious that it will be to the advantage of the individual to participate in the research. Perhaps the individual will benefit from extra nursing care or a special teaching program. Perhaps employees will reap the benefits of shorter working hours, less shift rotation, or improved supervision. Although this may be true, it is still the individual's right to decide. Thus, although the advantages of participation can be mentioned as part of the information needed for informed consent, the decision should never be made for that person.

Withholding Benefits from Control Subjects

This issue is particularly critical for studies in which the new treatment would be of value to all the subjects, including the control group, or when a control group is deprived of something the members of the group had access to earlier to obtain a more accurate assessment of the new treatment. Both instances provide ethical dilemmas for researchers. Remember, however, the majority of control groups suffer no deprivation.

Sometimes problems with control-group deprivation occur because of the overzealousness of an inexperienced researcher, when, in fact, they are not necessary. For example, in a study to test the effectiveness of a preoperative teaching program on postoperative anxiety, the nursing staff was told not to answer any questions from the participants in the treatment or the families in the control group. This overzealousness deprived the control group of expected privileges and introduced a new variable—withholding of information—which was not part of the research question. This kind of mistake can easily be identified in the proposal if the researcher addresses the topic of human rights for all subjects, including the control group.

In some experimental studies, the benefit of the experimental variable is so obvious that those who are cooperating with the researcher in carrying out the study will refuse to deprive the control group of the benefit. This kind of study is particularly difficult for nurses to carry out because their primary responsibility is the care of people and not experimentation. Dedicated nurses would find it difficult to deprive a group of individuals of an obvious beneficial treatment, such as a simple relaxation exercise that relieves postoperative pain. If this difficulty could be predicted, perhaps control data should be collected before introducing the experimental variable, thus avoiding the problem for the attending nurse.

Sometimes, withholding benefits from the control group can be rectified at the end of the experiment by making the benefits available at that time. A method of teaching diabetics that has proved to be immensely successful could be provided for the control patients after the data have been collected. Remember, however, that this effort must be planned in advance along with the actual experiment so that time and money are budgeted for carrying it out.

Invasion of Privacy

All research has the potential of being invasive, whether it is simple observation and recording of behavior or an experimental design. If you, the researcher, decide to take movies of persons leaving a bar, a church, or a jail, you may unintentionally be taking movies of people who don't want others to know where they were. When you show these movies publicly, you are invading the privacy of the persons you have photographed. When you go to people's homes for interviews, particularly when the topic is sensitive, you are again invading individuals' privacy. These persons have a right to refuse to participate in your research or to have all identifying data about themselves removed from your study.

Another violation of privacy is observing individuals on units when they are living in a healthcare facility such as a long-term or continuing care institution. These individuals have as much right to privacy in the hospital as you do in your home. Because their privacy is limited, it must be protected even more. Hospital records are private documents—not to be shared for the sake of curiosity. As private citizens, we have the right not to have our private lives spread all over the front page of a newspaper or be placed on TV for the purpose of research. Without our permission, researchers simply don't have the right to violate that principle.

Informed Consent

Just as all patients entering the healthcare delivery system have the right to know what will happen to them and to sign a consent form for any procedures, so do the participants in a research project. The protection of the rights of the research subject revolves around the concept of informed consent.

Informed consent has three major elements: the type of information needed by the research subject; the degree of understanding required of the subject to give consent; and, finally, the fact that the subject has a free choice in giving consent.

Information

All research subjects need to know in full detail what will happen to them during the research project. To receive consent, the researcher must explain the study and the subject's participation in the study. Therefore, the informed portion refers to the amount and type of information that should be given so that the research subject is thoroughly oriented. The information needed by research subjects includes the nature, duration, and purpose of the study; the methods and procedures by which data will be collected; how the data will be used; all the inconveniences, potential harm, or possible discomforts that may reasonably be expected from the research protocol; the benefits to be gained from the study; the results, effects, and side effects that may come from participation in the study; and the alternatives available to the subjects. In addition, the researcher must inform the subjects that they may withdraw from the study at any time without prejudice. Subjects should also be told if they will receive any compensation for being in the study and, if so, what, and how any injuries resulting from participation will be treated (Code of Federal Regulations, 1978). In an experimental design in which the researcher manipulates the independent variable (such as in a clinical trial or clinical experiment), subjects must be told about the entire experiment, including the risks and benefits, and that they may be assigned to either the control or the experimental group. To give consent as informed, knowledgeable subjects, participants need as much data as possible to make a decision. Just imagine how you would feel if you were a research subject and found out about the hazards of the research later!

The information given to the research subject must be presented in such a way that the subject can understand the study in its entirety. The researcher, therefore, is obligated to inform the potential research subject about the research so that the subject fully understands all the ramifications of the study. To do this, subjects must be informed in their own language, at their own level of understanding, and in their own common vocabulary. When healthcare professionals explain to individuals that they must void or have an EMG right after they have been prepped, they are not communicating in terms that most people would understand unless they too were healthcare professionals. Therefore, all research or medical jargon should be eliminated from the information given to the potential subject. In experimental designs especially, language that is loaded in favor of consenting to participate in the study should be avoided as much as possible because biased language does not provide the balanced explanation needed for full comprehension. Lay terminology, rather than professional jargon, must be used to describe the study.

Free Choice

This last aspect of informed consent implies that the subject should not be coerced, in any way, to participate in the study. Coercion in this sense ranges from mild coercion, such as the offering of remuneration that may be irresistible, to severe coercion, such as threat of failure in school, refusal of treatment, physical punishments, and so on. When an individual feels coerced or threatened, choice is not free. Similarly, excessive rewards limit freedom of choice. The subject may feel constrained to act in one way or another. For this reason, subjects must be told that they are free to withdraw at any time before or during the study. In this way, the subject is ensured freedom of choice.

When you plan your research project, consider the issue of informed consent in your research proposal. Write down exactly how you intend to tell the research subject about the study. Write out what you will say in simple language and look up synonyms for words you think may not be clearly understood. As you write your explanation, make sure that the nature and amount of information your subjects will be given, as well as the steps you intend to take to ensure freedom of choice, are present in the informed consent portion of your proposal.

Obviously, not all research meets the criteria for informed consent. Many studies fail in one or more of these areas to protect the subjects' rights fully, often because completely informed consent is impossible. The reasons vary—from using data from deceased subjects to giving subjects incomplete information so as not to bias the data. Whatever the reason and however sound, just, and reasonable it may be, all violations of the basic right of subjects to informed consent result in ethical problems for the researcher. These problems must be attacked in the proposal and may be so pervasive that the researcher should consider abandoning the study.

Proxy Consents for Research

Ethical guidelines for research demand that the subject's informed consent be based on enough information, comprehension of that information, and freedom to choose. There are certain groups in society who do not meet these basic criteria for informed consent. Those who are cognitively impaired may lack the ability to comprehend. Children, because of their parents' legal rights, may lack the right to make a free choice. Other groups who cannot meet one or more of these essential criteria are comatose individuals and fetuses. The researcher who wishes to study these groups has an additional burden to assume—that of assuring that the human rights of the subjects will be protected and obtaining legal permission (usually by proxy from a parent or guardian). Federal guidelines require that consent be obtained from the subject and permission be obtained from the guardian, if possible. If the subjects are children, the researcher must explain the study, at the appropriate level so that the child understands the explanation, and obtain consent from the child as well. Similar guidelines apply to the cognitively impaired. If the subject cannot understand either the spoken or the written word, then only the permission of the guardian is required.

Balancing Potential Benefit Against Actual Cost

In all disciplines, scientists must develop new knowledge through research. In any research proposal, the researcher is obligated to weigh the potential contribution of the research, both to the discipline and to society, against the costs to participants in the study. In some cases there is no problem. Full, informed consent can be obtained from the participants. They can make a free choice based on sufficient information. In other cases, because of the nature of the question and the procedures necessary to elicit the required data, there is some violation of the rights of the subjects. The benefits of the research must be carefully examined in light of the cost of these subjects.

The process of weighing the costs and benefits is always a subjective one. The investigator will always be slanted in favor of the research. To reduce subjectivity, three areas should be addressed: potential contribution to knowledge, practical value to society, and benefit to the subject. The first includes the development of theory to explain nursing practice and an improvement in the consumers' understanding of healthcare delivery. The second involves improvement in the delivery of health care to the public and improved assessment of the healthcare needs of ethnic minorities. The third might be more rapid recovery from illness because of improved nursing care or increased understanding of preventive health measures. Addressing one or more of these three areas should produce substantial evidence to balance the potential cost to the subject.

The process of balancing potential benefits and costs requires analysis of degree as well as benefit or cost. How important is the problem under study? It is frequently difficult to say. Questions about current issues in nursing will assume more relevance and importance than those of interest only to the researcher. The same question can be asked of the potential cost to the subject. How serious is the potential infringement on the subject's rights? How much harm might it do? Is it likely to be fleeting or lasting? Answers to these questions will meet with considerable disagreement among colleagues. Once again, the researcher is likely to be biased in favor of the research. Therefore, all possible resources should be used to help make the decision to go ahead.

Consultation can be obtained from a number of sources to evaluate the protection of the rights of subjects in the proposal. People who are interested in the same or similar research area are a valuable resource. You may obtain helpful advice on how to proceed from other researchers who have faced the same dilemma. There is one shortcoming to using colleagues: they may be as biased as you are in favor of the proposed research. Because it is difficult for one who is closely involved in the field to be objective about balancing pluses and minuses, there may be a tendency to view the potential contribution as much more valuable than would be the case by someone not involved in the research subject.

Persons with different backgrounds, from other disciplines, and even lay people can help to assess the importance of both the contribution of the study to society and the potential effect on the subjects. Many nursing studies would also benefit from consultation with potential subjects regarding their view of the dilemma.

Medical centers, schools, universities, and many hospitals have formed committees to review research proposals for the purpose of monitoring the protection of subjects' rights. These committees must approve proposals before research can be carried out and often provide consultations to researchers relative to protecting the rights of subjects. Accustomed to reviewing proposals, these committees can sometimes help to put the study in proper ethical perspective for the researcher.

There are no easy rules for solving the ethical issues in planning research. The major consideration must always be the safety and well-being of the participants. After this, the research question should be looked at in relation to the rights of the subjects. When there is a conflict, priority must be given to protection of the subjects.

Maintaining Anonymity and Confidentiality

As a researcher, you may find yourself in the position of having to promise confidentiality and anonymity to your subjects before they sign a consent form. The meaning of these terms is important. Confidentiality implies that you will keep all records closed and that only persons involved in the research will have access to them. Therefore, only you, the investigator, your research committee, and other researchers who wish to replicate your findings can have access to the raw data. Thus, your promise of confidentiality implies that you will screen individuals before they have access to the data. Anonymity means that you will not publish the names and addresses of your data sources and that you will make every attempt to group your data so that personal characteristics will not become known. Basically, you promise to publish or report your findings in such a way that the subjects will remain anonymous.

When promising subjects anonymity and confidentiality, it is wise to plan ahead for problems that might prevent you from keeping these promises. For example, the institution where you plan to collect the data may expect you to share them with their administration. Parents may expect to have access to research data involving their children. Other researchers may request your data to use in their own research. None of these possibilities become a problem if you have planned ahead. The institution must understand and agree that it will have access only to the summarized results and not to the raw data. If this is not acceptable, either do not promise anonymity to the subjects or select another institution. Whatever the request for access to the data might be and however innocuous, no information should be released without the subject's permission.

All researchers should be aware that confidentiality of research data is not recognized by law. This means that research data can be subpoenaed for use in court and that a researcher may be required to testify about people who have been research subjects. When your subjects are heroin addicts, child abusers, and others who may have broken the law, you need to consider the possibility that you may be required to surrender your records or to testify against your subjects.

Before they consent to participate, your subjects need to be told that you intend to publish the results of your study. In studies of groups of people, it is frequently impossible to maintain anonymity of the group when publishing your findings. It may be the only group of its kind, so that, even disguising names and location, it is possible to identify the members. This possibility can prove to be embarrassing to the individual members, and they need to be aware of it before they can give full consent to participate in the study.

Your method of data analysis can cause loss of anonymity for your subjects if you are not careful. If, for example, you are reporting findings in an attitude study of staff nurses, and you cross-tabulate them by shift, unit, and position, you may find that there is only one RN on the night shift of a particular unit, and her responses will be easily identified. To maintain anonymity, you may be required to omit some of your data analysis from the published report.

These potential difficulties in maintaining confidentiality can be avoided by planning ahead. It is not enough just to avoid promising what you can't deliver. The onus is on the research to inform the subject that some or all of the data will become public knowledge or that some individuals other than the researcher will have access to them. Otherwise, the subject has the right to assume that all data will be kept confidential.

Federal Guidelines on the Submission of Proposals for Review ___

When you have written your research proposal, you probably will be asked to submit it to the institutional review board (IRB) at your institution. If you plan to collect data in a hospital setting or in the community, you will have to submit your proposal to those IRBs as well. All review boards have the same general guidelines based on the federal guidelines; you need to be aware of these guidelines and how to incorporate them into your research plan.

In the United States, the National Institutes of Health sponsored the development of the first Public Health Service Policy on the Protection of Human Subjects issued in 1966. At the outset, the policy applied only to extramural research but was later expanded to include all research involving human subjects either conducted or supported by the Department of Health, Education, and Welfare (HEW). In 1974 the National Research Act was passed requiring HEW to develop a code that would be the basis of federal regulations for the protection of human subjects in research.

At the same time the National Commission for the Protection of Human Subjects of Biomedical and Behavioral Research was formed to evaluate the existing HEW system. This body issued a number of reports, including the Belmont Report of 1979, a landmark document that outlined the distinction between therapeutic medicine and research, identified three ethical principles for the protection of human subjects, and demonstrated how these should be applied to research involving human subjects. In 1981, the new Department of Health and Human Services (HHS) approved Title 45, Code of Federal Regulations, Part 46 Protection of Human Subjects (45 CFR 46) (Code of Federal Regulations, 1978). Although at the outset these regulations were applicable only to HHS conducted or supported research, in June, 1991, 45 CFR Part 46 was revised and extended to govern all federally supported research. This continues to be applicable to research sponsored by the federal government.

You are responsible only for submitting your proposals to the IRBs that are relevant to your research, following their requirements for submission. The regulations unequivocally state that only proposals funded by a federal agency must be reviewed. In the past, all research conducted in a setting funded by federal grants was reviewed, whether directly funded or not. Second, broad categories of certain behavioral and social science research have been exempted from review. These studies "normally present little or no risk or harm to subjects" (Hastings Center Report, 1981, p. 3). The exempted categories include research on normal educational practices and surveys, interviews, or observation of public behavior that does not in any way identify the subjects or place them at risk if their participation becomes known or that does not involve some sensitive aspect of behavior. The collection of available data, such as documents, records, pathology reports, and diagnostic specimens, is exempted if the information recorded maintains the privacy of the subject.

Certain categories of research that can be processed via an expedited review process include the collection of nail clippings or human hair, excreta, dental plaque, records of routine noninvasive clinical procedures, moderate exercises on normal, healthy subjects, as well as individual or group behavior or characteristics of individuals, such as studies of perception, cognition, game theory, or test development (Hastings Center Report, 1981).

The regulations place the burden of protecting human rights on the investigator rather than on the IRB, thus reopening the question of who is to decide whether a research proposal is ethical (Veatch, 1981).

If there is an IRB at your institution, ask for its guidelines on protection of human subjects and incorporate the relevant guidelines to protect your research subjects. If you are using animals in your research, you need to know how they are protected, and your institution will also have those federal regulations.

In Canada, the Tri-Council Policy Statement: Ethical Conduct for Research Involving Humans is used in a great many Canadian agencies as the policy governing health research. It is based on similar ethical principles as are used in the United States and the international community.

Ethical Principles Underlying Protection of Human Subjects

Three major ethical principles guide researchers: autonomy, beneficence, and nonmaleficence. Each is important, and each must be valued by the researcher. Different researchers, however, will emphasize one principle over the others or will rank order them according to their importance in a particular piece of research. In the following paragraphs, the three principles are defined, then examples are given as to their use by different researchers.

Autonomy refers to the individual having the right to self-determination. People are considered to be individuals and not just members of a group. Individuals are not interchangeable. Each has worth, and each has the freedom to decide whether to participate in a research project.

Beneficence is the principle of doing good for another. Doing good for another person requires that someone make the decision that the act will be good for that individual. Someone needs to decide. The principle is fairly clear in a simple description of parent–child interaction. The parent teaches the child about dental hygiene to prevent tooth decay. The parent is doing good for the child despite the child's attempts to avoid the daily scrub. Our society also has decided that it is good for its citizens to be protected from infectious diseases. Some individuals, however, are allergic to vaccines. In medical research, beneficence includes developing new treatment procedures as well as preventive interventions. These are all intended to benefit the patient.

Nonmaleficence, or do no harm, requires that the researcher do no direct harm, although indirect and unanticipated harm may occur. This concept is specific to experimental designs in which the experimenter cannot intend harm to either the experimental or the control group. The Willowbrook and the Tuskegee studies described earlier are examples of maleficence—the experimenter directly harmed the research subjects to see what would happen to them. In the Willowbrook case, the children were infected with hepatitis, and in the Tuskegee case, the patients with syphilis were untreated. In both cases, there was direct harm to the subjects. At the same time, the researchers sincerely believed that they were acting on the principle of beneficence—doing good—by studying the effects of these diseases in a controlled experiment. Today, studies like the Tuskegee case are not allowed because we know the outcome of untreated syphilis.

The question posed by human subjects review committees is, Can the information be found from any other source or with any other research methods than the one in which there is direct, anticipated harm to the subjects?

These three ethical principles form the basis of ethical review of research proposals. Each is weighed against the other two. Assuming that the research protocol is sound, approval of the research will depend on the degree to which the investigator plans to protect the rights of subjects.

In an analysis of all professional codes of conduct, Veatch (1989) concluded that the Code of Ethics for Nurses developed by the American Nurses Association was heavily influenced by the principle of autonomy, whereas medicine and dentistry were more influenced by nonmaleficence. Just as professional codes of conduct emphasize one ethical principle over another, so do research review committees.

From these three ethical principles, the following research issues are derived (see Table 11-1). The ethical principle of autonomy underlies several research issues. First is the issue of obtaining informed consent from the research subject by (1) providing adequate information so the subject is able to judge whether to participate and (2) providing that information in a form that is clearly understandable to the subject. The second research issue is that the subject must feel free to make the decision; there must be no known coercion to participate either overtly or covertly. There is an ordinal scale of pressure to participate, however, from mild pressure to extreme coercion. The committee needs to establish where on that ordinal

TABLE 11-1
Legal/Ethical Matrix

	Legal	Illegal
Ethical	Marriage	Rosa Parks
Unethical	Cheating on examinations	Murder

Source: Judith M. Saunders, RN, DNS, FAAN.

scale the particular proposal lies. Finally, issues of confidentiality and anonymity also are based on the principle of autonomy. A person has the right to privacy. Persons need to be told, if or when they lose their privacy, how this loss will be handled by the researcher.

The principle of beneficence underlies the determination of what good this study is going to do anyone. Is it going to benefit the research subject directly? If not, will anyone else benefit from the research findings? This determination is very important because if there is any harm at all to the research subject, the good must outweigh the harm. In medical research particularly, the risk–benefit ratio is critical.

The principle of nonmaleficence simply reaffirms that no research shall be undertaken that has direct harm to the research subject as its primary goal. Although this may sound somewhat silly, an article in the *Western Journal of Nursing Research* by Hilda Steppe (1992) poignantly describes what happens to the ethics of nurses when they live and work in a totalitarian environment. There are oppressive environments in which nurses work every day. They may not be as blatant or as maleficent as the one described by Steppe, but they may be just as harmful to the patient.

Finally, the principle of social justice is beginning to be discussed in research circles. Feminists argue from this principle when they protest the lack of women in samples ostensibly on human beings. For years, drug companies have avoided including women as subjects in their drug trials on the assumption that they would skew the data. Many drug studies, therefore, were done on male-only samples and the findings generalized to females. Feminists assert, rightly, that women have as much right to know what will happen in their bodies when they take a certain drug as men do. This is the principle of social justice. The operationalization of this principle is to include both men and women in any study of human beings.

Bibliography

American Nurses Association. (1968). The nurse in research: ANA guidelines on ethical values. *American Journal of Nursing. 68*(7), 1504–1507.

Anema, M. G. (1989). Ethical considerations in conducting clinical research. *Dimensions of Critical Care Nursing, 8*(5), 288–296.

Arford, P. H. (2004). Working with human research protections. *Journal of Nursing Scholarship, 36*(3), 265–271.

Beauchamp, T. L., & Childress, J. F. (2001). *Principles of biomedical ethics* (5th ed.). New York: Oxford University Press.

Beauchamp, T. L., & Walters, L. (Eds.). (1999). *Contemporary issues in bioethics*. Belmont, CA: Wadsworth.

Belmont report: Ethical principles and guidelines for the protection of human subjects of research. Report of the National Commission for the Protection of Human Subjects of Biomedical and Behavioral Research, Department of Health, Education, and Welfare, Office of the Secretary. *Federal Register, 44*(76), 23192–23197.

Bindless, L. (2000). Identifying ethical issues in nursing research. *Journal of Community Nursing, 14*(4), 26, 28, 30.

Capron, A. M. (1991). Human experimentation. In R. M. Veatch (Ed.), *Medical ethics* (pp. 125–172). Sudbury, MA: Jones and Bartlett.

Code of Federal Regulations. (1978, November). 45 CFR 46 protection of human subjects. *PRR Reports*. New York: Holt, Rinehart and Winston.

Cowles, K. V. (1988). Issues in qualitative research on sensitive topics. *Western Journal of Nursing Research, 10*, 163–179.

Creighton, H., & Armington, C. (1973, August). *Legal concerns of research and nurse researchers. Issues in research: Social, professional, and methodological*. Selected papers from the ANA Council of Nurse Researchers Program Meeting, 18–30.

Davis, A. J. (1989). Informed consent process in research protocols: Dilemmas for clinical nurses. *Western Journal of Nursing Research, 11*(4), 448–457.

Davis, A. J., Aroskar, M. A, Liaschenko, J., & Drought, T. S. (1997). *Ethical dilemmas and nursing practice* (4th ed.). Stamford, CT: Appleton & Lange.

Dobratz, M. C. (2003). Issues and dilemmas in conducting research with vulnerable home hospice participants. *Journal of Nursing Scholarship, 35*(4), 371–376.

Fleming, J. (1973, August). *Human rights and ethical concerns of scientists. Issues in research: Social, professional, and methodological*. Selected papers from the ANA Council of Nurse Researchers Program Meeting, 36–49.

Hastings Center Report. (1981). New human subjects research regulations effective in July. *Hastings Center Report, 11*(2), 3.

Ingelfinger, F. J. (1981). Informed (but uneducated) consent. *New England Journal of Medicine, 287*(9), 465–466.

Interagency Advisory Panel on Research Ethics. (2005). *Tri-Council policy statement: Ethical conduct for research involving humans.* Retrieved November 10, 2009, from http://www.pre.ethics.gc.ca/english/policystatement/policystatement.cfm

International Council of Nurses. (2000). *The ICN code of ethics for nurses.* Retrieved November 10, 2009, from http://www.icn.ch/icncode.pdf

Kite, K. (1999). Anonymising the subject: What are the implications? *Nurse Researcher, 6*(3), 77–84.

Koivisto, K., Janhonen, S., Latvala, E., & Vaisanen, L. (2001). Applying ethical guidelines in nursing research on people with mental illness. *Nursing Ethics, 8*(4), 328–339.

Lutz, K. F., Shelton, K. C., Robrecht, L. C., Hatton, D. C., & Beckett, A. K. (2000). Use of certificates of confidentiality in nursing research. *Journal of Nursing Scholarship, 32*(2), 185–188.

Mabunda, G. (2001). Ethical issues in HIV research in poor countries. *Journal of Nursing Scholarship, 33*(2), 111–114.

Mapes, T. A., & Zembaty, J. S. (Eds.). (1996). *Biomedical ethics.* New York: McGraw-Hill.

Noble-Adams, R. (1999). Ethics and nursing research 1: Development, theories and principles. *British Journal of Nursing, 8*(13), 888–892.

Noble-Adams, R. (1999). Ethics and nursing research 2: Examination of the research process. *British Journal of Nursing, 8*(14), 956–960.

Northrup, C. (1981). Data collection: Human research and the law. In S. D. Kramptiz & N. Pavlovich (Eds.), *Readings for nursing research* (pp. 75–79). St. Louis, MO: Mosby.

Orb, A., Eisenhauer, L., & Wynaden, D. (2001). Profession and society: Ethics in qualitative research. *Journal of Nursing Scholarship, 33*(1), 93–96.

Polit, D. F., & Beck, C. T. (2004). *Nursing research: Principles and methods* (7th ed.). Philadelphia: Lippincott.

Ramos, M. C. (1989). Some ethical implications of qualitative research. *Research in Nursing and Health, 12*(1), 57–63.

Rankin, M., & Esteves, M. D. (1997). Perceptions of scientific misconduct in nursing. *Nursing Research, 46*(5), 270–276.

Smith, L. (1992). Ethical issues in interviewing. *Journal of Advanced Nursing, 17*, 98–103.

Steppe, H. (1992). Nursing in Nazi Germany. *Western Journal of Nursing Research, 16*(6), 744–753.

US Department of Health and Human Services. (2004). *Guidelines for conduct of research involving human subjects at the National Institutes of Health.* Retrieved November 10, 2009, from http://ohsr.od.nih.gov/guidelines/GrayBooklet82404.pdf

Veatch, R. M. (1977). *Case studies in medical ethics.* Cambridge, MA: Harvard University Press.

Veatch, R. M. (1989). Medical ethics: An introduction. In R. M. Veatch (Ed.), *Medical ethics* (pp. 1–26). Sudbury, MA: Jones and Bartlett.

Veatch, R. M. (1981). Protecting human subjects: The Federal Government steps back. *Hastings Center Report, 11*(3), 9–14.

Veatch, R. M. (2000). *Basics of bioethics.* Upper Saddle River, NJ: Prentice Hall.

Visscher, M. B. (1981). Medical research on human subjects as a moral imperative. In T. A. Mapes & J. S. Zembaty (Eds.), *Biomedical ethics* (pp. 148–150). New York: McGraw-Hill.

Planning for Analysis of Data

➤ **LEARNING OBJECTIVES**

- Understand the basic features of descriptive analysis.
- Choose appropriate ways to analyze structured and unstructured descriptive data.
- Understand the principles of inferential analysis.
- Review appropriate data analysis techniques for each of the three levels of research question.

The goal of data analysis is to provide answers to the research questions. The plan for data analysis comes directly from the question, the design, the method of data collection, and the level of measurement of the data. The choices you have made in these areas will both direct and limit what you can do to analyze your data.

The basic differentiation in plans for analysis lies between descriptive and inferential analysis. Descriptive analysis provides a description of the data from your particular sample. Therefore, your conclusions must refer only to your sample. Inferential analysis, on the other hand, provides statistical support for the answer to your research question, allowing you to draw inferences about the larger population from which your sample is drawn.

Descriptive analysis includes content analysis of unstructured data, which results in summarizing the data into categories. It also includes presenting categories of data in tables or graphs that provide a pictorial description of the sample, the use of descriptive statistics to further describe individual variables, and the use of statistical analysis for the purpose of looking for relationships among categories or variables.

Inferential analysis always involves the use of statistical tests, either to test for significant relationships among variables or to test for differences between groups in an experimental or quasi-experimental design. In either case, your purpose is to support your explanation of the relationships among your variables, or differences between groups, thus testing the conceptual or theoretical framework behind your study.

The data analysis is intended to provide the answer to your research question. Thus, it must be planned ahead along with the rest of your study. Too often, researchers stop planning after they complete their plans for data collection, thinking that the analysis can be done later. Later may bring a rude awakening when you suddenly discover that the data collected will not provide the answers needed. Then it is too late to plan the analysis. Keep in mind that you want to answer your question. Critically examine your data analysis plan with this thought in mind, and you will not become bogged down in masses of irrelevant statistics.

This chapter will present descriptive analysis, followed by a discussion of inferential analysis. Because there are many excellent references for the actual performance of statistical tests, the tests will be discussed here only as they relate to answering the research question, and then only in general terms.

Descriptive Analysis

Within descriptive analysis there is a wide range of choices for planning the analysis of the data, from simple to complex. But descriptive methods all have one thing in common—they summarize the data. Summarization ranges from the use of content analysis to organize the data into categories so that you can use descriptive statistics, such as frequency distributions and measures of central tendency. A descriptive analysis might also include looking for statistical relationships among categories or variables.

The type of analysis you choose depends on how precisely you were able to measure your variables, the level of question you asked, and the number of subjects in the sample. Very imprecise, crude measurement is apt to be nonquantifiable or quantifiable only at the nominal level. Therefore, the analysis is limited to depicting the data summary in charts or graphs. You can categorize, list, and describe your findings, giving a graphic representation of how your sample might fall in each category. Then all that is left for you to do when you have collected your data is to describe how each case was different from or similar to each other case and on what dimension.

For some studies, this analysis technique is sufficient, particularly if you are using a new or different way of categorizing and describing your variable, or if you are describing something for the first time. On the other hand, you might want to investigate which categories are most frequently associated with others, which always stand alone, and which seem to vary depending on the interaction with one or more factors. Because you are exploring relationships, all possible combinations of these relationships need to be described and given some kind of rationale. Exploratory studies require the most time-consuming and detailed analysis of data of any research. Do not be fooled by the simplicity of the design; the analysis is the hardest part of this type of study simply because you know so little about what you are studying. And, obviously, from the literature review, neither does anyone else. Therefore, it is up to you, the one who asked the question, to describe in detail everything you observed so that your study is informative and capable of being replicated.

The time and effort involved in the analysis of exploratory studies cannot be overemphasized. The simplicity and flexibility of the design lead many novice researchers to think that exploratory studies are the easiest to conduct. These people obviously have not considered the analysis of data. Take, for example, an exploratory study of stress reactions of hospitalized children. This study can be likened to a series of in-depth case studies of individuals undergoing the stress of hospitalization. Initially, the subjects are chosen for their similarity to one another; they are all children, and they are all hospitalized patients. Perhaps they even have similar diagnoses. However, as soon as you begin to observe them in depth, differences begin to emerge. The more you observe, the more differences you see. When you have finished data collection, there will be a tremendous volume of material describing a lot of different children and their reactions to a stressful situation. These data could be reported as a series of case studies in story form with no analysis on your part. But as an exploratory researcher, you are obligated to organize the data from these individual children in such a way that the similarities and trends can be examined as well as any differences. Further, when differences are described, they must be looked at in terms of other descriptive characteristics of the children so that tentative hypotheses can be formulated for further study.

In descriptive analysis, the process is very similar in all types of studies, but more precise measurement enables you to use more techniques in your analysis. The choice always depends first on your question and then on the type of measurement you plan to use.

Structured Versus Unstructured Data

When you plan your data collection procedures, you choose one of the major methods of data collection: questionnaires, interviews, physiological measures, available data, or observation. Your plan for data collection becomes more structured at each level of design, so that no matter which method you choose, the level of design influences the structure of your data. At Level I, when you are doing exploratory descriptive studies, your data are predominantly descriptive and unstructured. At Level II, when you are comparing and contrasting two or more variables, your data must be far more structured, although you might have some unstructured data as well. At Level III, the experimental or quasi-experimental design calls for highly structured data collection techniques. If any unstructured data are collected, they will not be central to the hypotheses. The degree of structure of the collected data influences the ease and rapidity of data analysis. The more structured the data, the more likely it is that there will be a statistical program that is just right to answer your question. The less structured your data, the more likely it is that you will have to spend time introducing order to the data so that they make sense. Unfortunately, no one will be willing to read all your field notes, diaries, and interviews to find out what you studied. You must condense all that unstructured material into a summarized form so that it can be communicated to others.

Content Analysis: Structuring Unstructured Data

One of the most difficult steps in data analysis is to structure unstructured data. Whether the data are a result of participant observation techniques, projective tests such as Goodenough draw-a-man, or open-ended interviews, the process is the same—to develop categories of answers and either describe those categories or make frequency tabulations of them. Structuring unstructured data takes both an extremely creative mind and an extremely analytical one. The fields of biology and anthropology have been based on this type of research. Sometimes, there is no preset structure into which to place the data; sometimes there is. When you categorize unstructured data, you are following in Darwin's footsteps. Darwin compiled an extensive collection of observations of the plants and animals he saw around the world. The categories developed from these observations formed the basis for the science of biology, provided the basic biological taxonomies used today, and represented the beginning of his theory of evolution. Collecting unstructured data still has a place in scientific circles, but knowing what to do with the data is what separates the scientific, analytical mind from the simple observer.

The process of structuring unstructured data is called content analysis. Because all unstructured data are subject to content analysis, you need to be aware of the complexity of this process when you are planning your study. If the process of content analysis does not appeal to you, then plan your data collection procedures so that you do not need to collect unstructured data. Whether your unstructured data are the result of participant observation, interviews, or available data, the process of analysis takes the same form.

The first step in the process is to look for themes in the data. What are the groupings of similar data that fall into mutually exclusive categories? The term "theme" is used to denote the fact that the data are grouped around a central theme or issue. When you are looking over your data, sometimes these themes arise naturally out of the data themselves. Other times, you must make some decisions about how to organize the content.

In a study of the way in which the media portrayed nurses during the SARS crisis in Toronto, the researchers first developed a comprehensive summary of the media portrayal of nurses during the crisis. During the first round of analysis, these materials were categorized according to their main topics. Some articles covered more than one topic, and these were included under multiple codes. Data within each category were then explored in depth, according to how the media accounts presented various aspects of the SARS crisis. The researchers identified six themes: (1) changing schemas of nursing practice: the new normal; (2) barriers to relational nursing work; (3) the process of events; (4) nursing virtue: nurses as heroes and professionals; (5) paradoxical responses to nurses from the community; and (6) leadership in nursing during the SARS crisis (Hall, et al., 2004).

These themes represent categories that are mutually exclusive, nominal scale categories. Interestingly enough, the actual categories developed from unstructured data are dependent on the point of view and personality of the researcher. Another person or group could group the data in an entirely different way. In this study, however, several researchers agreed on the themes that were selected, which gives a stronger sense of validity.

Another example of content analysis can be found in a study of personal understandings of illness among people with type 2 diabetes in which Hornsten and her colleagues interviewed persons who were diagnosed with diabetes during the previous two years. These interviews focused on the patients' experience as depicted in their stories about their experience. Content analysis of the text of the interviews began with the research team reading the text several times and discussing what they read. They then proceeded to divide the text into meaning units, or statements that related to the same central meaning, using a software program to code these units. Using the software program, the codes were then sorted into tentative categories and subcategories and then organized in relation to the course of the disease. Six categories and 16 subcategories were the outcome of this process. The main categories were labeled image of the disease, meaning of the diagnosis, integration of the illness, space for the illness, responsibility for care, and future prospects (Hornsten, Sanderstrom, & Lundman, 2004).

The last step in structuring unstructured data is to develop frequency tabulations for the categories you have developed. Frequencies indicate for each category how often that response occurred, how many subjects gave that response, and how many times each subject gave that response. Now you have completed the circle—from reams of data to a few categories. Your data can now be described in terms of how many times each response occurred. These frequencies can then be looked at in relation to the characteristics of the subjects.

One of the reasons this discussion on data reduction has been extensive is that many beginning researchers think that qualitative research is the easiest form of research, so they set out to ask open-ended questions of many people. But they don't know what to do with the reams of data they collect. To prevent you from making the same mistake, we may have provided an overly detailed description of the difficulties involved in content analysis. However, if you limit your sample size to fewer than 20 and limit the number of open-ended questions to fewer than 15, then you have a manageable first study. This type of study is exciting and fun to do if it remains of manageable size. When it becomes unmanageable, it is less likely you will finish the analysis.

Reliability and Validity in Content Analysis

The subjective nature of developing categories for the data underscores the need for reliability as the responses are placed in the categories. The definition of each category should be clearly different from those of all other categories, and the results should be mutually exclusive. The simplest measure of reliability of this process is to ensure agreement between two or more persons analyzing the same data. These persons should agree which category best describes each response. It is up to you to develop the categories and to define them, after which anyone should be able to categorize the data. To establish the reliability of the content analysis, you need to have a random sample of your data analyzed by one or more people. This procedure is a type of equivalency similar to that used in estimating the reliability of instruments.

Validity in content analysis refers to the extent to which the categories represent the theme or concept on which they are based. In studies where the categories come from a theoretical or conceptual framework, their content validity must be established. This is done by explaining where they came from, why they fit the theory or concept, and how they measure a single theme or concept. If you are classifying nurses' responses to physicians as assertive, passive, and aggressive, you must first relate the three categories to your conceptual framework and then show that they are on a continuum measuring one dimension of the theme and not three independent concepts.

Most exploratory studies do not have theoretical or conceptual frameworks. Therefore, it is not possible to establish more than face validity for the categories. This is done by developing a rationale for the categories and their definitions and by showing that they are appropriate to the data. Face validity is further supported by the ease with which the responses can be classified into the categories and the apparent relevance of the categories to the research question. Further studies using these categories add support to their validity.

Structured Data: Statistical Analysis

A major concept in statistical analysis of data is the use of a frequency distribution to predict the probability that a specific event will occur. Descriptive statistics are used to communicate the results when there is no intent to generalize beyond the study sample. Inferential statistics are intended to determine the likelihood that the results of the study could have happened by chance (Norman & Streiner, 2008).

Descriptive Statistics

The various methods of summarizing numeric data for descriptive purposes are only briefly discussed here because they can readily be found in any statistics text.

Measures of central tendency—mean, median, and mode—isolate one response that is representative of the sample. Each requires a specific level of measurement. To have a meaningful measure of central tendency, the appropriate one must be used. The mean requires interval or ratio data; the median requires ordinal data; and the mode requires nominal data.

To arrive at a mean, the scores of the sample are totaled and the sum is divided by the number of scores. The mean represents the average score of the sample. You can use the mean with physiological variables, such as blood pressure, pulse, and blood volume, or with age, income, time, and other measures.

The median is meant to be used with ordinal data, although you can certainly use it with interval and ratio data, as well. The median is simply a point on a scale where half of the scores fall above and half fall below. You can use the median with any rating scale.

When the measurement scale is nominal, the mode is the only appropriate measure of central tendency. The mode indicates the category that occurs with greatest frequency. In Table 12-1 the categories of anesthetic and no anesthetic were nominal data. The measure of central tendency from the data in that table indicates that no anesthetic is the modal category because the majority of subjects fall in that category.

Measures of variation describe how widely the individuals in the sample vary. Are your subjects quite similar to one another or is there a great diversity among them? The most often-used measures of variation are the range, the quartile range, the standard deviation, and the variance.

The range shows the highest and lowest scores in the group, or the extremes of variation. The range can be used with ordinal, interval, or ratio data. As an example, you might say, The ages of the subjects ranged

TABLE 12-1
Frequencies of Nonverbal Indicators of Stress and Use of Local Anesthetic

	Anesthetic	No Anesthetic	Total
Relaxed	47	35	82
Tense	5	21	26
Total	52	56	108

Chi-square = 11.5, d.f. = 1, p = .01

from three months to 97 years. As you can see, the range is affected by extreme cases and gives no indication of what lies between the highest and lowest scores.

The quartile range gives the middle points between which half of the subjects fall. For example, if the ages of subjects range from three months to 97 years, the quartile range might be from 45 to 60 years. That tells you that one-fourth of the sample is below 45, one-fourth is above 60, and the remaining half is between 45 and 60. Now you have a much better picture of the age range than you did before.

The standard deviation, on the other hand, is a measure of the average distance of each subject from the group mean. Like the mean, the standard deviation requires interval or ratio data. The standard deviation derives from the normal curve, so you know that approximately 75% of the sample falls within two standard deviations above or below the mean. Thus, if the mean age is 52 years and the standard deviation is four years, you know that 75% of the sample is between 44 and 60 years of age (eight years, or two standard deviations, above and below the mean age of 52).

If you have nominal data, the number of categories needed to represent a theme or concept indicates how much variation there is in the sample. If two diagnostic categories are sufficient to represent the range of diagnoses in the sample, that indicates less variation in diagnoses than if several are required.

Table 12-2 clarifies the different types of statistics used in descriptive studies and relates them to the level of measurement of the data. It will help you choose the appropriate methods of describing your data in Level I and Level II studies.

Cross-Tabulation

The old saying that a picture is worth a thousand words describes the reason for developing tables. A cross-tabulation is simply a tabular presentation of data, either in frequency or percentage form, or both, in which variables can be examined for any relationships among them. Cross-tabulations enable the researcher not only to look at the relations among variables but also to organize the data into a convenient form for statistical analysis.

The variables used to cross-tabulate the data are either the categories resulting from content analysis or the variables found in the purpose of the study. Although cross-tabulations are used mainly with nominal data, they can also be used as a first step in more complex analysis.

Imagine a descriptive study of stress in which the purpose is to describe patients' reactions to stress while in the dental chair. Data will be collected by observing nonverbal behavior and by measuring blood pressure, pulse, and palmar sweat volume. Data will be compiled on the procedures and instruments used by the dentist, the length of the procedures, and demographic variables from the patients. In this descriptive study, you know in advance what you will observe, how, and what instruments you will use to collect data. Most of the data will be in numeric form. In developing a plan to analyze the data from this study, you would start by cross-tabulating the variables.

The simplest cross-tabulation is a 2×2 table. In the dental patient study, look at nonverbal behavior (relaxed or tense) according to whether or not the dentist used an anesthetic (see Table 12-1).

In this example, the categories are set up using variables found in the purpose of the study. In another study, they could just as easily be the categories that result from content analysis. The categories used in cross-tabulation must meet the same criteria as those developed in content analysis; they must be independent, mutually exclusive, and constructed so that there is a category for all observations. (In Table 12-1 there is no category for general anesthetic, so it is possible that it does not meet all the criteria.)

TABLE 12-2
Selecting the Appropriate Descriptive Statistic

Type of Statistic	Level of Measurement	Statistic
Measures of central tendency	Nominal scale	Mode
	Ordinal scale	Median
	Interval/ratio scale	Mean
Measures of variation	Nominal sale	Number of categories
	Ordinal scale	Range
	Interval/ratio scale	Standard deviation
Tests of relationships	Nominal data	Chi-square (X^2)
	Ordinal data	Spearman rank
	Interval/ratio data	Pearson r

Cross-tabulations can be used to describe three or four variables, each one of which has multiple categories. Theoretically, it is possible to cross-tabulate any number of variables, but when more than three are used, the table becomes confusing to read and loses its major value, simplification of the data.

Table 12-3 illustrates the cross-tabulation of three variables. In this case, increase in apical pulse is used as a measure of patient stress during dental work and is examined in relation to the age and gender of the patients.

It is now possible to compare males and females in each of the age groups on apical pulse increase. This can be done for any number of sets of variables you wish to examine. Statistical analyses of data, including descriptive statistics, are usually carried out on a data analysis software program.

If cross-tabulation is appropriate to your study, it must be planned in advance. As pointed out in the discussion on sample size, the number of variables you plan to cross-tabulate can affect your sample size. Therefore, it is wise to plot out your tables ahead of time. Make up some fictitious data while you are planning your tables. This will give you a good idea of what your results will look like so you can be sure that you will be able to answer the research question.

Parametric and Nonparametric Statistical Tests

Every statistical test is based on certain assumptions that set out the conditions under which the test is valid. The line between parametric and nonparametric statistics is somewhat fluid. Parametric tests generally are based on strong assumptions about the population from which the observations (measurements of the variable) were drawn. If the population meets these assumptions, the parametric test is very powerful and,

TABLE 12-3
Relationships among Age, Sex, and Average Increase in Apical Pulse during Dental Work

	Males			Females		
	20–30	31–40	41–50	20–30	31–40	41–50
Apical pulse increase						
> 10/min.	25	60	10	30	40	25
< 10/min.	75	40	90	70	60	75

hence, the most likely to reject a null hypothesis when it is, in fact, false. Nonparametric tests are based on fewer assumptions and are less powerful. They can be used to analyze data from populations about which very little is known. Because the nonparametric test is less powerful, it is sometimes safer to use with data from unknown populations because the risk of error will be smaller. This is particularly true when the sample size is small.

The parametric test can be used if the population meets the following assumptions:

- Known distribution: The distribution of the variable in the population is known. For many tests, the variable must be normally distributed in the population. The sample must be randomly selected so its distribution is the same as that for the population.
- Equal variances: When two or more groups are being compared on a particular variable, variances of scores are assumed to be the same among the groups. In other words, the variances are homogeneous from group to group.
- Equal intervals: Because of the arithmetic operations used in computing parametric tests, the variables are usually measured on an interval or ratio scale. Ordinal scales are also acceptable under certain conditions.

Since the 1940s, researchers have insisted that measurements using parametric tests must be used with interval or ratio scale data. However, use of these tests with ordinal scales has not made a significant difference to the results of data analysis (that is, it has not increased the likelihood of a Type II error) and so it is now considered quite acceptable to use parametric statistics for ordinal data as well (Cohen, 2001). However, caution should be exercised in the case of ordinal data collected from a small sample (less than 30). Here, nonparametric statistical tests should be used. In this text, we continue to discuss the equivalent nonparametric test whenever appropriate so that in the event you are working with ordinal data but a small sample, you will know which test to choose.

Nonparametric tests do not specify conditions about the parameters of the population from which the sample was drawn. They are sometimes said to be distribution free and thus can be used when you do not know the distribution of the population. Also, there are nonparametric tests for use with nominal data. In behavioral research, we frequently measure variables on nominal scales. Therefore, nonparametric tests assume a prominent role in data analysis.

Looking for Relationships

In descriptive studies, the plan is to describe the variables and also to look for significant relationships among them. For example, you may wish to know if patients' ethnic backgrounds are related to their responses to group therapy. Or you may wonder if education and income level are associated with career choice in high-school students. You may have a long list of demographic variables and want to know if any one or a combination of these variables is related to a student's success in nursing school.

There are several statistical methods of showing the relationships between variables, and some of the more commonly used ones will be discussed. Remember, however, that in descriptive studies, no attempt is made to draw conclusions about causal relationships from the data. Rather, hypotheses are formulated from statistically significant relationships, and these relationships are later tested in more controlled studies from which causal relationships might be developed.

Chi-square analysis is designed for analyzing categories of nominal data that have been set up in cross-tabulation form. The chi-square test is based on the assumption that if there is no relationship between two or more variables, then the likelihood of the individuals in your sample falling into the various categories of each variable is a chance occurrence. For example, in Table 12-1, if there is no relationship between stress (as measured by relaxed or tense) and use of local anesthetic, then the 52 subjects who received local anesthetic should have an equal chance of falling into either category of stress; this chance would be the same for the no anesthetic group. The chi-square test picks up the significance of any true departures from the frequencies that would be expected by chance alone. When you find significantly more subjects in one category than would be expected by chance alone, you can interpret this finding as an association between the two variables being tested.

In Table 12-1, a chi-square analysis was done using the method described by Siegel and Castellan (1988). The results indicate that there is a significant relationship between local anesthetic and nonverbal indicators of stress. The probability of the sample falling into the categories of relaxed and tense, as they would simply by chance alone, was less than 0.05 (the actual probability was 0.01). Therefore, the results are considered to be statistically significant.

If your data consist of pairs of numbers (that is, two variables have been measured for each subject in your sample), then a measure of correlation can be used to tell if these variables are related to each other. For example, you might be planning to measure IQ and attitude toward women's rights, blood pressure and temperature, or self-image and body weight. A correlational test will tell you whether these pairs of variables have a tendency to vary together. Does blood pressure increase (or decrease) as the body temperature goes up? Is a negative self-image related to being overweight, and, therefore, does self-image go down as weight goes up? If the direction of the relationship is positive (both variables increase or decrease together), the numeric value of the correlation will be positive (somewhere between 0 and $+/-1$). If the direction of the relationship is negative (as one variable increases, the other decreases), the correlation will be negative (somewhere between 0 and -1). The strength of the relationship between the two variables is greater as the correlation approaches $+/-1$, so that a correlation of 0.9 is much stronger than a correlation of 0.3.

All measures of correlation require at least ordinal data. If you plan to have nominal data for one or both of your variables, use a chi-square analysis instead. Ordinal measurements require at least a three-point scale to qualify as an ordinal scale for statistical testing. A scale that measures old–young or pass–fail, therefore, must be used as a nominal scale even though it has some degree of quality or quantity to its measurement.

If your variables are measured on ordinal, interval, or ratio scales, you will be able to test for correlation between your variables. The usual parametric test of correlation is the Pearson product moment correlation (r). The correlation coefficient (r) obtained with this test tells us the extent and type of relationship that exists between two variables (that is, somewhere between $+1$ and -1, and either positive or negative). When you have obtained the correlation coefficient, a further test can demonstrate whether or not the coefficient you obtained is significantly different from what you would find from chance alone. If you use a statistical computer program, the level of statistical significance will be given to you automatically. If not, you will find tables in most statistics books in which you can look up the "Critical Values of the Correlation Coefficient." A rule of thumb to keep in mind to clarify the meaning of correlation coefficients is that the coefficient squared (r^2) is a measure of the shared variance between your two variables. Thus if $r = 0.5$, $r^2 = 0.25$. You can interpret that to mean that one of your variables accounts for 25% of the variance of the other. This is a considerable amount but still leaves 75% variance unaccounted for. This illustration demonstrates why relationships between variables, even when statistically significant, do not support cause and effect. There are still other factors influencing these variables that are not part of your study.

If you wanted to do a nonparametric test of correlation, the Spearman rho or the Kendall tau would give you a correlation coefficient similar to that of Pearson r. If you are hand calculating your own statistics, you will find Spearman's rho easy to do by hand. Kendall's tau, on the other hand, is available as an integral part of an SPSS software program.

Inferential Analysis

In Level III studies, it is not enough to describe the data. You are expected to draw conclusions from those data. Statistical inference, based on probability theory, is the process of generalizing from samples to whole populations. The tools of statistics help identify valid generalizations and those that are likely to stand up under further study.

Statistical techniques are designed to objectively evaluate the outcome of a study and help the researcher to decide whether or not the results occurred by chance. Probability theory is the basis for this evaluation. Look at the following example:

> Each research subject is seated in a room with two doors, one blue and one yellow. For ten minutes, loud music is played over the intercom. Then a voice tells the subject to leave the room. The researcher notes which door each subject chooses. When this experiment was done with ten subjects, seven subjects chose the blue door. The researcher concluded that loud music causes people to choose a blue door over a yellow one.

Is this a valid generalization? Of course not. The fact is that those results could be purely chance happenings.

Now consider another experiment in which a drug was injected into ten healthy subjects. Within five minutes, seven subjects were vomiting and the other three apparently were fine. The researcher concluded that the drug causes vomiting. Recalling the previous experiment with the blue and yellow doors, would you argue that the results of this experiment could also easily have occurred by chance? Let's examine the probabilities.

In the first experiment, each person had a 50–50 chance of choosing the blue door, without the music being a factor in the choice. Seven out of ten is not enough to show a relationship between music and the color of the door when five of the ten are expected to choose either door by chance. In the drug experiment, however, the chance that seven out of ten persons would have started to vomit without exposure to the drug is extremely slim.

Therefore, seven out of ten in this case may be conclusive evidence that the vomiting was caused by the drug. The results of these two experiments must be measured against different probabilities. Statistical analysis provides the means of eliminating most of the subjectivity that goes into the researcher's conclusions, thus separating science from opinion. This is done by using statistical models against which the results of research can be compared.

Because statistical procedures dictate some of the conditions for collecting the evidence, they must be part of the research plan. If planning data analysis is left until after the data are collected, often the optimal statistical technique cannot be used because some necessary condition of data collection was overlooked.

The basic steps in planning data analysis are summarized in Table 12-4.

Testing Hypotheses

The overall aim of experimental or quasi-experimental research is to determine the acceptability of hypotheses. The outcome of the study may be to accept or reject the hypothesis and the theory from which it was derived. To reach an objective conclusion, there must be an objective

---

TABLE 12-4
Basic Steps in Planning Data Analysis

Level I

Step 1: Content analysis of unstructured data.

Step 2: Descriptive summaries of data categories.

Step 3: Placing the data in charts, graphs, and tables.

Step 4: Tests of association between sample characteristics and data categories.

Level II

Step 1: Placing the data in charts, graphs, and tables.

Step 2: Correlational analysis of relationship among the variables.

Level III

Step 1: Placing data into charts, graphs, and tables.

Step 2: Analysis of the differences among the groups on the dependent variable.

procedure for either rejecting or accepting that hypothesis. This procedure is based on the data to be collected and on the amount of risk the researcher is willing to take that the decision to accept or reject the hypothesis will not be correct.

The Null Hypothesis

The first step in planning a decision-making statistical procedure is to state the null hypothesis. Null hypotheses usually state the opposite of what you expect to find, which means stating that there will be no relationship between the variables. The reason for using null hypotheses is that statistical tests are designed to reject rather than accept hypotheses. In this sense, rejection is an action word, whereas acceptance is a passive one. Active rejection of the null hypothesis is as close as you can come to proving your hypothesis. You never actively reject your research hypothesis because it is never directly tested; only the null hypothesis is directly tested. Your goal in statistical analysis is to reject the null hypothesis, thus giving support to your research hypothesis as the alternative. Failure to reject the null hypothesis means only that you failed to support your research hypothesis in this particular study, leaving the door open for you to test it again under other circumstances.

If your hypothesis states, During dental procedures, those patients given a local anesthetic will exhibit less stress than those not given a local anesthetic, the null hypothesis would be written as: There will be no difference between the stress exhibited by patients receiving local anesthetic and the stress exhibited by patients not receiving local anesthetic during dental procedures. There are two possible alternatives to this null hypothesis:

- Patients given a local anesthetic will exhibit more stress than those not given a local anesthetic.
- Patients given a local anesthetic will exhibit less stress than those not given a local anesthetic.

Because this latter alternative is the one predicted by your research hypothesis, you will apply a one-tailed test, which will reject the null hypothesis only if there is less stress among the local anesthetic group.

Two types of error can be made when testing the null hypothesis. The first, called Type I error, is to reject the null hypothesis when it is actually true. The level of significance that you select for your statistical analysis is the probability that Type I error may occur. If the level of significance is 0.05, the researcher runs the risk that five times out of a hundred the null hypothesis may be rejected when it is actually true. You always determine the level of significance in advance so that the decision to reject or accept the null hypothesis remains objective.

The second type of error (Type II) is to accept the null hypothesis when it is actually false and should have been rejected. The probability of committing a Type II error can be decreased by increasing the sample size (which is another reason for having as large a sample as possible).

Choosing a Statistical Test: What Does Your Hypothesis Ask?

Although the field of statistical analysis is quite complex, you can use some simple guidelines to help you choose the appropriate technique. The best indication of what general technique to use can be found in your own hypothesis. Look at what it says. Are you looking for a significant difference between two groups or among several groups? Are you interested in significant correlations between (or among) variables? Or are you trying to estimate what the population is like from findings in your sample? The technique you choose will depend on which of these questions your hypothesis is asking. Let's look at each one individually.

Difference Between Two Groups

In some studies the subjects are randomly assigned to two groups, one of which is subjected to an experimental independent variable. In other studies, the sample is selected from two populations—for example, two ethnic groups or two educational groups. Both types of studies are interested in the same kind of data analysis. They ask, Is there a difference between the two groups?

The t-test is the classic technique for analyzing the differences between the means of two groups. It is a powerful parametric test, and thus, the data must meet the following four assumptions:

- The dependent variable is normally distributed in the population.
- There are equal variances between the two groups (that is, they represent a single population).
- You are using interval data.
- The two groups are independent (that is, a single subject will not be in more than one group).

If your data do not meet these assumptions, a nonparametric test such as the Fisher exact probability test or the Mann-Whitney U test can be used to test for a significant difference between the two groups.

Sometimes you have two sets of scores from the same group, such as before-and-after measurements of some variable. In this case, you are looking for a change in scores from one measurement time to another, and you want to know if the change is statistically significant. Often a difference score will be obtained for each subject by subtracting one measurement from the other. The t-test can be used to test for the significance of the difference if the assumptions are met. When the t-test cannot be used, nonparametric tests for ordinal data include the Sign test and the Wilcoxon signed rank test. The McNemar change test can be used with nominal data. These tests are all designed to analyze the significance of the difference in two sets of scores from the same group of subjects.

Difference Among Multiple Groups

In reality, there are few studies that compare only two groups. A study is more likely to involve several groups, particularly if it is an experimental or quasi-experimental design. Your study may be comparing several groups on a particular measure and determining whether the groups vary from one another in the way they score on that measure. For example, you might include four groups receiving different patient teaching strategies and compare their postoperative anxiety levels. This could be tested using several t-tests, but running multiple tests increases the possibility of a Type I error. To avoid this possibility, you can examine the differences among the groups through an analysis that looks at variation across all groups at once. This test is the analysis of variance (ANOVA). The resulting F-test indicates whether any of the groups are significantly different from the others. It does not, however, tell us which of the groups being compared is different from the others. For that, further analysis is required, and several tests are available to clarify the source of the difference, for example, the Tukey test for multiple comparisons or the Scheffé test. ANOVA can be used for groups numbering from two upward (for two groups it will provide the same results as a t-test). The ANOVA tests whether group means differ from one another. It requires that the independent variable be at the nominal level and the dependent variable be interval or ratio level. The null hypothesis assumes that all groups are equal, that is, drawn from the same population.

The usual assumptions for parametric tests are required for analysis of variance. If these do not hold, there are several nonparametric tests from which to choose. For nominal data, the chi-square test can be used with multiple groups. Table 12-5 gives an example of what the chi-square table might look like. The chi-square test tells you whether certain ethnic

TABLE 12-5
Frequency of Selecting a Private Physician, Government System, or Health
Maintenance Organization by Subjects from Five Ethnic Groups

Healthcare System	Caucasian	Asian	Black	Native American	Hispanic	Total
Private physician	14	12	10	2	6	44
Government system	1	2	11	25	4	43
Health maintenance organization	3	14	20	20	1	58
Total	18	28	41	47	11	145

groups choose any of the healthcare systems more often than would be expected by chance alone.

If the data are on ordinal scales, and you have small groups (15 subjects per group), the Kruskal-Wallis one-way analysis of variance by ranks can be used. This technique tests the null hypothesis that the groups come from the same population or from identical populations with respect to the variable being measured. It is the most powerful of the nonparametric tests for independent groups.

Correlation Between Variables

In Level II studies, the purpose is usually to find out if a significant relationship exists between two or more variables. The Pearson product moment correlation coefficient (r) is used when two or more variables have been measured on each subject and the goal is to test for a significant relationship among them. For example, in a study of obesity, you might be interested in the relationship between body mass index (BMI) and amount of daily exercise in your subjects. It is possible to use any level of data when calculating r. Even nominal data can be coded for use with r. Meeting the assumptions of the test, however, will ensure that the results can be generalized beyond the sample, which, after all, is the main purpose of a survey design.

The assumptions are first that the sample is representative of the population from which it was selected. Next, the variables (e.g., BMI and amount of exercise) must each have a normal distribution, and their scores must have equal variability. Thus, for every possible BMI score, the distribution of exercise scores must have approximately equal variability. Lastly, the relationship between the variables must be linear so that when they are entered into a graph they would tend to form a line, rather than a clump or a curve.

The results of the Pearson r will provide you with indicators of the direction (plus or minus) and the strength of the relationship between the two variables, along with a measure of the exact probability of this r correlation occurring by chance. The significance of a correlation coefficient increases dramatically with the sample size, so that in a very large sample, a small correlation may well be statistically significant. The correlation itself may not be meaningful because it may not explain much of the variance in the two variables. To counteract this possibility, the coefficient of determination (r^2) is calculated to provide a measure of the meaningfulness of r because it approximates the shared variance between the two variables. If the correlation between BMI and exercise were 0.7, for example, r^2 would be 0.49, and we could say that exercise accounts for half of the variance in BMI. The other half would presumably be explained by many other factors, such as genetics, age, or diet, making the relationship between BMI and exercise a powerful one.

In addition to testing the relationship between two variables, one independent and one dependent, correlation can be extended to measure the relationship between one dependent variable and several independent variables, simultaneously. In multiple correlation, the statistic R can range from 0 to 1, and R^2 represents the amount of variance accounted for in the dependent variable by all the independent variables together. These tests of correlation are among the most commonly used techniques for the analysis of data in nursing research. With ordinal data and small samples, the nonparametric test called Spearman rho will provide a good test of correlation, and chi-square is often used for nominal data to establish whether or not the observations could have occurred by chance.

Estimation of Population Parameters from Sample Data

Your hypothesis may predict a population parameter (such as the mean or variance) from the sample statistic. For example, you might plan to use the mean IQ from a sample of registered nurses to predict the IQ of the whole population of registered nurses. An ideal estimator provides an unbiased estimate of the unknown population parameter. As such, it will correspond closely to the population value when a large number of sample estimates are averaged.

All the descriptive statistics discussed in the previous section are examples of sample statistics that can be used to predict population parameters (such as means, medians, and standard deviations). An individual estimate obtained from one sample, however, will not necessarily be an accurate estimate of the population parameter. It usually is necessary to take the average mean from a large number of samples to get an accurate estimate of the population mean. Because you will not generally use a large number of samples, you must establish the accuracy with which your sample statistic predicts the population parameter. This is done by the use of a confidence interval.

A confidence interval gives you a range of values within which the true value of the population parameter is estimated to fall. You decide in advance how confident you would like to be in your estimate (say, 95% or 99%). Then, instead of saying that the population mean is 80, you will say that you estimate the population mean to be somewhere between 75 and 83 and that you are 99% certain your estimate is correct. The range between 75 and 83 is your confidence interval.

Confidence intervals for the mean and standard deviation can be obtained using the versatile t-test, provided that the observations come from a normally distributed population with equal variances and are measured on an interval scale. Nonparametric tests for establishing confidence intervals include Tukey's confidence interval for the median and the binomial test for the confidence intervals of quartiles.

Be Sure You Can Answer Your Question

The brief discussion of statistical analysis presented here has been for the sole purpose of guiding you to plan a simple analysis for a simple question. The major criterion for analysis technique is that the results provide the answer to the question. It follows from this that you must understand the technique. If you choose a technique that is beyond your understanding, it will be difficult to interpret the results of your study. It is better to be simple and sure than complex and incomprehensible.

The Answer Is in the Question

The plan for data analysis is intended to provide support for one answer to your research question. As we have emphasized throughout this book, the type of answer you require depends on how you asked the question. Look again at the table in the front of the book that outlines the three levels of studies. Now is the time to review your plan to make sure that it logically follows one of the three levels and that the answer you have planned will be the answer to your original question. If your plan is consistent and logical, the data analysis plan will help you distinguish the best answer among possible alternatives. So look now at your stem question because it specifies the answer you need.

Level I Questions

As you have seen, Level I questions lead to exploratory descriptive research designs that, in turn, dictate primarily unstructured data obtained from small convenience samples. The quality of the answer you obtain depends on how successfully you have mastered the steps in data analysis.

You will have masses of data, both structured and unstructured, and your primary task will be to order those data into some form that can be described, tabulated, and perhaps even subjected to tests of association. Therefore, unlike the other two levels of research, Level I studies have at least two (and sometimes three) steps to the process of data analysis.

The two basic steps in the analysis of data at Level I are those of content analysis and frequency tabulations. You must make some sense out of the data and subject them to categorization of some sort. These categories usually will be scaled on a nominal scale, although occasionally an ordinal scale might be developed. As you develop the categories, you must define them carefully so that you know they are mutually exclusive.

After development of the categories, your content analysis will not be complete until you have verbally described what you found. This is called a descriptive summary of the data. You may want to go on to the next step and develop charts and graphs that further describe what you found. These charts usually include a summary of the characteristics of your sample as well as frequency tabulations based on your categories. These visual pictures of your results can help clarify your description of the data. These charts and graphs can include descriptive statistics so that the reader will have an even better idea of the sample characteristics (such as mean age and education level). To do this, you must have collected some structured demographic data on your sample, so be sure to plan for this information even if the rest of your data are unstructured.

When you have completed these two steps, structured your data into categories, and compiled frequencies and descriptive statistics, you may attempt to do some tests of association if you feel this will enhance the answer to your question. (See Table 12-2 for the appropriate test of association for your level of data.)

Level II Questions

Questions at Level II ask about the relationship between (or among) variables and lead to descriptive survey designs and to structured or quantitative data. Answers at Level II require statistical analysis to determine the significance of the relationship between the variables.

The first step in the analysis of Level II data involves placing the results into tables, charts, and graphs. It is the same process as the second step of the analysis of unstructured data. At Level II, you always present a cross-tabulation of your variables, which would look somewhat like the following chart for the relationship between anxiety and pulse rate in preoperative patients.

In this cross-tabulation, you need only fill in the number of patients who were highly anxious and had a high pulse rate and those with low anxiety and a high pulse rate. Then fill in those with high anxiety and a low pulse rate and those with low anxiety and a low pulse rate. Now you have a complete picture of the relationship between these two variables. A test of association will tell you if the relationship is significant. The tests of correlation in Level II studies involve both parametric and nonparametric tests, depending on the level of measurement of the variables.

At Level II, you have two steps in the data analysis. The first is to put the data into tables for descriptive statistics; the second is to test for the significance of the relationships.

Level III Questions

At Level III, your original why question leads to an experimental or quasi-experimental design for which you have developed hypotheses. Data analysis at Level III focuses on testing the hypotheses.

An experimental design provides at least two groups of subjects, and the hypotheses predict how these groups will respond in the experimental situation. The data analysis must test for the difference between (or among) groups. No matter what the original question asked, the analysis at this level will always examine the difference between or among groups, and this difference will relate only to the dependent variable. The independent variable has been manipulated by you, in that you have applied it, in its various forms, to the experimental and control groups. You have controlled extraneous variables through sample selection. Now you are ready to test your hypothesis: are the measurements of the dependent variable significantly different between the groups in the design?

The type of statistical test you will choose at Level III, as at Level II, depends on the level of measurement of the dependent variable and whether or not you can assume a normal distribution from your sample. These factors affect your choice of a parametric or nonparametric test. Table 12-6 will help you to select the best technique for data analysis.

TABLE 12-6
Selecting the Appropriate Test for Statistical Analysis

Parametric tests	Nonparametric tests
Assumptions: The distribution of the variable in the population is known.	Assumptions: Thought to be "distribution-free." Parameters of the population are unknown.
Variables are measured on either interval or ratio scales.	Used with nominal and ordinal data, as well as with interval scales.

Difference between Two Groups

t test	Fisher exact test (small groups) (nominal data)
	Mann-Whitney *U* test (ordinal data)

Two Sets of Scores for the Same Group (Before and After)

t test	McNemar Chi-square test for nominal data
	Sign test or Wilcoxon test for ordinal data

Differences among Multiple Groups

One-way analysis of variance (*F* test)	Chi-square test for nominal data
	Kruskall-Wallis one-way analysis of variance for ordinal data

Correlations between Variables

Pearson *r*	Chi-square test (nominal data)
	Spearman rank correlation (ordinal data)

Bibliography

Abdellah, F. G., Levine, E., & Koop, C. E. (1994). *Preparing nursing research for the 21st century: Evolution, methodologies, challenges.* New York: Springer.

Abraham, I. L., Nadzam, D. M., & Fitzpatrick, J. J. (1989). *Statistics and quantitative methods in nursing: Issues and strategies for research and education.* Philadelphia: W. B. Saunders.

Brandt, P. A., Kirsch, S. D., Lewis, F. M., & Casey, S. M. (2004). Assessing the strength and integrity of an intervention. *Oncology Nursing Forum, 31*(4), 833–837.

Clarke, L. (1995). Nursing research: Science, visions and telling stories. *Journal of Advanced Nursing, 21*, 584–593.

Cohen, M. E. (2001). Consive review: Analysis of ordinal dental data: Evaluation of conflicting recommendations. *Journal of Dental Research, 80*(1), 309–313.

Colling, J. (2004). Demystifying nursing research. Coding, analysis, and dissemination of study results. *Urologic Nursing, 24*(3), 215–216.

DeVon, H. A., Block, M. E., Moyle-Wright, P., Ernst, D. M., Hayden, S. J., Lazzara, D. J., et al. (2007). A psychometric toolbox for testing reliability and validity. *Journal of Nursing Scholarship, 39*(2), 155–164.

Eaton, N. (1997). Parametric data analysis. *Nurse Researcher, 4*(4), 17–27.

Fink, A. (1995). *How to analyze survey data.* Thousand Oaks, CA: Sage.

Hall, L. M., Angus, J., Peter, E., O'Brien-Pallas, L., Wynn, F., & Donner, G. (2004). Media portrayal of nurses' perspectives and concerns in the SARS crisis in Toronto. *Journal of Nursing Scholarship, 35*(3), 211–216.

Hornsten, A., Sanderstrom, R., & Lundman, B. (2004). Personal understandings of illness among people with type 2 diabetes. *Journal of Advanced Nursing, 47*(2), 172–182.

Krippendorf, K. (1980). *Content analysis: An introduction to its methodology.* Beverly Hills, CA: Sage.

Lehmkuhl, L. D. (1996). Research forum. Nonparametric statistics: Methods for analyzing data not meeting assumptions required for the application of parametric tests. *Journal of Prosthetics and Orthotics, 8*(3), 105–113.

Lewthwaite, B., & Klassen, F. (1997). The cycle of life: An experience with qualitative data analysis. *The Canadian Nurse*, 24–26.

Martin, C. R., & Thompson, D. R. (2000). *Design and analysis of clinical nursing research studies.* New York: Routledge.

Miles, M. B., & Huberman, A. M. (1994). *Qualitative data analysis: An expanded sourcebook.* Beverly Hills, CA: Sage.

Munro, B. H. (1997). *Statistical methods for health care research* (3rd ed.). Philadelphia: Lippincott.

Norman, G. R., & Streiner, D. L. (2008). *Biostatistics: The bare essentials* (3rd ed.). Whitby, Ontario, Canada: PMPH-USA.

Notter, L., & Hott, J. R. (1994). *Essentials of nursing research* (2nd ed.). New York: Springer.

Oliver, D., & Mahon, S. M. (2005). Evidence-based practice. Reading a research article part II: Parametric and nonparametric statistics. *Clinical Journal of Oncology Nursing, 9*(2), 238–240.

Pagano, R. R. (1998). *Understanding statistics in the behavioral sciences.* Pacific Grove, CA: Brooks/Cole.

Polit, D. F., & Beck, C. T. (2004). *Nursing research: Principles and methods* (7th ed.). Philadelphia: Lippincott.

Reid, B. (1983). Potential sources of type I error and possible solutions to avoid a "galloping" alpha rate. *Nursing Research, 32*(3), 190–191.

Rempusheski, V. F. (1991). Research data management: Piles into files—locked and secured. *Applied Nursing Research, 4*(3), 147–149.

Siegel, S., & Castellan, N. J. (1988). *Nonparametric statistics for the behavioral sciences* (2nd ed.). New York: McGraw-Hill.

Sweeney, M. A., & Olivieri, P. (1981). *An introduction to nursing research: Research, measurement, and computers in nursing.* Philadelphia: Lippincott.

Vojir, C. P., & Hudson-Barr, D. (2005). Scientific inquiry: Hypothesis testing and power in research. *Journal for Specialists in Pediatric Nursing, 10*(1), 36–39.

Waltz, C. J., & Bausell, R. B. (1981). *Nursing research: Design, statistics, and computer analysis.* Philadelphia: F. A. Davis.

Watson, H., & McFadyen, A. (1997). Nonparametric data analysis. *Nurse Researcher, 4*(4), 28–40.

Writing the Research Proposal

➤ **TOPICS**

➤ **LEARNING OBJECTIVES**

- Review the structure of a research proposal.
- Describe the essence of the introductory section.
- Understand the relationship of the research problem to the rest of the proposal.
- Review the format of the research design, sample, and methods sections.
- Integrate the discussion of reliability, validity, and data analysis into the proposal.
- Review the ethical considerations in a research proposal.

From the beginning of this book, you have read over and over again that the research plan is the most critical phase of the research process because it forms the basis for the rest of the process. As you know, it is easier to change a plan before you have started than it is to change an almost finished product based on a faulty plan.

Now that all the parts of the research plan have been considered, all that is left is to write a final proposal. All research requires a written proposal before it is undertaken. Every part of research, from the beginning question to the final report, needs to be written down. Therefore, a research plan that is not written into a proposal is not complete.

You may be asking how we differentiate research plan from research proposal at this late date. In our opinion, the difference between the two is as great as that between your initial working definitions and your final operational definitions. The research plan is the basic outline of your entire research idea, with your references, your working definitions, and so on. Your research proposal is the essay that fills in all the gaps of the outline, makes all the logical transitions for the reader, and shows the consistent development of the idea from question to answer.

The art of writing the proposal in such a way that someone else can follow your train of thought requires serious consideration. You don't want your project to be lost at this stage simply because you were inarticulate. This final step is worth the effort.

Every research proposal has a slightly different character, as you will notice when you look over those in the Appendixes. The reason is rather basic—a research proposal reflects the personality of the writer. Although the basic parts of a proposal are identical and include every major point in this book, the way that you write each aspect of the proposal is a reflection of you.

There are two major parts of any research plan, whether you write it for yourself, for a class, or for a grant proposal: the introductory matter and the research design. Both parts are always present, though the titles may differ. Each part has its particular components, though they too may have different terms. Both the structure and the components within the structure are derived from the research question.

Chapters 1, 2, and 3 described the process of converting the topic of your research question into the problem of the research proposal. Because the research question is the basis for your research plan, and because the problem is the foundation of the rest of the research proposal, the emphasis on these two areas was quite deliberate.

Your research question is your guide to the entire process, including what you have to do and think and read and plan to arrive at your research proposal. Your question is an activity guide; your proposal is the end product. Put another way, your question is the process; your proposal is the content.

The process of developing a research proposal is similar to using the nursing process to develop a nursing care plan for a patient. You begin the nursing process with a question such as, What care will this patient need? You begin by gathering information from the patient, the patient's chart, and available resources on the pathology and medical interventions and by looking up medications and treatments with which you are not familiar. You then put these data together, analyze them, and arrive at your final formulation of the patient's problems and needs. The culmination of all your questioning, reading, and analysis is written in a final form called the nursing care plan. You didn't write down your entire step-by-step process; you wrote only the end result.

The same process is used for the research proposal. The question guides and directs your activities; the proposal is your end result.

The basic structure and the components of the research plan are fairly standardized across many disciplines, and each component is based on the previous ones, thus we will discuss each of the basic components in turn. In addition, the concepts of reliability and validity of the research and the protection of human rights for the people involved also will be discussed even though their placement in the proposal is not standardized. Omitting them from the proposal would seriously jeopardize your chances of eventually doing your project.

The Introductory Section: Research Problem

The introductory section is the place where you introduce your readers to the research you are proposing to do. It is often titled "The Research Problem," but it can also be something like "The Problem," "Introduction," "Rationale," "Conceptual (or "Theoretical") Framework," or even "What This Study Is All About." Whatever the title, the purpose of the first section is to introduce the reader to the subject matter of the research. This part of the proposal should always include the problem, the purpose (or hypotheses), and definitions of terms. The order may vary, but not the content. We recommend that you use no title at all. The title of the proposal serves as the title for the introductory matter and is placed at the head of the first page of the proposal. Following the proposal title is an essay about the topic, the format of which is discussed in the next section.

When choosing a title for your project, try to be brief and to the point. In nursing research, there is a tendency to write what we call "colon-ized titles" or titles with colons. There is no good reason for this practice. A thoughtful researcher can write a straightforward title for a research project that is brief and informative. Novice researchers tend to put everything into a title, which may take up half a page. You can see many examples of colonized titles in the bibliography at the end of each chapter. Many of these titles could be a single, brief, descriptive title had the researcher taken a little time and effort. Remember, you can usually follow the title with an abstract if you want your reader to know more about your research at the beginning.

Form of the Final Research Problem

The first portion of any proposal introduces the subject matter of the research, the rationale for selecting the problem, the literature to substantiate the rationale, and the direction the study will take. As you have seen, the problem is derived from the topic of the research question. If you have thought through your problem well, the theory and the literature will substantiate your choice of topic. You don't need to be repetitive to get your point across. You can, however, subhead your problem according to the different theories or concepts that relate to your subject. This is often done, particularly when more than one theory is used to form a theoretical framework, but a well-written problem can introduce the entire research plan under one heading.

Whether you end up with one page or 26, the form and shape of the full and final research problem will be the same. Like an essay, article, or term paper, the research problem has an introduction, a middle part, and a conclusion. In fact, your final problem has the same requirements as a good essay: you introduce your question, you point out the pros and cons for your argument, and you end with the statement of what you are going to study and why. The rest of the research plan is an expansion of the problem and focuses on the activities you will carry out to find the answer to your question.

Your research plan is only as good as your research problem. If you have a strong method but a weak problem, you will have a weak piece of research. Although the reverse is just as true, it's easier to salvage a weak method than a weak problem. There is nothing worse than using a sophisticated method to answer a trifling question. If anyone reads it, few will use it, and all your work is wasted. And because usability is a keynote for nursing research, you don't want your efforts to be considered irrelevant. So, for now, concentrate on writing the best possible problem. Not only will you have a sense of satisfaction, but your credibility will increase enormously.

The Introduction

Regardless of the length of your problem, you need to introduce your topic to the reader. This should occur at the very beginning of your proposal. All introductions follow the same pattern and include the same kinds of information. Your introduction does not need to be any longer than one paragraph—and a short one at that—but if it isn't there, it's like trying to read a road map before you know where you are going. The introduction is the preparation for the rest of your discussion.

Introductions are exactly what you think they are; they introduce the subject under discussion. The first sentence in the introduction sets the general tone and direction for the subject matter. The middle sentence (or sentences) narrows the focus. The last sentence begins with such words as "Therefore" or "Finally."

We recommend that you use your original question as the first sentence of your introduction. This immediately sets the tone for the paper and lets the reader know exactly what your proposal is all about. You can rephrase your question or use it as written, but if you begin your paper with your question no one needs to hunt for your topic. Follow your question with a few brief statements about what your study is about and then state your intention to answer this question in your study.

One function of the introductory paragraph is that it tells the reader what the rest of the research problem will discuss; it is the abstract of your problem. The rest of the problem flows from the introductory paragraph in which each sentence will be substantiated, argued, and supported. When you are writing your research problem, write the body first, then go back and write the introduction.

The Body

The body of the research problem is where you present arguments for your project, supported by your cited literature. Subtitle your problem according to the concepts you are discussing, or have one long uninterrupted series of arguments from general to specific. Whether you use subheads or not is up to you, but use descriptive labels for the content. Avoid terms such as "conceptual framework" and "theoretical framework" as your headings or subheadings. They are simply labels and do not describe the content you are using. Your problem could be headed with the terms you used for your topic in your original question, and your subheadings can reflect the different areas you have looked up in the literature to support your choice of topic. Look at the way other students have headed their content areas in the proposals at the end of the book. Build up to your major point. Be sure that you account for the three major elements of the problem: rationale, literature review, and theoretical–conceptual framework.

Use your theory or concept outline and your references here. This is not the place to describe your sample or your methods of data collection. Both topics are dealt with elsewhere in the proposal, under their own headings, so do not waste this precious space detailing the method of data collection used by someone else. You may introduce it, of course, along with methods used by others, but the full exposition of your methods, the specific instruments, and who developed them and what they found is left to the design section. Fill in the outline with your reading. Paraphrase as much as possible. There is nothing more boring than reading a series of quotations. The readers want to know what you think and what your argument is; if they want other opinions, they can check the sources you have cited. Write this section as much as possible in your own words. When you cannot improve or paraphrase an author's statement, then quote, but only sparingly. When you are quoting (copying work verbatim) from one published source or document, you are allowed to quote up to 300 words, total, throughout your paper without requesting permission, but for anything more than that you must ask permission to reprint from the publisher. When received, the permission is then cited as an acknowledgement at the beginning of the paper or at the end.

Use repetition only for emphasis. If you want to emphasize a point, paraphrase several authors who make the same statement. Or quote one, paraphrase another, and list several others who have said essentially the same thing. But use this technique only to emphasize major points. Otherwise, quote or paraphrase the originator of an idea or research and then simply list the authors who agree. You can type pages and pages of everyone's position on the same idea, but all that work will go unread.

Because you are using references to substantiate your points, you may find yourself beginning each statement with "Jones said," or "Maxwell stated," or "According to Pinchpenny." Don't worry about it as you are working on the first draft of your problem, but never let it stand that way. After you have finished writing the body and have exhausted every single argument for every part of your question, go back and rewrite every sentence that begins with "Jones stated" or "A comment by Jones et al." Reference Jones at the end of the quotation or at the end of your paraphrased paragraph. The whole point in the body of your problem is to maintain the flow of ideas, not to list sources. When you introduce each sentence with a source, you are essentially writing a Who's Who in the literature, not a statement of your argument. The difference is critical.

This section of the proposal is also called an integrated literature review. All of the relevant literature is integrated into an interesting explanation of why this project is necessary and appropriate.

The Rationale for Your Research

Every research proposal, whether for a student thesis or dissertation or for a major national grant, has an explanation of why the research is being conducted. Grant funding agencies entitle this section of the proposal "Significance." Student theses and dissertations have two sections: "The Problem" in Chapter 1 and "The Literature Review" in Chapter 2. Both sections are required in the traditional format. Whatever the label, this section supports the entire research process. This section explains why the research is being conducted in the way it is being conducted; why the variables were chosen for study; why the variables are expected to vary; and why the research instruments, the sample, and the data analysis are right for the study. In other words, the researcher's decision on what and how to do this piece of research is supported by relevant literature. The researcher writes what is known as an integrated literature review to support the rest of the proposal.

An integrated literature review is really an essay about the topic chosen for the research supported by the relevant literature. The title for this section is not "The Integrated Literature Review"; rather, the title should reflect the major conceptual topic(s) dealt with in the project, such as "Self-Concept" or "Uncertainty." Look at the proposals at the end of the book. Notice how the titles of the proposals reflect the topic of the research. The titles are not all "Proposal." The same idea applies to the problem segment of the proposal. Label it by the content area and give the reader an idea of what is to come. Leanne Fontanie's proposal is on the use of the partograph as a tool to prevent maternal death. Her problem statement, supported by an integrated literature review, should have that heading or something that reflects that content. When the reader sees this heading, assumptions are made about what the literature will cover. We can assume that Leanne will discuss the literature relating to maternal mortality and the development and use of the partograph. Had she simply entitled this section "Literature Review," we would have no clear idea of what she plans to talk about.

As with an essay, there is a logical flow between paragraphs. The researcher takes us through a chain of thinking demonstrating how the research is an integrated whole. A mistake that novice researchers make is to write an annotated bibliography rather than an integrated literature review. An annotated bibliography is a summary of each relevant article, with one article summarized per paragraph, strung together under a single topic heading. Sometimes the student arranges these summaries by date of publication, sometimes in alphabetical order by author. This is not the correct form to present the literature base for the research.

The integrated literature review should include all the literature used to build the argument for the study being proposed. This will not be all the literature you may have read about your topic because much of it is likely not directly relevant. To make the review representative, you will have gone through an analytical process of culling literature that is not relevant, is redundant, or is based on secondary sources. You want the strongest argument for the study, so use the strongest literary support for the argument. The strongest literature review uses a variety of sources, not just one journal or medium, and represents the characteristics of the primary research.

One way in which researchers arrive at an integrated review is through the use of a conceptual map. (Some people find that mapping the concepts in the research question helps them to visualize the entire process.) Begin by writing the central concepts on a large sheet of paper. Then try to indicate, by arrows, how each concept interacts with the other concepts. The concepts are represented by circles or squares, which are arranged in order of their importance to the project: central variables in the middle of the page, extraneous variables on the edges of the page. Then each variable is connected. Sometimes central variables are represented by large circles, with smaller supportive variables inside the circle. Use whichever way you find easiest to visualize how your concepts and variables work together in your research plan.

When you have the basic visual map, list the articles dealing with those concepts and variables under that concept. (Some students find that putting these sheets of paper on the walls of their study room is extremely helpful. By doing so, for example, they may find that they have read a great deal on one variable but very little on the others.) The articles can be listed either alphabetically or chronologically. Sometimes the same article will be listed under more than one topic heading.

Another step in the process is to use a spreadsheet format (Table 13-1) with headings such as author, date of publication, source, variables studied, purpose and hypothesis, methods, instruments, sample, data analysis, and major findings and conclusions. As each article on the topic is read, it is entered into the database. When viewed in the spreadsheet format, similarities in certain articles become immediately apparent. Articles can be grouped according to methodologies or designs, sample sizes or characteristics, date of publication, author(s), major references, variables studied, or findings and conclusions. With every rearrangement, you can see more clearly new insights that were not possible when simply reading one article after another. These insights might be explicitly stated in yet another column of the spreadsheet. These rearrangements form the basis for the integrated literature review. If you used a bibliographic software package for your literature review, you will have downloaded the results of the search of the various databases into the software package, and it is then available for you to sort in any of the ways previously described. This will greatly simplify the process of integrating your literature review.

Sometimes a single author or researcher appears to be overly represented. In reading that person's work, you may find that the person has quoted him- or herself extensively. This may be because he or she is the only person writing on the topic, or this person coined the term or created the area. If, however, you find many other authors writing on the same topic but this one author rarely cites the other authors, you may feel free to question this author's scholarship and include or not include his or her work in your review. (These issues become very clear if you have a heading for the major references listed.)

Each of us has a different visualization process. You may have created a conceptual map of the variables and concepts in your research at the very beginning and used this as a basis for your literature review. You may have found that as you read, you had to expand (or contract) your conceptual map. The most complex maps to draw are, of course, the maps for experimental designs. That's because so much research has been previously done. Your independent and dependent variables form the center of the map, with an arrow indicating which variable influences the other and indicating the direction of the influence. You know you must survey all the available literature on each variable and the literature on all research that

TABLE 13-1
Integrated Literature Review Spreadsheet

Author(s)	Journal	Year	Purpose/ Hypothesis	Variables	Design	Sample	Methods	Reliability/ Validity	Analysis	Major Findings

studied the two variables together. From that research, you discovered all the intervening variables that are to be accounted for in your study. You may have a separate column for these in your spreadsheet. You also map them. You need to indicate how and when these variables intervene in the action of the primary variables and how they influence and counterinfluence one another. The intervening variables must also be included in your integrated literature review. The next step is to map the extraneous variables in your study—those that may or may not influence the action of the independent on the dependent variable but that are not of direct interest to the research design. If you planned ahead, you have a column for these in your spreadsheet. If not, you can always add a column. These variables also need to be discussed in the literature review. (Recall that the extraneous variables often include the research environment or type of sampling.)

Whatever your method of mapping or visualization, this process will help you to see what you need to include in your literature review and how to organize it logically.

As you develop the body of your problem, remember to leave the strongest, most central point for last. You are leading the reader along the path of your logic, and you want to make your strongest point just before the conclusion. You want to leave the impression that there is not one single i that has not been dotted, a single comma left out, nor a point neglected. You have used and manipulated each point in your outline to its fullest extent, and you have led up to your research question—again.

The Conclusion

Like the introduction, the conclusion should be no more than one paragraph in length. Unlike an essay, in which the conclusion moves from the specific to the general for closure, the conclusion of the research problem serves as the introduction to the rest of the research plan. Your conclusion pulls all the strands of your argument together and ties up loose ends. It ends with your revised research question written as a statement. Your question is better rewritten as a statement introduced by "Therefore, this study," or "For this reason, this study," or "As a result, this study."

Your conclusion places your rationale, thinking, and arguments into one neat package. You want to leave the reader—and yourself—with the feeling that there is nothing further to be said, explained, or argued about your choice of topic. You have closed the door on this aspect of your proposal.

One way of writing a conclusion is to rephrase the introduction. Because the body of the problem simply expands and explains the introduction, the conclusion can restate the introduction with authority. In this way, the conclusion ties in with both the introduction and the problem, and the sense of completeness is achieved.

At the same time, the conclusion also leaves the reader on a high note, with a sense of anticipation of what is to come. This is achieved through the restatement of the research question that appeared in the introduction. Although this brings the reader full circle from question back to question, the answer and how it is to be reached are yet to come. The reader is fully aware of this if your problem is well written.

So, keeping in mind that you don't need to repeat everything you have already said, use your conclusion to pull together all the major points covered in the body of the problem and lead directly into the research question. Remember, keep it brief, keep it to the point, and keep it interesting.

Statement of the Purpose of the Study

After you have written the problem of your study in full detail, you need to state the purpose of the study in a separate section entitled "Purpose of the Study." Simply head this section and write your purpose as shown in Chapter 5. Don't introduce your statement of purpose. Your problem has already done this, and another introduction would be redundant. Just state your purpose under its own heading.

This is also the place in which you are required to write the hypothesis (or hypotheses if you have more than one) that you intend to test. Write your hypothesis as a research hypothesis, not as a null hypothesis. When you write the data analysis section of the proposal, you may rewrite your hypothesis as a null hypothesis, but under the section entitled "Purpose of the Study," simply state: "The purpose of this study is to test the following hypothesis."

The statement of the purpose of your study is as simple as that. Set it off and state your purpose as a declarative statement (Level I), as a question (Level II), or as a hypothesis (Level III).

Definition of Terms

The next step in your proposal is the section entitled "Definition of Terms." Here you will list the variables you intend to study (one or more) and operationally define them as you learned to do in Chapter 6. The definition of terms always follows the statement of purpose of the study so that the reader knows exactly what you mean by the key variables in your purpose and how you intend to measure them. Check and double-check your definitions to be sure that you have included what you mean by the term and how you intend to measure the variable. Many proposals fall short at the operational definitions.

When you are at a Level I exploratory descriptive study, you will usually have one variable that needs to be defined—the central variable you are studying. You may find that the one variable has several components that also need definition. Go ahead and include all the operational definitions you think are necessary for the clarity of your proposal. When someone looks over your final proposal for you, he or she will tell you whether you are being unnecessarily exhaustive.

At Levels II and III you need to define each variable completely, particularly at Level III. In fact, this is probably the most precise point of definition in Level III studies, and you will need to concentrate heavily on this aspect of your proposal. The definitions must fit with your theoretical framework.

You have now finished explaining your problem and have convincingly argued for the way in which you will study the variables. The logic of your conclusion will be clear. You have introduced your research topic and explained the reasons for your choice; you have described whom you are studying; and you have explained the theoretical basis for your study and how you will measure your terms. You are now ready to proceed to the research design.

The Research Design

You may have noticed in the table of contents that the chapter on research design is subtitled "Blueprint for Action." That's exactly what the design is all about. It is your blueprint, or guide, to your activity. If you have ever seen the blueprint or plan for a house, you know that on one page is a master print of the building, which shows the number of stories and their basic outlines. You can see the number of rooms on each floor, the relationship of the rooms to one another, the placement of doors and windows, and so on. Succeeding pages deal with each room separately. The smaller the area being planned, the more specific the detail. Your research design follows the same principle. Your problem statement is the master plan; you are now going to deal with each section separately and in detail.

Although not required, it is often helpful to introduce the design with a general statement about what it will encompass. Frequently, this introduction states the general direction the research will take. When you identify and label your design, give it the appropriate title: exploratory, descriptive, correlational, comparative, quasi-experimental, experimental, historic, and so on. If you are not using all the required elements of a particular design, it is best to use a more generic label for the design. When you say, "This is a Level II design" you are misusing the concept of levels. The level refers to the level of knowledge and/or theory about the topic, which in turn directs and guides the thinking and planning for the research. A level is not a name of a design. This introduction puts the reader in the right frame of reference and also makes you, the researcher, more careful in handling the rest of your proposal.

You should be aware at this point that the level of study you have chosen to do will be reflected in the amount of detail that goes into the research proposal. At Level I, when you may have only a vague idea of what you will find because you are doing an exploratory study, your proposal will not have the detail based on research findings that you will need for Level II. Level III studies are the most highly detailed and exhaustive in the review of literature and in relation to the experiment itself. Therefore, the design discussion of the proposal must be meticulously written and referenced, more so than at either of the other two levels. The reason becomes very clear after you have had some actual research experience. At Level I, most of the work of the research goes into the content analysis of the data and the final write-up of the project. At Level III, most of the work goes into the proposal because everything must be planned in advance. If you keep this in mind as you write your proposal, you will find it easier to understand what you have to do for each level.

The Sample

Following the introduction of the research design, you may describe either the sample or the methods of data collection. However, your design section will flow better if you describe the sample next because it will be easier to discuss methods and procedures of data collection just prior to data analysis.

The heading for this section of the proposal can simply be "The Sample." Other headings just as acceptable are "Criteria for Sample Selection," "Sample Selection Procedures," and "Sample Selection."

Target Population

When you describe your sample, begin with a description of the population from which you intend to draw your sample. Describe the population in great detail, discussing who they are, where they are located, and when they can be found. Here is where you will probably mention whether or not there is a listing of your population anywhere and if that listing is available to you.

If you are doing a Level I study, describe your target population in as much detail as you possibly can. Because you may be doing a convenience sampling technique, your reader needs to know what you know about your population and just how representative your sample may or may not be. If you know nothing about your sample except what you have read in the literature, be honest and say so. If anyone knows the population you are referring to, it will be obvious in reading your proposal that you have no firsthand information. Don't try to fake it; just tell what you know. If you know anything at all about the people, describe them as best you can according to age range, gender, educational level, and so on. The demographic characteristics of a population need to be included here—if you have those data. If you are studying burn patients on X hospital ward, say so. If you are investigating runners, dieters in Weight Watchers, crystal meth addicts, or staff nurses, say exactly who it is you are studying.

Where you intend to study your population is also important information. If you intend to sample from the entire country, you need to let the reader be aware of the population to which you wish to generalize. If you are limiting your target population to a particular city, school, or hospital, say that too, because that is the population to which you generalize.

Give the time frame for your study here because sometimes you will have to stop a study before you have achieved your ideal sample. You may want to have a certain minimum number of people in your study, but if you cannot get that number in the amount of time you wish to spend collecting the data, say so. Because your proposal will be reviewed more than once for different purposes, have as much information as possible in it about your population so that you don't have to write several different drafts.

Sample Selection

When you have exhausted the subject of the population from which you plan to select your sample, you can discuss the sample selection techniques. Because you have been precise about your description of the population, you have little left to do by way of description. At Level I, you will mention your sampling technique and specify the number of research subjects or time limits of the study. At Level III, you will need to justify the sample size you have chosen, and you will spell out exactly what your method of assigning the subjects to groups will be. Whether you are conducting your experiment in one setting or several, you will have to describe the procedures explicitly and in detail, clarifying the number of experimental and control groups, how you intend to do the random assignment, how many you need in each group, what you intend to do about replacement, and so on. If you are using a matched sampling technique, you must detail the process of matching and on what variables. Again, precision and clarity are key at Level III.

If you are at Level II, remember that the method of sample selection is critical to generalizing your findings back to the population. The ideal method on which survey designs are based is the probability sample. Be sure when you are describing your sample selection procedures that you identify what type of probability sample you plan to use—simple random, stratified random, multistage, or cluster. Give your reason for the choice, state the sample size you intend to obtain, and identify the percentage of the population it represents. There are statistical programs available for estimating the power of your sample size. Be sure to include all the information you have. Then specify how you intend to go about obtaining the sample. It is not enough to say what the sample will be; you must describe your procedures for getting subjects. Describe the numbering used in your list—and whether you will use those numbers or will assign new numbers—and then tell how you will make your selection—computer generated or by hand using a table of random numbers. It sounds tedious, but the more detailed your procedures are during the planning, the less error in the end. If you are not using a probability sampling method for your Level II study, you must explain why you are not and point out to your readers that this is a limitation of your study.

You will need to discuss the concept of replacement at Level II or III. You want to have a specified number of people in your sample. What will you do about dropouts, no-shows, and people who refuse permission? Will you replace them, or will you go on without them? Here is where you discuss your method of obtaining an alternate list for dropouts using the same probability sampling technique you used to obtain the original sample. We recommend that you plan to use approximately 10% more subjects than you need as replacements. These issues must be discussed here along with the rationale for your decision.

It is easier to be detailed in the proposal stage than to make these decisions later in the study when the usual disasters occur. Obtaining the sample is usually the most troublesome step in carrying out a research project, so try to imagine what might go wrong. If you plan ahead for your sample, for every possible contingency, and write it down in your proposal, you have a guide for yourself to follow if things go wrong. So be precise, be detailed, and be complete.

Methods and Instruments

You should now describe the method or methods you intend to use to collect your data. These include anything from observations, questionnaires, and interviews to physiologic measures or laboratory tests. If you are using more than one method, you will need to explain your rationale for each method, how the methods interrelate, and why they are appropriate in view of your sample selection.

Your methods must be consistent with your sample. On the basis of the method selected, you are now ready to discuss which research instrument you have chosen to collect the data from your sample. You will need to explain why you have chosen this instrument, discuss its strengths and weaknesses, and outline what tests of reliability and validity have been done on the instrument and on what populations it has been used before. If you have decided to develop your own instrument, the same type of rationale must be presented. Always keep in mind that the instruments must be consistent with the methods.

Here again, you will need to have reviewed the literature thoroughly to present the arguments for your choice of instruments with an authoritative voice.

Reliability and Validity

When you are discussing your research instrument or instruments, incorporate your discussion of reliability and validity testing in that section. Entitle that section "Procedures for Establishing Reliability and Validity of X Instrument," and then describe what you will do and how you will do it. If you are planning to do a test of internal consistency by a split-half correlation, describe how you will do it, which test you will use, and what correlation you will accept. The same would be true for an alternate form test or a series of repeated observations or test–retest situations. Establishing face and content validity is accomplished by a review of the literature and the use of a judge panel to determine completeness of content. Concurrent validation procedures are described by contrasting your instrument with the research findings from another instrument. If you are using an instrument that only has face validity, you will need to judge its content validity and perhaps test its concurrent validity and establish why the test is as good as the one you used for comparison. If you prefer, you may have a separate section just for these issues, particularly if you are planning to develop your own research instrument. If you are doing participant observation, describe how you will attempt to ensure that your research instrument is reliable, valid, or both. It's easier to discuss reliability and validity of data collection when you are using someone else's instruments. Simply describe how those were tested, if you know, and indicate how you intend to test them for your study.

In Level I studies, you will need to discuss reliability and validity issues in content analysis. You may discuss this subject either under the heading "Data Analysis" or under a separate heading. The choice is up to you.

Level III experimental designs provide a test of the theory underlying the experiment, and a discussion of the reliability and validity of the instruments is a major focus of the proposal. You can still decide whether to discuss these concepts separately or in conjunction with the data collection procedures. If you deal with them separately, you may find that you have a more complete discussion of both the instrument and its tests. If you discuss them together, you may overlook certain details critical to your plan. But again, it is up to you.

Remember that a discussion of reliability and validity refers to the way in which you will attempt to eliminate or minimize error in data collection or to account for the error that will occur. So when you are writing your proposal, this section is a very important one that needs particular attention.

Data Analysis

This is probably the easiest part of the research proposal to write because it usually follows the section on data collection. Because data analysis procedures follow directly from sample selection and data collection techniques, by now you should know precisely which analytical technique you will use. You can either describe the steps in detail or name the analytical tools you will use and provide a brief justification for your choice. As long as you know in advance how you will analyze your data, and say so, you are in fine shape. Although this might be the hardest part of the proposal for you to do, it's probably the easiest to write. Go back to the tables in Chapter 12 on data analysis (Tables 12-4 and 12-6), check how many steps are involved at each level of research design, look up the measurement scale you intend to use, and find the appropriate research data analysis technique.

Ethics

This last section of your research proposal should describe in detail exactly how you intend to protect the rights of the participants in your study. You need to include statements on how you intend to obtain their informed consent to be research subjects, how you intend to protect their anonymity as research subjects (make sure that no one can possibly know who they are), and how you intend to explain your research to them so that they can understand it. Here you will probably want to write a complete statement of what you will say to them, beginning with "Hello, my name is."

If you are a student, you may be asked to submit your research proposal to your institutional review board (IRB), or ethics review board (ERB) in Canada, for the protection of human rights. If you are a staff member, your hospital or agency will have an IRB to which you will be expected to submit your research proposal. The IRB will have specific requirements for the format of your submission because they usually do not want the entire proposal submitted to them on its own. Always follow their format to describe the protection of human rights for your sample. You may also be asked to attach your entire research proposal in case they have questions about your procedures. In some institutions, you will be asked to attend an ethics committee meeting at which your proposal will be discussed so that you can answer questions from committee members.

One of the key issues on which IRBs base their decisions is weighing the benefits against the risks of a study. This is an aspect of your statement of the protection of human subjects that you simply cannot neglect. If you can see no possible benefit to humanity from your study (except to yourself because you will get your degree from it), no one will approve it. A no-benefit study cannot possibly outweigh even the slightest risk. Remember, every time you do research, you are posing some degree of risk to someone in your sample because you are intruding in their life. No matter how slight, it is still a risk. Any kind of risk needs to be counterbalanced by some kind of benefit, so don't neglect this aspect of your proposal. The knowledge gained from your study must, at minimum, be seen as having the possibility to improve the situation for future people in the target population.

You will need to include a copy of the informed consent form that your subjects will be asked to sign or a complete transcript of an oral informed consent statement and an explanation of why you will not have it signed. Because requiring signatures is the norm, an exception must be made for any study where the researcher will not be obtaining signatures. The rationale must be sound and well explained.

In Summary

You now have completed the basic outline for the research design section of the proposal. You will have noticed that each section follows directly from the previous ones. Over and over you keep reading that this must be consistent with that. Because each section is based on the previous ones, they must be logically related and you must show this relationship. You must make the connection and close any gaps. In other words, don't throw something into a section because it looks sophisticated. If it doesn't fit, don't use it. If it wasn't introduced, it doesn't belong.

And, finally, you will have noticed that from time to time in this book a reference was made to looking up something in the literature. You weren't really finished with your literature review when you wrote your problem. Every item in your proposal should command authority. If you don't know enough about reliability and validity, look them up. If you don't know which method of data analysis to use, look it up. If you don't know anything about your sample or your methods, go to the literature. No one else can do this for you. Because you need a rationale for every part of the proposal, make sure your rationales are based on fact, not hearsay. By the end of your proposal you are not just an expert in your content area; you are an expert on the people you are studying, the particular method and design, and a specific form of data analysis. And by becoming an expert, you have developed credibility. You will be sought out by your peers and by employers because of your expertise. And you will have developed self-confidence as a nurse researcher.

Variations in the Proposal Format

The proposal outline you have just read is suitable for a number of functions. It is, first and foremost, the model for every proposal you will write now and in the future. You should retain this proposal in a form where it can be accessed for other purposes.

Second, if you do not deviate substantially from the proposal, you may use it as the basis for the first article you write for publication after completing your study. All you have to do is change your future tense to past; update and abbreviate your problem essay to four typed pages or less; make changes in the proposal that reflect the changes you may have made during the course of the study (in the actual sample, data collection process, and data analysis); enter your findings and conclusions; and presto! you have an article for publication in the approved format for a nursing research journal.

Thesis or Dissertation

If you are using this proposal as the basis for a thesis or dissertation proposal, talk to your advisor and find out the approved format at your school. Then alter this proposal to suit that format. For example, some schools require master's and doctoral students to present the first three chapters of their thesis or dissertation to their committee and are orally examined on those chapters prior to entering the data collection phase. In this instance, the first three chapters, references, and appendices would include the following information:

- Chapter 1: This is the problem chapter that includes the introduction with a very abbreviated literature review to substantiate the choice of this problem. This follows with a paragraph called "The Problem," which is an expanded statement of purpose followed by hypotheses or a list of research questions that further expand on the problem.
- Chapter 2: This chapter is the literature review, which is, in essence, an expanded version of your problem essay. More detail is given and more references are cited here than we have recommended in our abbreviated proposal. Your committee may want a justification for not using other theories, concepts, or methods in addition to those you have chosen to support your study. This is an area you should discuss with your thesis advisor.
- Chapter 3: This chapter is design and methodology. Here you simply put everything else in your proposal: design, sample, methods, data analysis, reliability and validity, and protection of human subjects.
- References: Here you need to use the style required by your institution and call it a bibliography or a list of references according to the style your school requires.
- Appendixes: These will be presented in the format required by your school. Each appendix will be given a different letter (beginning with A) and grouped by content: human subjects forms, letters of agreement from agencies stating they will let you do research at their institution, maps of the region if needed, copy of the data collection instrument(s), and so on.

Grant Proposals

If you are writing a grant proposal, the granting agency's requirements determine how you will alter your original proposal. If you are submitting to a foundation or private agency, write and ask for their guidelines on how they like to have proposals submitted to them. In other words, ask for their proposal specifications and then follow that format. Sometimes it is a simple matter of abbreviating the proposal you have just written. Foundations frequently want a brief summary of your idea first, and then if they are interested in the study you will be asked to submit a more detailed proposal. Requirements and forms for grant applications are usually on the Web site of the funding agency. Some agencies require that you submit the application online using a form as provided.

If you are planning to write a federal grant, the requirements are fairly standard. The grants office in your college or university may provide support services that will assist you to meet the guidelines. However, these proposals all follow the same basic format and include the following:

Abstract of Research Plan

A. Specific Aims

B. Significance

C. Preliminary Studies

D. Design and Methods

E. Ethics

F. Consultants

G. Collaborations

H. References

I. Appendix

There will be a separate form for submission of a budget and personnel requirements.

If not submitted online, this material is to be printed (using a letter-quality printer) within the margins specified, using the recommended font size, on copies of the sample page.

The Web site for the National Institute of Nursing Research (www.ninr. nih.gov/) gives detailed information about the submission of grants in the various categories for which funding is available. The appropriate forms are provided and can be printed from the Web site.

The Finished Proposal

The difference between the first draft of a research proposal and the final, polished version is enormous and generally reflects the amount of time spent on it.

Students usually have a limited amount of time for learning how to write a proposal, performing all the steps involved in the research process, and actually submitting that proposal. As a result, the submitted product is often a first draft—rough, awkward, and almost inarticulate.

To minimize these defects, we suggest that a friend review the first draft before you submit it to the instructor. Have the friend describe the project to you. This will tell you if the proposal is clear and logical. On the basis of this initial critique, changes should be made in the paper prior to submitting it. If your friend doesn't understand what you are doing, it is likely that your instructor won't either.

If possible, put your first draft of the proposal away and let it sit for a period of time (days, weeks, or months). You will be amazed at what happens to your thinking when you can see what you have written with a critical, analytical eye—not the eye of a fond parent. Your mistakes will loom before you—now your sentences seem muddy, your logic obscure, and your ideas poorly articulated. Now you are ready to polish the first draft. This is simply a matter of editing and rewriting. Now is the time to clarify your ideas, write transition sentences, make the tenses consistent, clean up typographical errors, and so on. You may end up revising the entire proposal, but better that than having it turned down because it failed to communicate your ideas.

Check Your References

When you write a research proposal, you are expected to be accurate in all details, major and minor. But most important is to be accurate in your referencing. Nothing is worse, especially in research, than misquoting, misreferencing, or failing to give proper credit.

Unfortunately, human beings tend to make errors. To be sure that you have listed all the references cited in the body of the paper, reread your entire proposal just for the references, and check each one against your list. Time consuming? Yes. Worth it? Definitely. You are required to give proper credit to the authors whose work came before yours and provided the foundation for your proposal.

One of the most difficult things to remember when writing from your notes is where those notes came from. They may have come from a lecture, a letter, a book, or a reading—in fact, any source for someone else's ideas. We all do this; it's not at all unusual. In fact, that's the way some people do all their writing. But when you do this, you run the risk of being accused of plagiarism. Plagiarism means using someone else's work without acknowledging the source. Using someone else's work refers to using their ideas, literally copying their words, or following their phraseology without acknowledgment. It is insufficient to say "Some authors" when, in fact, the idea came from one specific source. So keep your notes as complete as possible at the time you take them. You will be very glad later as you write your finished proposal.

Polishing the Draft

The finished proposal should have a sense of closure and completeness about it. All parts are present and accounted for, including the title page.

Completed proposals look good. They are printed double-spaced and have page numbers. Handwritten proposals simply are not acceptable, nor are proposals that have been edited so much that they are practically handwritten. Clean, neat proposals are not just pleasing to the eye; they also create a positive impression on the reader. Don't let typographical errors stand uncorrected in the final copy. By all means, correct your typos. If you have too many, reprint the page.

Your finished proposal, ideally fewer than 25 typed pages, is what you will present to your instructor at the end of the course or to a thesis committee. It will also serve as the basis for any grant proposal you may decide to write later. Most importantly, however, it also will guide you through the rest of the research process. Because it serves so many functions, make more than one copy of the proposal and back up your computer files; consider how you would feel if it were lost. Also, make sure everything you need for your future research is included in the proposal, because that is probably all you will refer to, rather than your stacks of notes and papers. If you keep the uses of the proposal in mind, you may consider brevity a virtue—and, indeed, it is. Be as brief as possible without losing your train of thought or neglecting an important point.

The final polish includes reviewing the manuscript for grammar, style, and appropriate language. Some of us persist in the use of sexist language and language that is not politically correct, forgetting the subtle influence of language in our lives and in our thinking. Biased language needs to be ruthlessly abandoned in our research. Not all humans are he and not all nurses are she. Simply eliminate these pronouns from a sentence by rewriting it. Avoid words such as "should," which is a moralistic judgment, and substitute "could," which indicates possibility. Sentences that either begin with or include clauses such as "it has been stated that," "it is assumed that," or "it is clear that" use up a number of words to sound scholarly. Rewrite them to eliminate everything from "it" to "that" and begin with the next word. Or just say "clearly." Other editing hints refer to sentences that use phrases such as "the findings of this study reveal that" or "the findings state." Cut your sentences to say something like "the findings were" or "the study resulted in" and let it go at that. The more you attempt to sound scholarly, the more ponderous you become.

As your write up your final proposal, try to remember that what you are writing about is what you intend to do in the future. Therefore, your proposal should be written in future tense. Write clearly, with as little superfluity, pomposity, and garrulousness as possible. Some people believe that a scholarly proposal is unintelligible to the general reader. This does not have to be true. Write it so you can understand it; when you read it a month or two later, you will remember what you were thinking about and can go on from there.

The finished research paper, whether written by one person or a group, is a reflection of the time and thinking that went into the plan from question to proposal. The finished proposal marks the end of one phase of research—it is a milestone achieved.

Bibliography

American Psychological Association. (2001). *Publication manual of the American Psychological Association* (5th ed.). Washington, DC: Author.

Artinian, B. M. (1982). Conceptual mapping: Development of the strategy. *Western Journal of Nursing Research, 4*(4), 379–393.

Boyd, C. O., & Munhall, P. L. (2001). Qualitative research proposals and reports. In P. L. Munhall (Ed.), *Nursing research: A qualitative perspective* (3rd ed.). Sudbury, MA: Jones and Bartlett.

Clare, J., & Hamilton, H. (Eds.). (2003). *Writing research: Transforming data into text.* Edinburgh, Scotland: Elsevier.

Cooper, H. M. (1989). *Integrating research: A guide for literature reviews* (2nd ed.). Newbury Park, CA: Sage.

Epstein, D. (2005). *Writing for publication.* London: Sage.

Ganong, L. H. (1987). Integrative reviews of nursing research. *Research in Nursing and Health, 10*, 1–11.

Gillham, B. (2000). *The research interview*. London: Continuum.

Higgins, J., & Green, S. (2008). *Cochrane handbook for systematic reviews of interventions*. Hoboken, NJ: Wiley-Blackwell.

Holliday, A. (2001). *Doing and writing qualitative research*. London: Sage.

Huberman, A. M., & Miles, M. B. (2002). *The qualitative researcher's companion*. Thousand Oaks, CA: Sage.

Kane, M., & Trochim, W. M. K. (2007). *Concept mapping for planning and evaluation*. Thousand Oaks, CA: Sage.

Lester, J. D., & Lester, J. D., Jr. (1999). *The essential guide to writing research papers*. New York: Longman.

Oermann, M. H. (2002). *Writing for publication in nursing*. Philadelphia: Lippincott Williams and Wilkins.

Payne, L. V. (1965). *The lively art of writing*. New York: Mentor.

Slade, C. (2003). *Form and style: Research papers, reports, theses* (12th ed.). Boston: Houghton Mifflin.

Strunk, W., Jr. (2007). *The elements of style*. Boston: Allyn and Bacon.

Tornquist, E. M., & Funk, S. G. (1990). How to write a research grant proposal. *Image: Journal of Nursing Scholarship, 22*(1), 44–51.

Woods, P. (2006). *Successful writing for qualitative researchers*. New York: Routledge.

Appendix Contents:
Sample Research Proposals

LEVEL I

An Exploratory Study

Appendix B: The Experience of Nurse–Midwives in Ghana with the Use of the WHO Partograph. By Leanne Fontanie

A Descriptive Study

Appendix C: The Incidence of Acute Stress Disorder Among Parents of Premature Infants Admitted into the Neonatal Intensive Care Unit. By Jocelyn M. Jubinville

LEVEL II

Survey–Relationship Designs

Appendix D: Nausea and Vomiting Following Posterior Fossa Surgery: Determination of Incidence, Risk, and Protective Factors in Children. By Susan M. Neufeld

Appendix E: The Impact of Older Maternal Age at First Birth on the Risk of Spontaneous Preterm Birth in Northern and Central Alberta. By Safina Hassan McIntyre

LEVEL III

True Experiments

Appendix F: Maintaining Catheter Patency Using Recombinant Tissue Plasminogen Activator. By Colleen M. Astle

Appendix G: Standardized Telephone Triage Practice: Impact of Protocol Implementation on Reported Job Stress and Satisfaction by Nurses in a Pediatric Oncology Outpatient Setting. By Karina Black

The Experiences of Ghanaian Nurse–Midwives in Utilizing the Partograph

Leanne Fontanie

Introduction

Maternal mortality remains a global concern, with women in low-income countries bearing the greatest burden. Every year, an estimated 536,000 women die from complications of pregnancy and childbirth, 99% of which occur in low- and very-low-income countries (Obaid, 2007). The Safe Motherhood Initiative was introduced in 1987 as an international campaign to reduce maternal mortality (AbouZahr, 2003). This campaign was the first of its kind to recommend that all pregnant women in labor be managed by appropriately trained personnel using practical and relevant and evidence-based technology, including the partograph (Chalmers, Mangiaterra, & Porter, 2001). The partograph is an assessment tool used by birth attendants to monitor both maternal and fetal well-being during the labor process. Previous research conducted in Ghana concluded that there appears to be a disconnect between the reported value of the partograph and the buy-in of those who provide the intrapartum care (Gans-Lartey, 2006). Further research on the utilization of the partograph by the nurse–midwives is recommended. This study will examine the experience of nurse–midwives in the use of the partograph with the hope that more effective use of this tool can be promoted in the future.

The partograph needs widespread acceptance by its users to be successfully implemented within the system and effectively utilized. In addition to monitoring maternal and fetal well-being during active labor, the partograph can be used to diagnose prolonged and obstructed labor, which is one of the main causes of maternal death in sub-Saharan Africa (Ronsmans & Graham, 2006). Obstructed labor, if left untreated, can lead

303

to sepsis, ruptured uterus, postpartum hemorrhage, and obstetric fistula (Arrowsmith, Hamlin, & Wall, 1996; Hofmeyr, 2004). All of these, except obstetric fistula, are associated with maternal death.

Women with fistulas experience many physical impairments, including urine and feces incontinence. If the fistula is not repaired, serious social problems may develop, including isolation from family and friends, exclusion from activities, increased poverty, and lifelong suffering (Arrowsmith, et al., 1996). In addition to increased severe morbidity and mortality for women, improper usage of the partograph can lead to an increase in unnecessary interventions (Groeschel & Glover, 2001).

The death of a mother has a negative effect on the health of her children and other family members. Motherless children die more frequently, are at an increased risk of becoming malnourished, and are less likely to enroll in school (World Health Organization [WHO], 2005). The future health of the children is directly associated with the health of their mother. In 2000, the United Nations developed the Millennium Development Goals (MDGs) and identified improving maternal health as Goal 5. The partograph, when used effectively, is a tool that can help prevent the tragic death of women in labor and in turn enable progress toward MDG 5. Findings from this study will be used to aid the nurse–midwives in overcoming barriers that inhibit the effective implementation of this safe motherhood initiative and to develop strategies that will facilitate its use.

Literature Review

The strategy used for the literature review included searching the following databases: CINAHL, MEDLINE, Global Health, PubMed, EMBASE, Scopus, and Google Scholar. The keywords searched were maternal health, maternal mortality, partograph or partogram, World Health Organization, nurse, midwife, safe motherhood initiatives, Africa, and Ghana. These words were searched separately and in various combinations. The use of the partograph has not been studied extensively, and limited research articles are available. I have noted a gap in the literature that this research proposal will address. No qualitative research study was found that exclusively examines the factors that inhibit and support the use of the partograph from the perspective of the nurse–midwife.

Maternal Mortality

According to the ICD-10 definition by the WHO (2004), maternal death is defined as the death of a woman at any point during her pregnancy to less than one year after the termination of the pregnancy. Maternal death is any death directly or indirectly related to the pregnancy or its management, but it is not from accidental or incidental causes. The main causes of direct maternal deaths in low-income countries include hemorrhage, sepsis, hypertensive disorders, obstructed labor, and complications from abortion. Indirect causes of death include existing medical conditions, such as HIV–AIDS, tuberculosis, and malaria, that complicate pregnancy (Ronsmans & Graham, 2006; WHO, 2005).

The highest maternal mortality ratio is found in sub-Saharan Africa, where there are 900 maternal deaths for every 100,000 live births (WHO, 2007a). Of the estimated annual 536,000 maternal deaths, 270,000 occur in the sub-Saharan Africa region. The adult lifetime risk of maternal death is highest in Africa at 26 (WHO, 2007a). In other words, for every 26 women in this region, one will die of maternal causes. In Ghana, the adjusted maternal mortality ratio is 560 deaths per 100,000 live births (WHO, 2007b). To put this in perspective, the maternal mortality ratio in Canada is 6.1 deaths per 100,000 live births (Health Canada, 2004). The stark contrast in maternal mortality ratios between low- and high-income countries are outstanding and demonstrate the greatest global health disparity.

The Partograph As a Safe Motherhood Initiative

The first graphical representation of labor progression was developed in the United States and included plotting cervical dilatation against the number of hours a woman was in labor (Friedman, 1955). This seminal work was the basis for further development of the partograph in 1972 as a tool to assess and manage the progress of labor (Lavender & Malcolmson, 1999). Philpott and Castle further developed the partograph in 1972 as a tool to assess and manage the process of labor. In the partograph, they included an area to record the woman's cervical dilatation, presenting part and station, presence of caput or molding, timing of uterine contractions, and fetal heart rate (Groeschel & Glover, 2001; Philpott & Castle, 1972). The WHO (1994b) adapted their own version of the partograph from the work of Philpott and Castle (1972) and currently promotes its use worldwide in all hospitals and healthcare centers that have skilled attendants and educational materials available. Their partograph consists of three sections: the fetal condition, the maternal condition, and the progress of labor (WHO, 1994b). This partograph assesses the same areas as the original partograph developed by Philpott and Castle with a few additions that include assessment of membranes and amniotic fluid, maternal vital signs and urine analysis, drug administration, maternal positioning, and behavior.

The partograph allows for a graphic recording of cervical dilation in centimeters against the number of hours a woman is in labor. The alert and action lines were placed on the partograph to help identify maternal or fetal risk factors and/or labors that do not progress within normal parameters or are obstructed (Groeschel & Glover, 2001). The first stage of labor has two stages: latent and active. The healthcare provider should not begin using the partograph until the woman is in active labor, which is defined as being three centimeters dilated and contracting regularly. If the cervical dilation moves to the right of the alert line on the partograph, the healthcare provider is aware that the labor is progressing slowly and the woman should be monitored closely. If the action line is crossed, an intervention should occur, such as starting an oxytocin augmentation, artificially rupturing the membranes, or completing a cesarean section if necessary (Dangal, 2007).

The partograph provides objective data that is required to make clinical decisions by presenting a continuous pictorial overview of the well-being of both the fetus and the mother (WHO, 1994b). The effective use of the partograph ensures that there is a comprehensive monitoring of the progress of labor as well as maternal and fetal well-being. It is then possible to address in a timely manner the complications that arise (WHO, 1994b). The introduction of the partograph led to a reduction in prolonged labor, augmentation, and cesarean section rate (Studd, 1973; WHO, 1994a). While effective assessment could theoretically increase rates of induction and operative birth as a response to obstructed labor, it is possible that these contradictory findings were the result of not implementing necessary interventions.

In a UK survey of midwifery views regarding the partograph, midwives (n = 71) were asked if a partograph was necessary; 97.2% agreed that it was and acknowledged the benefit of "being able to see at a glance what is happening" (Lavender & Malcolmson, 1999, p. 24). They concluded that although the partograph is an effective tool, it should not prevent midwives from using their own judgment and clinical skills. In a qualitative Angolan study, participants (n = 11) found the partograph valuable in guiding decisions, helpful in providing continuing care, and a useful document in liability cases (Pettersson, Svensson, & Christensson, 2001).

The partograph was originally designed for use in low-income countries. However, it has been effectively utilized in higher-income countries since 1980 and is part of routine obstetrical care provided at healthcare centers in Canada (Lavender & Malcolmson, 1999; Liston & Crane, 2002). Although there are many medical and nonmedical determinants of maternal mortality, a discrepancy between high- and low-income countries is clear. To improve maternal and newborn outcomes, the partograph is a valuable resource for low- and very-low-income countries, such as those in sub-Saharan Africa.

Partograph Utilization in Africa

There is some evidence that healthcare professionals in Africa are not using the partograph consistently or correctly. A pilot study was conducted in Zambia to examine the routine care of women experiencing normal deliveries; it was found that the use of the partograph was not adequate in any of the healthcare settings, including a university teaching hospital, two urban healthcare centers, and eight rural hospitals (Maimbolwa, Ransjo-Arvidson, Ng'andu, Sikazwe, & Diwan, 1997). A round partograph was introduced in rural Burkina Faso and compared to the WHO partograph (Wacker, Kyelem, Bastert, Utz, & Lankoande, 1998). It was reported that only 46.6% of the partographs were properly completed despite the continuous supervision given during the study period.

In a Tanzanian study (n = 196), it was concluded that although the partograph was available for most eligible deliveries in the three hospitals studied, "the overall proportion of satisfactory implementation was only 58%" (Bosse, Massawe, & Jahn, 2002, p. 244). Unsatisfactory fetal and maternal outcomes were associated with poor partograph-based monitoring. In a Nigerian study (2004 to 2005) it was found that overall only 39 out of 216 (9.8%) healthcare professionals routinely used the partograph (Oladapo, Daniel, & Olatunji, 2006). A quasi-experimental research study conducted in Angola examined the use of the WHO partograph in a peripheral delivery unit following an educational intervention (Pettersson et al., 2001). The researchers found that although documentation of the partographs by midwives was adequate, the information gathered was not consistently utilized as evidenced by a high number of missed transfers. In another Nigerian study, researchers found that 95% of physicians (n = 200) and 84% of midwives (n = 163) had heard of the partograph, but 75% of midwives and 40% of physicians could not provide a correct definition (Umezulike, Onah, & Okaro, 1999).

The Ghanaians adopted the use of the WHO partograph in labor wards throughout the country in 1990 with the intention of improving maternal health and reducing maternal and perinatal mortality (Gans-Lartey, 2006;

Seffah, 2003). Few studies were found where the use of the partograph in Ghana was examined. Only 64 women of 384 (16.7%) who were referred during labor to the Korle Bu teaching hospital in Accra came with a partograph (Nkyekyer, 2000). When the incidence of ruptured uterus was compared to whether or not the partograph was used, Seffah found that the partographs were not being utilized effectively (2003). For example, it was reported that 49% of the women had uterine rupture after the action line was crossed, indicating the length of time for normal labor was exceeded and that labor was possibly obstructed. It can be inferred from this finding that the provider was unable or unwilling to initiate an intervention after a risk was identified. Only 17% of births in healthcare facilities at the primary care level met the criteria of good practice, and midwifery assistants attended as many as one-third of hospital births without supervision (Hussein, et al., 2004 as cited in Koblinsky, et al., 2006).

Consistent with the other African studies, Gans-Lartey (2006) found that despite having access to the partograph, the nurse–midwives at a national teaching hospital were not using the partograph adequately. Of the 1845 charts reviewed, 472 (25.6%) of the partographs were correctly filled out in accordance with WHO guidelines, and 1373 (74.4%) partographs were incorrectly filled out. In 464 charts (25.1%) where the action line was crossed, an intervention was not implemented in a timely manner for 238 charts (51.3%).

The research conducted by Gans-Lartey is alarming because the partograph had been implemented 16 years prior to her study, yet the majority of providers for charts reviewed were not effectively using this tool. Only 25.6% of the partographs were filled out correctly. More importantly, when the action line was crossed on the partograph, more than half of the charts showed that an intervention was not being executed. The partograph is a valuable tool that is not being utilized in the largest and most advanced hospital in Ghana. The development of technology to improve maternal health is important, but "it must be adapted to each country's context in order to be of optimal value to the users" (Pettersson, et al., 2001, p. 110). As a result, further research is recommended to examine the buy-in of the partograph by nurse–midwives.

Why the partographs are not utilized effectively was briefly addressed. It was reported that the time it took to complete the partograph was a factor in its poor utilization (Wacker, et al., 1998). Maternal cervical dilatation upon admission to the hospital is a factor because when women arrived at the institution fully dilated, a partograph obviously cannot be started. Awareness and utilization of the partograph among study participants in one study was low, and lack of continuing education and lack of quality assurance measures on the unit were identified as probable reasons (Oladapo, et al., 2006). In another study, the unavailability of the partograph was identified as a reason for its low usage (Umezulike, et al., 1999).

Equity Framework

The global inequity in maternal health between low- and high-income countries is internationally recognized, yet the appalling disparity still exists. The maternal mortality ratio is the main health indicator that reveals the greatest gap between rich and poor women (Obaid, 2007). Maternal health is directly linked to poverty and gender inequality. Efforts to reduce maternal mortality must also consider social and cultural factors that affect women's health and access to services (Filippi, et al., 2006). Women will have increased access to maternal healthcare services and a lower risk of maternal death if the education of women is improved, employment opportunities are created, and women are involved in deciding key aspects of their lives (Yinger, 2007). Therefore, improving maternal mortality directly links to four other Millennium Development Goals: MDG 1, poverty reduction; 3, women's empowerment; 4, child survival; and 6, infectious diseases (Filippi, et al., 2006; United Nations, 2006). To ensure the health of future, the largely preventable and unnecessary deaths of so many socially and economically disadvantaged mothers, especially those living in poverty in low- and very low-income countries, need to be eliminated. To survive pregnancy is a basic human right for all women.

Purpose

The purpose of this research project is to understand the factors that influence the effective use of the WHO partograph by nurse–midwives in Ghana, Africa. The acceptability of the partograph among the nurse–midwives will be explored, as well as insights that increase our understanding of facilitators of and barriers to its utilization.

The research question is as follows:

> What is the experience of the Ghanaian nurse–midwives with the WHO partograph? More specifically, an understanding of facilitators of and barriers to the effective use of the partograph by nurse–midwives in Ghana will be gained. This will provide insights into how the partograph can be more effectively implemented into birthing centers and will identify the areas that need to be addressed within the centers to ensure consistent and correct use of the partograph by nurse–midwives.

Design

Ethnography

A focused ethnography is proposed as the qualitative research methodology that is best suited to answer the research question. Ethnographic methods can be implemented to describe a specific culture or way of life; patterns of behavior can be examined to understand why people do what they do (Creswell, 1998; Roper & Shapira, 2000). Ethnography emerges from a naturalist perspective or the assumption that people are best studied in their natural setting (Hammersley & Atkinson, 1995). Traditionally it was used by anthropologists to explore cultural groups and societies, and the word "ethnography" was defined as a "portrait of a people" (Burns & Grove, 2007, p. 69), in this case the culture of Ghanaian nurse–midwives. It is important to point out that culture is defined broadly and can relate professional groups or other groups with shared beliefs within a given society. Ethnography allows the researcher to explore a culture's customs, beliefs, and traditions that in turn influence its behavior. It is a means to learn about people by learning from people (Roper & Shapira, 2000). The process of ethnography is inductive because there are no predicted outcomes, only an interest in gaining insights into the values and beliefs of a specific culture (Morse, 1991).

Culture is the central concept of ethnography, and its definition requires exploration. In 1960, Leininger, a nurse anthropologist, defined culture as "the learned and shared beliefs, values, and lifeways of a designated or particular group that are generally transmitted intergenerationally and influence one's thinking and action modes" (Leininger & McFarland, 2002, p. 9). Culture is found in any group of people, including those in a classroom, a hospital unit, or a religious ceremony, and it is not limited to an indigenous community traditionally studied by ethnographers. The culture under study in this research is Ghanaian nurse–midwives in intrapartum practice settings. It is an assumption of ethnography that a group of humans situated together for a length of time will develop a culture (Patton, 1989).

Roper and Shapira (2000) stress the importance of taking a holistic perspective of a culture to come to an understanding of the complexity of the community of people. They also conclude that it is imperative for the researcher to place all the information gathered in context to the larger perspective. In other words, how the people behave, the relationships that are formed, and the events they attend need to be analyzed with consideration and understanding of the people's meanings, beliefs, and historic influences. Consistent with all qualitative methods, it is assumed that multiple realities based on the context of one's life exist and there is no single truth (Mayan, 2007).

Focused Ethnography

Focused ethnography has the same core characteristics as a traditional ethnography but is completed in a shorter timeframe. To achieve this, a specific problem is identified and a research question is formulated prior to entering the field (Roper & Shapira, 2000).

When questions requiring an ethnographic approach are asked by nurses, it is common to choose *focused ethnography* (Roper & Shapira, 2000). Nurses are natural ethnographers in that there are parallels between the research methodology and the nursing process. Nurses need to have excellent assessment skills in their practice and gather information through dialogue and observation. The result of a focused ethnography in nursing is expected to have a useful and practical application for the healthcare professionals, particularly nurses (Meucke, 1994). The goal of all ethnographic research is to gain an "emic insight," that is, to understand from the point of view of insiders why people do what they do or believe what they do (Roper & Shapira, 2000, p. 9).

A focused ethnography is appropriate to address the research purpose of describing the influences that facilitate or create barriers to the effective use of the partograph by healthcare providers, specifically nurse–midwives in a low-income West African country where maternal mortality rates are high. Insights with respect to the context in which the partograph is utilized will be described.

Setting

Ghana is a low-income country situated in West Africa with a population of more than 22 million people (WHO, 2007). Ghana has been an independent republic since 1957 and is the most politically stable country in West Africa (Ghana Information Services Department, 1994). The health system in Ghana is in a state of change. A form of national health insurance was implemented in 2006, but the majority of Ghanaians do not have insurance for their health care. Similar to other low-income nations, there is a lack of available human resources to work within the healthcare system. In 2007, only 0.15 physicians and 0.91 nurses were available for every 1000 people in Ghana (WHO, 2007).

Sample

In ethnographic research, it is important to identify key informants and gatekeepers to gain access to the community (Creswell, 1998). A key informant is an individual who can provide useful insights into the group and can provide guidance and names of individuals to contact. I have identified two key informants for my proposed research, Florence Gans-Lartey and Dr. Beverley O'Brien. Ms. Gans-Lartey is the researcher who conducted the previous study on the use of the partograph in Ghana. She is a nurse–midwife who can introduce me to the key contacts at the hospital where my proposed research will occur. Dr. Beverley O'Brien is a professor on the faculty of nursing at the University of Alberta. She has an established relationship with the nursing faculty in Ghana, has supervised Florence Gans-Lartey, and has traveled to Ghana numerous times. I have established contact with both key informants. Gatekeepers can control access to the research site (Hodgson, 2001). Ms. Gans-Lartey has agreed to support me while in Ghana and introduce me to those who could potentially facilitate data collection.

In qualitative research the sample size must be large enough to identify themes and concepts within the data (Burns & Grove, 2007). The focus of qualitative methods is a phenomenon or event rather than a person, so the emphasis is on the quality of data obtained from carefully selected participants rather than the number of participants (Sandelowski, 1995). It is necessary to collect data until saturation occurs, that is, until no new themes or concepts emerge from the data (Gagliari, 1991, as cited in Roper & Shapira, 2000). Focused ethnographers typically recruit smaller samples than do traditional ethnographers.

The initial recruitment for the proposed study will be initiated with the help of the key informants, including Ms. Gans-Lartey. Posters will be placed on the unit in the study site to recruit nurse–midwives for the formal interviews. Initially, volunteers will be interviewed and it is hoped that will result in a snowballing technique to recruit the sample in a purposeful way (Roper & Shapira, 2000). It may be possible that, consistent with focused ethnography design, individuals other than nurse–midwives, such as students, physicians, or nurse–midwives from other health clinics, may participate if it is deemed that they are able to provide important insights that will increase understanding of the phenomenon. These individuals will be invited to participate in the interviews only if they approach the principal investigator either directly or express interest to a neutral person on the unit. My focus sample is the nurse–midwives, but I acknowledge that other people may have information that can enhance my research.

The sample size cannot be determined a priori in qualitative studies, but it is usually about eight to ten individual interviews to be included in a master's thesis. All participants will be given oral and written information about the study (see Exhibit B-1), and only those who sign an informed consent form, which will be signed by both myself and the participant, will be interviewed (see Exhibit B-2). All nurses who express interest will be eligible to participate, and I will collect demographic information, such as age range and number of years in practice.

Data Collection

Three data collection strategies are employed by ethnographers: participant observation, formal interviews, and examination of documents. Participant observation is regarded as central to ethnography and can range from complete observer to complete participant (Roper & Shapira, 2000). In this proposed research, I will be a complete observer and not a participant on the obstetrical unit. This is partially due to time constraints but is also related to the legalities to which I, as a nurse, can participate in the care of patients in another country. My role will be that of a researcher rather than a clinical nurse. An idea associated with participant observation is that an individual's actions probably tell more than their verbal accounts (Oliffe, 2005). It is imperative in ethnography to understand the observations within the context in which they occur and to not make assumptions that can discredit the data (Oliffe, 2005).

Ethnographers observe situations as they occur in the natural setting. I will initially observe clinical settings before focusing on selective observations. The exploratory phase allows the researcher to immerse herself into the setting and to observe the whole picture (Roper & Shapira, 2000). It also provides an opportunity for participants to become used to my presence in the research setting. I will be able to gain understanding on how the unit is organized and observe the nurse–midwives at work.

The selective observation period will allow me to observe the partograph in context. Because I will be in the field for a limited period of time, I plan to develop a checklist to use as a guide in the field to capture the activities related to the partograph. A checklist was identified by Roper & Shapira (2000) as a way to "capture behaviors and events systemically" (p. 71). The data collected during the exploratory phase will help direct the information necessary to include on the checklist. I anticipate some aspects of the checklist will include when the nurse–midwives chart on the partograph, how often they chart, the location of the partograph, how long after the alert line is crossed that an action is taken, and the resources that are available to the nurse–midwives. This checklist will be revised in the field as new knowledge is gained through interviews and through continued observation.

Field notes will be taken during both the exploratory and selective observations. Field notes are a written documentation of the events the researcher observed, conversations with and among people, interpretations for further questioning, and emotions that were felt (Roper & Shapira, 2000). I will follow the technique presented by Roper & Shapira (2000), where I will keep a notebook to record my observations and I will divide each page in half. On the left-hand side I will record the observed events as they occur, and the on right-hand side I will record my interpretations and comments.

To document conversations, I will place conversations in which I have direct recall in quotation marks, I will use apostrophes when paraphrasing, and I will not use any marks when I have a fair recall of the conversation (Strauss & Corbin, 1990). This will maintain the accuracy of the data and will be important for analysis. All entries will be identified by location, date, and time. When I am unable to complete full field notes, I will write partial notes and complete them as soon as possible following the event or conversation. Koch (1994) found that if she did not complete her notes daily, she was unable to accurately recall the event, which decreased the rigor in which the data were reported.

There are challenges to be addressed with participant observation. The presence of the researcher may affect the behaviors that are being observed (Creswell, 1998). For example, there is a potential to disrupt nursing care as well as make the nurses feel judged (Field, 1989). To address this challenge, it is recommended that the researcher spend time in the study setting before initiating the data collection. I will spend approximately two weeks getting to know the country of Ghana, the setting, and the nurses. The selection observation will follow this period of time and will occur for approximately one week. Therefore, it is not until three weeks into the process that I will begin to collect specific observation and interview information. I hope that this time will allow the nurses to become accustomed to my presence and to conduct their work normally, as if I were not present.

Another form of data collection that will be utilized for the proposed research is the interview. Semistructured interviews with open-ended questions will be conducted. It is anticipated that the interviews will last up to one hour. McCracken (1988), as cited in Oliffe (2005), states that the interview "is one of the most powerful qualitative methods which takes the ethnographer into the world of the participant and allows him/her to see the content and patterns of daily experience" (p. 397). Open-ended questions are utilized when the researcher wants participants to answer in their own words, and an interview guide ensures that specific content will be addressed (Burns & Grove, 2007). The questions that are initially formulated will continually be refined as new data are collected through observation and dialogue (see Exhibit B-3).

To conduct the interview I will utilize a constructivist approach, which is appropriate for ethnographic research. The notion is that the researcher and the participant are cocreating knowledge by engaging in a conversation. Therefore, knowledge is constructed, and both the researcher and the participant are changed from the interview (Mayan, 2007).

It is important that the interview occurs in a safe, private, comfortable, and mutually agreed upon location. If the nurse–midwife does not wish to discuss the partograph at her place of work, we will establish a private location, at her convenience, where we will not be seen or overheard. I will seek the assistance of Florence to establish such an interview location after I am in Ghana. The interviews will be audiotaped and transcribed. I will seek the assistance of a transcriber if my key informant is able to recommend an individual who is capable and willing to assist me in transcribing the interviews. I will ensure that this person does not have a conflict of interest prior to his or her commencement on the research and will sign a confidentiality agreement. If there is no such person available, I will transcribe the audiotapes myself.

The last method of data collection that I will use is an examination of related documents. I plan to read the educational materials on the partograph that are available to the nurse–midwives on the unit. I will also seek information on the obstetrical curriculum, including the partograph, taught to undergraduate nursing and midwifery students. I will read the hospital and unit policies on labor management and the use of the partograph, if available. I plan to examine partographs that are on the unit during the observation period. The purpose is so I can better understand the charting on the partograph and have an understanding of the information available to the nurse–midwives.

Data Analysis

A large amount of data will be collected from observations, interviews, and documents. The important aspect of analysis for ethnographers is to organize and understand the data during the research process because the analysis is driven by the data (Roper & Shapira, 2000). It is a continuous experience of gathering and analyzing data as opposed to collecting all the data and then analyzing it at a later time. I will follow the analytic techniques identified by Roper & Shapira (2000): coding the field notes, sorting to identify patterns, generalizing constructs and theories, and memoing to note personal reflections (p. 93). It is important to remember that this is not a linear process but rather an iterative process. The techniques can occur concurrently. I will analyze the data without the use of computer software.

Coding the data involves assigning broad descriptive labels to segments of words or sentences (Miles & Huberman, 1994). I will use the data I collect by interview, observation, and personal field notes to direct the labels I need to create. I will underline keywords in the data and identify in the margins any repeated terms I observe, which in turn will become my codes.

I will then place the descriptive labels into groups to sort for patterns in the data. At this point I may develop an initial understanding of the connections between the data I have collected, which then can direct the remaining observations and interviews (Roper & Shapira, 2000). It is important to identify outliers in the data, or any information that does not fit with the rest of the data. If this is present in the data, I will use them to "test the rest of the data" because they may enhance the analysis and create a better explanation of the findings (Miles & Huberman, 1994, p. 269).

I will also record any reflective insights I have about the data, which Roper & Shapira (2000) refer to as "memoing" (p. 101). These memos may be questions or ideas that can lead to theoretical understandings (Miles & Huberman, 1994). It is important to distinguish these notes from the data so they are not placed in the text by mistake. I will organize my analysis by highlighting keywords in the text, writing patterns in the left margin, and recording reflections with a different color pen. This reflective analysis occurs at all stages of the research process and will be included in my field notes.

Rigor

Because participants are studied in their natural environment, it is important that the researcher ensures that participants are sharing the truth about their everyday activities (Roper & Shapira, 2000). I will spend time at the hospital with the participants, which will enhance my understanding of what actually occurs at the study setting. Participants may initially respond with the correct answer, but my presence over time will allow me to assess the accuracy of their responses and my analysis (Roper & Shapira, 2000). I will confirm the information I gather during the observation period with the participants in the formal interviews. I will also use the information gathered from the documents in both my observations and interviews. This will allow for triangulation, which enhances the rigor of the research. I will begin conducting the interviews approximately three weeks after I have begun the observation process.

The data collection method needs to be transparent in that the same or different researchers could replicate the method (Burns & Grove, 2007). The systematic process of ethnography fosters this type of reliability because the researcher has the opportunity to observe many events and to repeat interviews with participants, which increases the chance that the views of the group are represented (LeCompte & Goetz, 1982). To ensure interrater reliability, I will provide my supervisor, Dr. Beverley O'Brien, with the interview transcripts to confirm that she would categorize the data in a similar manner.

Other strategies I will incorporate into my research process to ensure rigor include both an audit trail and maintaining a journal. An audit trail is the record of the study that includes the details of the data analysis and information on how the researcher came to understand the findings in the results section (Wolf, 2003). It allows the auditor to locate the raw data that lead to interpretations in the analysis and vice versa. All decisions made during the research process for this study will be documented. The audit trail will help to establish credibility and ensure rigor within this qualitative study. I will send emerging codes and examples to my supervisor as I develop them so that she is able to ask questions and confirm the effectiveness of my audit trail.

The concept of reflexivity is instrumental in ethnography and also helps to achieve rigor within the research. Reflexivity infers that the researcher requires an awareness of how she affects both the research process and the outcomes (Pellatt, 2002). The researcher and the research are not separate identities because it is impossible for the researcher to put her own knowledge of the world aside to obtain objectivity (Pellatt, 2002). To obtain reflexivity, I will maintain a reflective journal, which will be different from my field notes and will be kept private. In this journal I will attempt to record a continuous self-critique by examining my thoughts and emotions to understand the impact my beliefs, interests, and values have had on the research (Mulhall, 1997). I will also identify any preconceived ideas and biases I have regarding Ghanaian nurse–midwives. This acknowledgement and personal awareness will help to enhance the rigor of the research.

Ethical Issues

The Health Review Ethics Board at the University of Alberta and the ethical review committee at the hospital where the research will be conducted will approve the proposed study prior to the commencement of data collection. There are several important ethical considerations. The first issue is the notion of *insider* versus *outsider* role, and the fact that I am not Ghanaian will separate me from the culture of the unit. I will work closely with the Ghanaians to understand their perceptions and beliefs. There is also the potential for the nurse researcher to experience role conflict (Baillie, 1995). Conflict can occur when incorrect nursing practice is observed or when the unit is short staffed and the researcher experiences guilt for not helping in the care of patients (Robertson & Boyle, 1984). Nurse researchers have a tendency to go into worker mode (Morse & Lipson, 1989). I am a registered nurse with labor and delivery experience, and I will conduct research in a different setting but within a clinical area that is familiar to me. I will be in the researcher rather than the nurse *role* while conducting this study. The dilemma occurs when these two roles are confused and the nurse researcher feels a need to advocate on a patient's behalf (Roper & Shapira, 2000).

The participants are nurse–midwives and not patients; however, my only role is to examine the partograph in its use. I will observe practice on the unit, and I may witness a situation that puts a patient at risk or be asked to participate in the care of a laboring woman during an emergency. I am then put in a situation to question my obligation and professional integrity. I will clearly define my role as nurse researcher and not participate in any clinical care. It is important to maintain a balance and to understand the role one has as a researcher to maintain the "scientific integrity of the study as well as the immediate safety of patients" (Baillie, 1995, p. 15). I will not be registered as a nurse in Ghana and thus not licensed to practice. It would be inappropriate to intervene in a professional nursing role.

Within the initial exploratory phase of observation, I will observe the nurse–midwives use of the partograph and gather information on the resources available on the unit. The partographs may be located in patients' rooms, and as a result I may overtly observe patient care. I will explain to the patient that I am a researcher working with the nurse and that I am not involved in her care. I will ensure privacy and confidentiality to the patient by not recording any identifiable information because it is not the intention of the research to focus on the laboring women.

Privacy for the participants is another issue to be addressed in the study. I will not name specific nurses during the observation period. However, I will meet with individual nurses who volunteer for the interviews. I will not use names but rather assign each nurse a number and keep the list of participants confidential. The interview will be held in a private location. All of my field notes, interview tapes, and transcriptions will be kept off-site in a locked cabinet at my accommodation, and I will have the key in my possession at all times. I will keep the consent forms in a sealed envelope separate from the data in a locked cabinet. Upon completion of the research, the data will be transported back to the University of Alberta in Edmonton, where it will be locked in a secure location for a total of seven years, when at that time the data will be destroyed.

The nurses who participate in the interviews will be given an honorarium at the end of the session. I will discuss what is appropriate to give the nurse–midwives with Ms. Gans-Lartey upon arrival in Ghana to ensure that the honorarium does not influence or coerce the participants in any way. The honorarium is given to thank the nurse–midwives for taking the time to commit to my project and share their knowledge.

Safety for myself, the researcher, is an ethical concern within this study. I will be in a setting that is unfamiliar to me in an area where I do not know many people. Upon arrival to Ghana I will register with the Canadian High Commission and provide them with updates on my location. I will maintain close contact with both of my key informants and with the other nursing graduate student from the University of Alberta, who will be in Ghana at the same time. If I need to conduct an interview away from the hospital, I will ensure someone knows the location and time-frame of the interview. I will have a cell phone with me at all times, both for safety reasons and to allow participants to contact me.

Dissemination–Knowledge Transfer Strategies

It is important to disseminate the knowledge obtained from the research back to the participants in the study. I will give a presentation to the unit on the preliminary results before I leave Ghana so the nurse–midwives have immediate feedback on my research. When the thesis is completed, I will prepare a report to be given to the hospital where the research is conducted. I will write a scholarly paper on what factors influence the use of the partograph and plan to publish the results in a nursing journal.

References

AbouZahr, C. (2003). Safe motherhood: A brief history of the global movement 1947–2002. *British Medical Journal, 67,* 13–25.

Arrowsmith, S., Hamlin, C., & Wall, L. (1996). Obstructed labour injury complex: Obstetric fistula formation and the multifaceted morbidity of maternal birth trauma in the developing world. *Obstetrics and Gynecology, 51,* 568–574.

Baillie, L. (1995). Ethnography and nursing research: A critical appraisal. *Nurse Researcher, 3,* 5–21.

Bosse, G., Massawe, S., & Jahn, A. (2002). The partograph in daily practice: It's quality that matters. *International Journal of Gynaecology & Obstetrics, 77,* 243–244.

Burns, N., & Grove, S. (2007). *Understanding nursing research: Building an evidence-based practice* (4th ed.). St. Louis, MO: Saunders.

Cartmill, R., & Thornton, J. (1992). Effect of presentation of partogram information on obstetric decision-making (see comment). *Lancet, 339,* 1520–1522.

Chalmers, B., Mangiaterra, V., & Porter, R. (2001). WHO principles of perinatal care: The essential antenatal, perinatal, and postpartum care course. *Birth, 28,* 202–207.

Creswell, J. (1998). *Qualitative inquiry and research design: Choosing among five traditions.* Thousand Oaks, CA: Sage.

Dangal, D. (2007). Preventing prolonged labor by using the partograph. *The Internet Journal of Gynecology and Obstetrics, 7*(1).

Field, P. (1989). Doing fieldwork in your own culture. In J. Morse (Ed.), *Qualitative nursing research: A contemporary dialogue.* Newbury Park, CA: Sage.

Filippi, V., Ronsmans, C., Campbell, O., Graham, W., Mills, A., & Borghi, J., et al. (2006). Maternal health in poor countries: The broader context and a call for action. *The Lancet, 368*(9546), 1535–1541.

Gagliari, B. (1991). The family's experience living with a child with Duchenne muscular dystrophy. *Applied Nursing Research, 4*(4), 159–164.

Gans-Lartey, F. (2006). *Relationship between the use of the WHO partogram and maternal/newborn outcomes.* Unpublished M'Phil thesis, University of Ghana, Legon, Ghana.

Ghana Information Services Department. (1994). *Ghana—a brief guide.* Accra, Ghana: Author.

Govindaraj, R., Obuobi, A., Enjimayew, N., Antwi, P., & Ofosu-Amaah, S. (1996). *Hospital autonomy in Ghana: The experience of Korle Bu and*

Komfu Anokye teaching hospitals. Accra, Ghana: School of Public Health, University of Ghana and Harvard School of Public Health.

Groeschel, N., & Glover, P. (2001). The partograph. Used daily but rarely questioned. *Australian Journal of Midwifery, 14,* 22–26.

Hammersley, M., & Atkinson, P. (1995). *Ethnography: Principles in practice* (2nd ed.). London: Routledge.

Health Canada. (2004). *Special report on maternal mortality and severe morbidity in Canada.* Ottawa, Ontario: Author.

Hodgson, I. (2001). Engaging in cultures: Reflections on entering the ethnographic field. *Nurse Researcher, 9*(1), 41–51.

Hofmeyr, G. (2004). Obstructed labour: Using better technologies to reduce mortality. *International Journal of Gynaecology & Obstetrics, 85*(Suppl. 1), S62–S72.

Koblinsky, M., Matthews, Z., Hussein, J., Mavalankar, M., Anwar, I., Achadi, E., et al. (2006). Maternal survival 3: Going to scale with professional skilled care. *The Lancet, 368*(9544), 1377–1386.

Koch, T. (1994). Establishing rigor in qualitative research: The decision trail. *Journal of Advanced Nursing, 19,* 976–986.

Lavender, T., & Malcolmson, L. (1999). Is the partogram a help or a hindrance? An exploratory study of midwives' views. *The Practising Midwife, 2*(8), 23–27.

LeCompte, M., & Goetz, J. (1982). Problems of reliability and validity in ethnographic research. *Review of Educational Research, 52*(1), 31–60.

Leininger, M., & McFarland, M. (2002). *Transcultural nursing: Concepts, theories, research and practice* (3rd ed.). New York: McGraw-Hill.

Liston, R., & Crane, J. (2002). *Fetal health surveillance in labour.* Ottawa, Ontario, Canada: Society of Obstetricians and Gynaecologists.

Maimbolwa, M., Ransjo-Arvidson, A., Ng'andu, N., Sikazwe, N., & Diwan, V. (1997). Routine care of women experiencing normal deliveries in Zambian maternity wards: A pilot study. *Midwifery, 13*(3), 125–131.

Mayan, M. (2007). Unpublished class PowerPoint presentation, INTD 560, University of Alberta, Canada.

McCracken, G. (1988). *The long interview.* Newbury Park, CA: Sage.

Meuke, M. (1994). On evaluation of ethnographies. In J. Morse (Ed.), *Critical issues in qualitative research methods* (pp. 187–209). Thousand Oaks, CA: Sage.

Miles, M., & Huberman, A. (1994). *An expanded sourcebook: Qualitative data analysis.* Thousand Oaks, CA: Sage.

Morse, J. (1991). Editorial: Evaluation of qualitative proposals. *Qualitative Health Research, 1,* 147–151.

Morse, J., & Lipson, J. (1989). Dialogue. In J. Morse (Ed.), *Qualitative nursing research.* Newbury Park, CA: Sage.

Mulhall, A. (1997). Nursing research: Our world not theirs? *Journal of Advanced Nursing, 25,* 969–976.

Nkyekyer, K. (2000). Peripartum referrals to Korle Bu teaching hospital, Ghana—a descriptive study. *Tropical Medicine & International Health, 5*(11), 811–817.

Obaid, T. (2007). No woman should die giving birth. *Lancet, 370,* 1287–1288.

Oladapo, O., Daniel, O., & Olatunji, A. (2006). Knowledge and use of the partograph among healthcare personnel at the peripheral maternity centres in Nigeria. *Journal of Obstetrics & Gynaecology, 26,* 538–541.

Oliffe, J. (2005). Why not ethnography. *Urologic Nursing, 25*(5), 395–399.

Patton, M. (1989). *Qualitative evaluation and research methods* (2nd ed.). Newbury Park, CA: Sage.

Pellatt, J. (2002). Ethnography and reflexivity: Emotions and feelings in fieldwork. *Nurse Researcher, 10*(3), 28–36.

Pettersson, K., Svensson, M., & Christensson, K. (2001). Evaluation of an adapted model of the World Health Organization partograph used by Angolan midwives in a peripheral delivery unit. *Midwifery, 16,* 82–88.

Philpott, R., & Castle, W. (1972). Cervicographs in the management of labour in primigravidae. *Journal of Obstetrics and Gynaecology of the British Commonwealth, 79,* 592–602.

Riley, R., & Manias, E. (2003). Snap-shots of live theatre: The use of photography to research governance in operating room nursing. *Nursing Inquiry, 10,* 81–90.

Robertson, M., & Boyle, J. (1984). Ethnography: Contributions to nursing research. *Journal of Advanced Nursing, 9,* 43–49.

Ronsmans, C., & Graham, W. (2006). Maternal mortality: Who, when, where, and why. *Lancet, 368*(9542), 1189–1200.

Roper, J., & Shapira, J. (2000). *Ethnography in nursing research.* Thousand Oaks, CA: Sage.

Sandelowski, M. (1995). Sample size in qualitative research. *Research in Nursing & Health, 18*(2), 179–183.

Seffah, J. (2003). Ruptured uterus and the partograph. *International Journal of Gynaecology & Obstetrics, 80*(2), 169–170.

Smith, F. (2002). Reflections on healthcare in Ghana. *The Pharmaceutical Journal, 268,* 278.

Strauss, A., & Corbin, J. (1990). *Basics of qualitative research: Grounded theory procedures and techniques.* Newbury Park, CA: Sage.

Studd, J. (1973). Partograms and nomograms of cervical dilatation in the management of primigravid labour. *British Medical Journal, 4*, 451–455.

Umezulike, A., Onah, H., & Okaro, J. (1999). Use of the partograph among medical personnel in Enugu, Nigeria. *International Journal of Gynaecology & Obstetrics, 65*(2), 203–205.

United Nations. (2006). *Millennium development goals report.* New York: Author.

Wacker, J., Kyelem, D., Bastert, G., Utz, B., & Lankoande, J. (1998). Introduction of a simplified round partogram in rural maternity units: Seno province, Burkina Faso, West-Africa. *Tropical Doctor, 28*(3), 146–152.

Wolf, Z. (2003). Exploring the audit trail for qualitative investigations. *Nurse Educator, 28*(4), 175–178.

World Health Organization. (1994a). Partograph in management of labour. *Lancet, 343*(8910), 1399–1404.

World Health Organization. (1994b). *Preventing prolonged labour: A practical guide. The partograph.* Geneva, Switzerland: Author.

World Health Organization. (2004). *Maternal mortality in 2000: Estimates developed by WHO, UNICEF, UNFPA.* Geneva, Switzerland: Author.

World Health Organization. (2005). *Make every mother and child count.* Geneva, Switzerland: Author.

World Health Organization. (2007a). *Ghana country profile.* Geneva, Switzerland: Author.

World Health Organization. (2007b). *Maternal mortality in 2005.* Geneva, Switzerland: Author.

Yinger, N. (2007). *Women deliver for development: Executive summary.* Retrieved from http://www.womendeliver.org/assets/Executive_Summary_English.pdf

EXHIBIT B-1
Information Letter

Title of Research Study

Attitudes and beliefs of Ghanaian nurse–midwives about the partograph

Principal Investigator

Leanne Fontanie, RN, BSN, MN candidate

Coinvestigator

Beverley O'Brien, RN, RM, PhD

Background

The partograph is used in many countries to monitor a woman's progress throughout labor. It is also used to monitor the well-being of a woman and her fetus. The partograph is used more in some countries than others. I want to learn more about how nurses and midwives in Ghana feel about it.

Purpose

You are being asked to be in a study to talk about your experience with the partograph, including what you like and what you don't like about it.

Procedure

If you decide to take part in this study, you will meet with the researcher, Leanne Fontanie. You will be asked to talk about the partograph and about how important you feel it is for your practice. The talk will not last for more than one hour. What you say will be tape-recorded so that later everything you say will be remembered. You can request at any time that the tape recorder be turned off. No one else will know what you say or even if you decided to take part in the study. We can meet in a private room in the hospital or somewhere near the hospital that is convenient for both of us.

Possible Benefits

Another possible benefit is that it is an opportunity to share your partograph experiences with others who may be able to recommend changes to fix problems that you identify.

Possible Risks

There are no known risks to being in the study.

Confidentiality

No one will know what you say or even if you decided to be in the study. Your name will not be linked to the information you share during the talk. It is possible that the study will be published in a journal. Leanne Fontanie will present what she learns to the nurses on the unit, but you will not be identified by name. What you say could be used in a future study. That can only happen if the appropriate ethics committee approves.

Voluntary Participation

You do not have to be in the study unless you want to be in it. You can stop being in the study at any time just by telling the researcher.

Reimbursement of Expenses

You will be given money to pay for your travel expenses and your time.

Contact Names and Telephone Numbers

If you have concerns about your rights as a study participant, you may contact:

Director
The Research and Development Office
Hospital where the research will occur
Contact name and number will be made available when in Ghana.

Please contact the following individuals if you have any questions or concerns. Contact Leanne Fontanie if you wish to participate in this study:

Dr. Beverley O'Brien
Mentor: Florence Gans-Lartey

EXHIBIT B-2
Consent Form for Participants

Title of Project: Attitudes and beliefs of Ghanaian nurse–midwives about the partograph

Principal Investigator: Leanne Fontanie
     Phone Number: Will be made available upon arrival in Ghana
Coinvestigator: Beverley O'Brien
     Phone Number: XXX-XXX-XXXX
Mentor (on-site): Florence Gans-Lartey
     Phone Number: XXX-XXX-XXXX

	Yes	No
Do you understand that you have been asked to be in a research study?	❑	❑
Have you read and received a copy of the attached Information Letter?	❑	❑
Do you understand the benefits and risks involved in taking part in this research study?	❑	❑
Have you had an opportunity to ask questions and discuss this study?	❑	❑
Do you understand that you are free to withdraw from the study at any time, without having to give a reason?	❑	❑
Has the issue of confidentiality been explained to you?	❑	❑
Do you understand who will have access to the information?	❑	❑
Do you understand that all records of the research will be kept for at least seven years in a locked cabinet at the University of Alberta in Edmonton, Canada?	❑	❑

This study was explained to me by: _____

I agree to take part in this study:

Yes ❑　No ❑

I agree that information from this interview can be used for secondary analysis if the appropriate ethics committee approves:

Yes ❑　No ❑

Signature of Research Subject: _____

Printed Name: _____

Date: _____

I believe that the person signing this form understands what is involved in the study and voluntarily agrees to participate.

Signature of Investigator or Designee: _____

Date: _____

The Information Letter must be attached to this consent form and a copy given to the research subject.

EXHIBIT B-3
Semistructured Interview Guide

Note: This guide will be revised during the observation period and initial interviews.

Tell me about your experience with the partograph.

Prompts:

What do you find helpful about the partograph? What do you find not helpful about using the partograph?

What can be done to make the partograph more useful for you?

Tell me about a time when the partograph made a difference in the outcome or care you were giving to a laboring patient. Can you think of a time when it did not make a difference?

Has your perception of the partograph changed since you first began to use it?

Who should use the partograph? How does the partograph influence decisions you make about the care needed by women in labor?

The Incidence of Acute Stress Disorder Among Parents of Premature Infants Admitted into the Neonatal Intensive Care Unit

By Jocelyn M. Jubinville

Introduction

Statement of the Problem

The experience of premature birth and subsequent admission into the neonatal intensive care unit (NICU) environment is considered to be a stressful, even traumatic event for parents. After the birth of a premature infant, parents are thrown into a world of the unknown. The NICU is a world where every beep and every light seems significant because parents may not understand the alarms and what they mean for their infant. Parental dreams of a perfect term infant are superseded by images of a tiny infant connected to wires, tubes, and machines. Physical separation from the infant occurs immediately after birth, and parental role adjustments have to be made because of their inability to hold or to provide care to their infant. Feelings of parental stress, detachment, helplessness, and increased anxiety are common (Miles, Funk, & Kasper, 1991). The time following the birth of a premature infant is a time clouded with parental uncertainty and most often one where the parents had little or no time to prepare. There are uncertainties regarding parental expectations after birth, such as the appearance and behavior of the infant and severity of illness. Uncertainties and fear of potential loss may contribute to feelings of stress for parents.

It has been proposed that the stress of premature birth can be defined as a traumatic stressor, one capable of having short-term and long-term effects on the emotional well-being of parents (Affleck & Tennen, 1991; Holditch-Davis, Bartlett, Blickman, & Miles, 2003; Kersting, et al., 2004; Peebles-Kleiger, 2000; Shaw, et al., 2006; Singer, et al., 1999). Barriers to parenting and emotional reactions to the environment may negatively influence the parent–infant relationship and the infant's developmental outcome (Affleck & Tennen, 1991). Extended emotional and psychological stress and postponement of parenting have been found to decrease emotional attachment to the infant (Shaw, et al., 2006). Symptoms of posttraumatic stress have been found in parents of premature infants immediately after discharge and in the months following discharge (Holditch-Davis, et al., 2003; Kersting, et al., 2004; Singer, et al., 1999). Symptoms of posttraumatic stress in parents have been associated with increased parental perception of stress from the NICU (Holditch-Davis, et al., 2003). Negative parental response to premature birth leading to posttraumatic stress symptoms has implications with regard to transition to parenthood and parental competency, which could have direct and indirect effects on the child later on in life (Pierrehumbert, Nicole, Muller-Nix, Forcada-Guex, & Ansermet, 2003).

It is proposed that stress symptoms typically emerge early in the NICU experience and can lead to the development of acute stress disorder (ASD). Shaw and associates (2006) performed one of the first studies describing evidence of ASD symptoms in parents of NICU infants. This retrospective study included all infants admitted to NICU and did not separate stress related to NICU admission from stress related to being parents of a premature baby. No previous literature has examined the impact of gestational age as a predictor of ASD. Parents of premature infants, regardless of gestational age, may be at risk for ASD symptoms; however, due to resources and time issues, this study will focus on parents of infants born less than 33 weeks gestational age.

Purpose of the Study

The overall purpose of this study is to determine if parents of premature infants within the study population have symptoms of ASD.

Study Objectives

The specific objectives of this study are (1) to measure the incidence rate of ASD among parents of premature infants admitted to the NICU; (2) to describe the symptom profiles of acute stress in mothers and in fathers of premature infants; (3) to examine the number and severity of

ASD symptoms from each of the following categories: intrusion, avoidance, hyperarousal, and dissociation; (4) to determine if the number of ASD symptoms reported in the first seven to ten days after birth (Time 1) diminish or persist one month following birth (Time 2); (5) to determine which factors are independently associated with the total SASRQ score; and (6) to determine the factors that may increase the risk of ASD among parents of premature infants admitted to the NICU.

Definition of Terms

For the purpose of this study, the following terms are defined as indicated:

Acute stress disorder (ASD): Experience or witnessing of an event that has been threatening to oneself or another person which involves a reaction of intense fear, helplessness, or horror. The response leads to the development of characteristic anxiety, dissociation, and other symptoms that occur during the period of time of 48 hours to 28 days posttrauma (Bryant & Harvey, 2000).

Posttraumatic stress disorder (PTSD): Experiencing of a serious threat to the physical integrity of self or others, which involves a reaction involving intense fear, helplessness, or horror with resulting characteristic symptoms present for greater than one month posttrauma (American Psychiatric Association, 2000).

Stress: A process in which environmental demands or experiences exceed the capacity of an individual to adapt, resulting in psychological and biological responses that may place an individual at risk for disease (Cohen, Kessler, & Gordon, 1997).

Stressor: A demand or experience that leads to a stress response.

Significance of the Study

Previous research has repeatedly shown that the birth of a premature infant and the many aspects of the experience creates parental stress, and in many cases extreme distress (DeMier, et al., 2000; DeMier, Hynan, Harris, & Manniello, 1996; Feldman Reichman, Miller, Gordon, & Hendricks-Munoz, 2000; Franck, Cox, Allen, & Winter, 2005; Jackson, Ternestedt, & Schollin, 2003; Miles, Carlson, & Funk, 1996; Miles, et al.,1991; Miles, Funk, & Kasper, 1992; Perehudoff, 1990; Reid & Bramwell, 2003; Shaw, et al., 2006; Singer, Davillier, Bruening, Hawkins, & Yamashita, 1996; Singer, et al., 1999; Spear, Leef, Epps, & Locke, 2002; Thomas, Renaud, & DePaul, 2004; Young

Seideman, Watson, Corff, Odle, Haase, & Bowerman, 1997). The psychological distress has been shown to persist in mothers of preterm infants even one year after delivery (Garel, Dardennes, & Blondel, 2006).

The birth of a premature infant is a potentially life-threatening event and has been defined as a traumatic stressor (Peebles-Kleiger, 2000). Feelings of anxiety, helplessness, and psychological distress are common in parents, which negatively impacts the parent–infant relationship (Jackson, et al., 2003) and impacts the infant's developmental outcome (Affleck & Tennen, 1991). Many of the symptoms reported by parents in the studies on parental stress previously listed are the same symptoms examined within ASD diagnosis. Thus, the emotional distress created by the traumatic event of premature birth and subsequent NICU hospitalization may be understood as an acute stress response. It is important to recognize that the traumatic event of premature birth may lead to the development of symptoms of ASD in parents of these infants. The association of increasing prematurity with higher anxiety and symptoms of depression in parents also substantiates the need to examine symptoms of ASD in parents of premature infants.

The proposed study will provide knowledge of the parental NICU experience and reaction to the birth of a premature infant by measuring the nature and severity of ASD symptoms within the time period defined for ASD by the American Psychiatric Association in the *DSM-IV*. The link between NICU hospitalization and ASD symptoms of parents has been studied very limitedly (Shaw, et al., 2006). To the author's knowledge at present, ASD symptoms have not been studied specifically in parents of premature infants. The identification of the incidence of ASD and the patterns and severity of ASD symptomatology in parents after the birth of a premature infant and subsequent admission to NICU will provide valuable knowledge of the parental experience and reactions to premature birth.

Although controversial, symptoms of ASD have the potential to predict further development of PTSD symptoms (Balluffi, Kassam-Adams, Kazak, Tucker, Dominguez, & Helfaer, 2004; Birmes, et al., 2003; Classen, Koopman, Hales, & Spiegel, 1998; Creamer, O'Donnell, & Pattison, 2004; Diefe, et al., 2002; Elklit & Brink, 2004). This increases the importance and significance of a study of this nature.

Gaining a greater awareness of the stress reactions of parents within the experience of premature birth may facilitate the development of appropriate screening and intervention strategies to assist parents who are at risk for psychological distress and parenting stress after birth.

Literature Review

The experience of giving birth to a preterm infant can be considered a traumatic event for parents. Current research studies are critically examined to provide evidence regarding the impact of the NICU experience on parents. This provides a starting point for grasping the rationale, significance, and gaps found within the literature related to parental stress, anxiety, and role adaptation within the NICU environment. Searching the literature to gain an understanding of parental stress will make evident the parallels of ASD symptoms and the reactions of parents after premature birth. The purpose of this literature review is also to identify, critique, and examine the results of studies on ASD in parents, as well as to explore how ASD is measured.

The key search terms utilized to compile this literature review were *acute stress disorder, premature birth, premature infant, parental stress, NICU environment, neonatal period, neonatal intensive care, pediatrics, pediatric intensive care, depression, parents,* and *posttraumatic stress disorder.* The following databases were explored from the years 1990 to 2007: CINAHL Plus with Full Text, Cochrane Database of Systematic Reviews, EMBASE, Evidence-Based Medicine Reviews (EBMR), Family and Society Studies Worldwide, Gender Studies Database, Health Source, Health & Psychosocial Instruments, Ovid MEDLINE, PubMed, Psychology & Behavioral Sciences Collection, PsycINFO, PsychiatryOnline, Scopus, and Social Work Abstracts. Secondary searches were also performed on the reference lists of potentially relevant literature.

The Parental Experience of Premature Birth

Statistics Canada reported 352,848 births in Canada from 2006 to 2007. Approximately 7.9% of these births can be defined as premature births occurring prior to 37 completed gestational weeks, according to 2004 national preterm birth rate (Statistics Canada, 2004). Advances in the management of high-risk pregnancy have increased the rate of premature birth (Singer, et al., 1999), and it has even been described as a silent epidemic. Medical advances in the NICU, such as assisted ventilation, surfactant therapy, and the increased use of antenatal steroid therapy, have increased survival rates of premature infants (Hack & Fanaroff, 2000). Survival has increased within the limits of viability, which is considered to be 23 to 24 weeks' gestation, contributing to a common occurrence of very low birth weight (VLBW) infants and extremely low birth weight (ELBW) infants within the NICU. The birth of a preterm infant commences a journey of struggle and survival, often described as a roller coaster ride of ups and downs for the infants, parents, and families of this population.

The technological advances within the NICU that are partly responsible for the improved survival rates of premature infants have been shown to affect the parental experience. In a phenomenological study it was found that the technological environment and equipment within the NICU had a negative impact on the experience by all the parents involved (Jamsa & Jamsa, 1998). These findings resulted from questioning parents about their experience within the NICU and the meanings these experiences created for them. Seven parents of full-term infants with unexpected illness and admission into the NICU were interviewed on four occasions prior to discharge and three times in the family home immediately following discharge. The parents considered the NICU environment to be shocking, oppressive, and a factor in their feelings of anxiety. The environment caused the parents to feel like outsiders in their parental role. There was evidence that the NICU environment caused fear and anxiety in parents and interfered with the holistic care of the infant. The importance of providing relevant information to parents to decrease fears was stressed by the researchers. The NICU environment did affect the parents of the term infants in this study. The unexpected admission to the NICU and the illness that precipitated the admission of these term infants played a factor in increasing the parents' feelings of anxiety.

Premature birth begins an often-unexpected journey into parenthood. It is a time of transition not only into parenthood but also into the role of the parent within the NICU environment. The experiences of parenthood over time were examined in a qualitative study by interviewing seven consecutive sets of mothers and fathers of preterm infants (Jackson, et al., 2003). The infants were less than 34 weeks gestation at birth and were defined, prior to enrollment, as having a good chance of survival. The timing of data collection was supported by previous research and occurred at one to two weeks after birth, at the time of discharge, at six months of age, and at 18 months. The phenomenon of parenthood within the NICU and after discharge home was examined. Over the span of data collection and analysis, synthesis of the interview information was verified and validated by a second author.

Being a mother and father was described as a process that changed over time, from feelings of alienation and responsibility to feelings of increased confidence and familiarity. Common themes of parental feelings of alienation, detachment, and ambivalence concerning parenthood and responsibility transpired during the phase that the infant–parent dyad was within the NICU environment. Parents were more likely to report feelings of confidence six months after discharge and familiarity at 18 months. The researchers provided clear conceptualizations of the experiences of mothers and fathers. Mothers reported more ambivalence, concern for the baby, and need to have control of the care of the infant, whereas fathers reported feelings of unreality surrounding the experience, concern for the baby, and wanting to transfer infant care to staff. Both parents reported feelings of responsibility and insecurity surrounding the discharge of their infant. The role of the NICU environment in creating these feelings was found to be an important consideration. Mothers expressed how the NICU environment reduced the possibility of participating in their infant's care, limited their privacy, and led to uncertainty in their maternal role. It is important to acknowledge that the parents were interviewed together, which created a risk of interference with mothers' and fathers' stories. Nevertheless, the qualitative nature of this research provided evidence that the parental experience within the NICU can be an influencing factor on how the experience of parenthood evolves.

Throughout the literature it appears evident that parental stress and anxiety are common reactions to the NICU environment and affect parental adaptation. Parental stress and parental anxiety are interrelated. In a quasi-experimental study, potential stressors were identified within the NICU environment and levels of stress that these experiences engendered were explored (Miles, et al., 1991). A convenience sample of 79 mothers and 43 fathers completed the Parental Stressor Scale: NICU (PSS:NICU) and the State Trait Anxiety Inventory (STAI) so the relationship between NICU environmental stress and parental anxiety levels could be explored. Both instruments had good internal consistency reliability as measured by Cronbach's alpha. Data collection occurred through interviews by trained data collectors following a set protocol.

Overall stress from the NICU environment was found to be low, and specific stress from the sights and sounds of the unit was perceived as low to moderate by the parents. It is important to note that 70% of the sample had prior exposure to intensive care units, which may have led to an underscoring of the perception of stress from the environment by parents. This suggests that exposure may be a potential factor in reducing stress from the NICU environment and one that needs to be further explored. In addition, parents in this study perceived the condition of their infant to be moderate to severe, which may have led to a general feeling of increased stress and anxiety. The appearance of the infant was identified as a moderate source of stress, which is congruent with previous research (Miles, et al., 1991).

Using Pearson's correlation coefficients, statistically significant relationships were found between the total stress and trait-state anxiety scores and between the PSS:NICU and the trait-state anxiety scores. Trait anxiety scores were similar to average adults; therefore, there was no need to separate the high trait anxiety group to control for baseline. State anxiety scores of the parents were similar to anxious adults. It is suggested that the environment of the NICU may be related to anxiety; however, it is plausible that more highly anxious parents view the NICU environment as more stressful. Parental role alterations were also found to be a moderate source of stress for parents. This included parental feelings of helplessness, separation, lack of ability to protect their infant, not knowing how to help their infant, and fear of holding their infant. These findings are consistent with the themes identified in the qualitative research studies described previously, even though the qualitative samples consisted of less ill infants. Clearly, having an infant in the NICU is a stressful time for parents.

Knowledge of parental stress and anxiety and how it is affected by parental role adjustments, by the infant, and by the NICU environment is just the beginning when exploring the nature of the parental experience within the NICU. Research on the psychosocial impact of premature birth is important, given that it has the potential to interfere with parental attachment.

A cohort longitudinal quasi-experimental study was conducted to explore the degree and type of stress experienced by mothers of VLBW infants, born less than 1500 g (Singer, et al., 1999). The intention was to determine if the degree of prematurity and severity of illness affects the degree of parental stress after birth. Three comparison groups consisting of mothers of high-risk VLBW infants with chronic lung disease (mean GA = 27 weeks, SD 2, n = 122), low-risk VLBW infants without chronic lung disease (mean GA = 30 weeks, SD 2, n = 84), and term infants with no medical condition (mean GA = 40 weeks, SD 1, n = 123) were recruited. Demographic homogeneity was found among the three groups. The following scales were used in this study: Brief Symptom Inventory Scale (psychiatric symptoms and patterns), the Parenting Stress Index (PSI, parental perceptions of the degree of stress related to the parenting role), Impact on Family Scale (maternal perceptions of the child's impact on the family), the Family Inventory of Life Events and Changes (to assess other life stressors potentially affecting the family), and the Bayley Scales of Infant Development (to measure infant cognitive development). Throughout the three-year study mothers of high-risk VLBW infants reported higher levels of psychological distress than mothers of low-risk VLBW infants and term infants. Nine percent of mothers in both VLBW groups reported severe symptoms of depression, defined as greater than 98th percentile for female norms. One month after birth, mothers of the high-risk VLBW infant group scored higher on dimensions of psychological distress, anxiety, depression, and obsessive-compulsive behaviors than mothers of term infants and low-risk VLBW infants. This supports the notion that higher infant risk is related to severity of psychological distress. Thirteen percent of mothers in the high- and low-risk VLBW groups reported severe symptoms of overall distress contrasted to 1% of term mothers. The severity of symptoms varied over time. By eight to 12 months after birth there were no differences among the groups, and the scores were within normal ranges, except 20% of mothers of high-risk infants continued to have significant symptoms of anxiety, which was much higher than the other two groups. Also, at two years, the high-risk group mothers were more likely to report symptoms of moderate depression, compared to none of the mothers of low-risk and term groups.

Significantly higher stress levels were evident in mothers of the VLBW high-risk infants as compared to mothers of the term infants. Symptoms of depression, anxiety, and obsessive-compulsive behaviors in mothers were most prominent during the neonatal period. Increased severity of maternal depression was related to decreased child developmental outcomes in the high- and low-risk VLBW infants, with no relationship in the term group. The researchers concluded that the psychosocial impact of VLBW birth on mothers during the neonatal period is significant and varies over time. It was concluded that the stress of premature birth does create psychological reactions and that there is a need to prepare parents for these reactions (Singer, et al., 1999).

Psychological Stress Reactions of Parents to Premature Birth

Studies have consistently shown that premature birth and the resulting admittance into the NICU environment results in a wide diversity of psychological stress reactions and physiological responses in parents. Gender differences seem to exist; however, research is limited. There is a relationship between parental stress and anxiety and the NICU environment, but more specifically, alterations in parental role and aspects of the parent–infant relationship are significantly correlated with increased perceptions of stress and anxiety. Knowledge of specific stress symptoms and associated risk factors will help the health professional to identify psychological stress reactions of parents. This will improve the ability to provide anticipatory guidance and support to parents during the stressful time of premature birth. Understanding of the family and their reactions to the stressful event of NICU hospitalization is important to the provision of family centered care.

The birth of a premature infant leads to many psychological reactions in parents identified within the literature. Feelings of helplessness and anxiety are common symptoms experienced by parents of premature infants (Affonso, et al., 1992; Brooten, et al., 1988; Carter, Mulder, Bartram, & Darlow, 2005; Doering, Dracup, & Moser, 1999; Doering, Moser, & Dracup, 2000; Feldman Reichman, et al., 2000; Franck, et al., 2005; Holditch-Davis, et al., 2003; Jamsa & Jamsa, 1998; Kersting, et al., 2004; Miles, et al., 1991; Miles, et al., 1992; Nystrom & Axelsson, 2002; Padden & Glenn, 1997; Pinelli, 2000; Reid & Bramwell, 2003; Shields-Poe & Pinelli, 1997; Singer, et al., 1999; Wigert, Johansson, Berg, & Hellstrom, 2006; Young Seideman et al., 1997). Depressive symptoms have also been found in mothers following premature birth, with estimates varying depending upon the scale used and timing of measurement (Brooten, et al., 1988; Davis, Edwards, Mohay, & Wollin, 2003; Doering, et al., 1999; Doering, et al., 2000; Feldman Reichman, et al., 2000; Kersting, et al., 2004; Miles, Holditch-Davis, Schwartz, & Sher, 2007; O'Brien, Heron Asay, & McCluskey-Fawcett, 1999; Singer, et al., 1999; Spear, et al., 2002). Davis and associates (2003) found 40% significant depressive symptomatology in mothers of very premature infants compared to 10 to 15% of the population norms. Maternal stress symptoms were the most significant variable associated with symptoms of depression.

According to Spear and associates (2002), there appears to be no relationship between infant illness severity (as measured by the Score of Neonatal Acute Physiology, SNAP) and depressive symptoms in parents. Other significant predictors of postpartum depression identified in the literature are prenatal depression, self-esteem, child care stress, prenatal anxiety, life stress, social support, marital relationship, a history of previous depression, infant temperament, maternity blues, marital status, socioeconomic status, and unplanned or unwanted pregnancy (Beck, 2001). Depressive maternal symptoms have been associated with infant cognitive and emotional delay and may affect child development (Grace, Evindar, & Stewart, 2003). Feelings of hostility and psychological distress have also been found in mothers of premature infants (Brooten, et al.,

1988; Doering, et al., 1999; Doering, et al., 2000; Feldman Reichman, et al., 2000; Singer, et al., 1999; Thompson, Oehler, Catlett, & Johndrow, 1993). Psychological distress in mothers has been shown to continue even up to one year after discharge (Garel, et al., 2006).

Davis and colleagues (2003) studied the impact of very premature birth on the psychological health of mothers. The EPDS scale, Depression and Anxiety and Stress Scales, Social Support Interview, Coping Health Inventory for Parents, the Nurse Parent Support Tool, and demographic data were collected on 72 mothers of premature infants (less than 32 weeks gestation). Gestational ages ranged from 24 to 32 weeks (mean 28 weeks, SD 2.4), with birth weights ranging from 513 to 2002 grams (mean 1088 grams, SD 359). There was a statistically significant relationship between maternal stress and depressive symptoms; each one-point increase in stress score increased the risk of depression by 14%. Gestational age was not found to be significant in this study; however, the small gestational age range of infants, 24 to 32 weeks, and the average weight being 1088 grams may have increased the fragility of these infants, making the difference between gestational ages unappreciable. The interview revealed that other concurrent life stressors (i.e., bereavement, financial, and work concerns) may have also contributed to maternal symptoms of depression.

Similarities have been shown between psychological stress reactions of parents of premature infants and symptoms of ASD (Shaw, et al., 2006) and PTSD (DeMier, et al., 1996; DeMier, et al., 2000; Holditch-Davis, et al., 2003; Kersting, et al., 2004), with ASD being the one less studied. Parental psychological reactions to premature birth compromise the emotional well-being of parents. Whenever parental emotional well-being is compromised, there is a potential effect on the infant, which makes this an important area of study.

Creedy, Shochet, and Horsfall (2000) studied 592 mothers of term infants and found that one in three women reported a stressful birth experience and three or more symptoms of trauma on the Posttraumatic Stress Symptoms Interview (measured four to six weeks after delivery). *DSM-IV* criteria for acute posttraumatic stress disorder were met by 5.6% of the mothers even though 75.6% of the women reported being well prepared for childbirth. Factors that contributed to acute trauma symptoms were level of obstetric intervention (emergency c-section), perception of partner support, and perception of skill of obstetric staff. Antenatal factors, such as obstetric risk, anticipatory anxiety, state anxiety, partner support, preparation for childbirth, and likelihood of birth complications, were not statistically associated with the development of symptoms.

Ayers, Wright, and Wells (2007) studied 64 couples (mothers and fathers) of term healthy infants and found symptoms of PTSD in the parents. All parents of infants transferred to NICU or stillborn were excluded. The Impact of Events Scale was used to measure traumatic stress symptoms, and greater than 20 symptoms were used to diagnose clinical PTSD (sensitivity of 0.94 and specificity of 0.33). Five percent of the parents studied had severe PTSD symptoms (greater than 20 symptoms) nine weeks after birth, which corresponds with previous research. PTSD symptoms were predicted by reports of birth complications, emotions during birth, and problems at delivery and were not associated by parent–infant bond or the relationship of the couples studied. It is suggested that when a birth is particularly traumatic it can affect both members of the couple.

Bailham and Joseph (2003) examined the literature to explore the relationship between the experience of difficult childbirth and the development of PTSD. The authors concluded that there is evidence that women who experience traumatic childbirth may exhibit clinical symptoms consistent with *DSM-IV* criteria of avoidance, reexperiencing, and increased arousal. This has implications for maternal well-being, relationships, and disruption in the maternal–infant bond. Risk factors for PTSD were evident; however, more longitudinal research is needed. It is important to acknowledge the complexity of the relationships among factors and individual differences that exist, which may give explanation for the development of PTSD in some women and not in others. Evidence for PTSD after a term delivery makes it even more plausible that the trauma of premature birth may also exhibit similar symptoms in parents of premature infants.

Findings by Kersting and colleagues (2004) support the notion that birth of the VLBW infant is an emotionally traumatic life event capable of producing psychological reactions in parents. Of 50 mothers studied comparing mothers of VLBW infants and control term infants, all mothers of VLBW infants experienced significantly more traumatic symptoms than control mothers. These mothers also had significantly higher rates of depression and anxiety two weeks after birth. Symptoms of posttraumatic stress were significantly higher during the initial period after giving birth and over a period of 14 months postpartum. Kersting et al. (2004) suggested that the response to the birth of a VLBW infant should be seen as an ongoing traumatic life event.

Holditch-Davis and associates (2003) used a convenience sample of 30 mothers of high-risk premature infants to retrospectively examine mothers' responses to having a premature infant in NICU. A descriptive, correlational design was used and interviews were analyzed for symptoms of the three major criteria of PTSD (reexperiencing the traumatic event, avoidance of thoughts of the traumatic event, and increased arousal level, such as insomnia, irritability, and difficulty concentrating). Data collection occurred before discharge and at six months corrected age. Mothers described emotional responses similar to a posttraumatic stress response. All mothers had at least one symptom of PTSD. A reexperience of aspects of the event through triggers and reminders of the NICU experience were reported by 80% of the mothers. Many spoke of avoiding aspects of the birth and hospitalization or being numb to the reminders. Feelings of overprotection of the infant; fears of infant death, illness, or injury; generalized anxiety; and sleep difficulties were described by 87% of the mothers, which fulfilled the criteria of arousal. Mothers with more PTSD symptoms at six months after discharge also reported greater perceived stress from the NICU environment (measured by PSS:NICU scale). Infant illness severity was unrelated to the number of posttraumatic stress symptoms. This is inconsistent with other studies that have found that severity of perinatal risk does increase the likelihood of parents developing posttraumatic stress symptoms (DeMier, et al., 1996; DeMier, et al., 2000; Pierrehumbert, et al., 2003). Different scales used to measure the severity of infant illness may have led to the inconsistency among studies, and other confounding factors may have been involved.

Pierrehumbert and colleagues (2003) reported similar findings in mothers and found that fathers also suffered from symptoms of posttraumatic stress. The Perinatal PTSD Questionnaire (PPQ) (sensitivity coefficient 0.89 and specificity coefficient 0.87) was used to examine PTSD symptoms in 50 families, which were split into low-risk and high-risk groups as determined by the Perinatal Risk Inventory (PRI). The 18 item PRI provides an indication of premature infant stress by describing infant–perinatal factors (birth weight, gestational age) as an index. It has been highly correlated with length of stay and intensive care procedures. A score of 0 to 4 was considered to be low risk, and greater than 4 was considered to be high risk, which was derived from clinical practice experience. Parents of premature infants were found to have high indices of posttraumatic stress reactions and an increased likelihood of developing PTSD as severity of perinatal risk increased. DeMier and associates (2000) also used the PPQ to measure postnatal emotional distress in mothers of premature infants and discussed an association among perinatal medical risk and maternal distress, poorer developmental outcomes, and disruptions in family functioning.

Acute Stress Disorder

The birth of a premature infant and subsequent NICU hospitalization can be paralleled with a traumatic event or stressor with the potential to affect maternal and paternal psychological well-being. The previously discussed studies provide evidence to support the occurrence of psychological symptoms in parents of premature infants consistent with PTSD symptoms (DeMier, et al., 1996; DeMier, et al., 2000; Holditch-Davis, et al., 2003; Kersting, et al., 2004; Pierrehumbert, et al., 2003). According to the APA's *DSM-IV* (2000) criteria, PTSD is defined as occurring at least one month or more posttrauma. There is preliminary evidence supporting ASD and symptoms of acute stress among parents of infants admitted into NICU (Shaw, et al., 2006).

ASD diagnosis, as described by *DSM-IV* criteria, is outlined by Bryant and Harvey (2000). According to the criteria, a prerequisite of the diagnosis of ASD is the experience of a precipitating stressor, either witnessed or experienced, that has been threatening to either himself or herself or to another person within one month of exposure (Criterion A). ASD is distinguished from PTSD by dissociative symptoms. To satisfy dissociative criteria of ASD (Criterion B), a person must display at least three dissociative symptoms, which are described as a subjective sense of numbing or detachment; reduced awareness of his or her surroundings; and derealization, depersonalization, and dissociative amnesia. The diagnosis of ASD also requires the reexperiencing of the trauma (Criterion C) through recurrent thoughts, images, dreams, illusions, flashback episodes, sense of reliving the experience, or distress when exposed to reminders of the traumatic stressor (Bryant & Harvey, 2000). There must be signs of avoidance of thoughts, feelings, or places that may remind the person of the traumatic event (Criterion D). Symptoms of anxiety or arousal after the trauma, such as restlessness, insomnia, irritability, and difficulties concentrating, are also evident (Criterion E). There must also be a clinically significant disturbance to social or occupational functioning (Criterion F) that must last for at least two days after the trauma (Criterion G) but not persist more than one month (after one month, PTSD is a more suitable diagnosis). The symptoms must not be due to a medical condition, drug or medication, or a preexisting mental disorder (Criterion H).

ASD diagnosis has not been without controversies since its introduction in 1994 in the *DSM-IV* by the American Psychiatric Association (Bryant, 2003). The reasons behind the development of ASD diagnosis were not based on empirical research but on the theoretical premise that a gap existed within the period of one month posttrauma where no diagnosis was available. Theoretical dissociative symptoms were also evident within this initial period of trauma response, setting the acute stress response apart from PTSD (Harvey & Bryant, 2002). With the development of ASD criteria and diagnosis, there was the intention of identification of the acutely traumatized individuals who would then go on to develop chronic PTSD. ASD diagnosis has triggered debate and criticisms due to equivocal data regarding the role of peritraumatic dissociation in the acute trauma response and the ability of ASD diagnosis to predict PTSD diagnosis (Harvey & Bryant, 2002). According to Harvey (2003), ASD has a reasonable ability to predict PTSD; however, there are also individuals who develop PTSD but do not meet all ASD criteria. The criteria for ASD diagnosis is not met when there is an absence of severe dissociative symptoms; however, research suggests that some of these individuals still go on to develop PTSD symptoms. Higher rates of dissociative symptoms have also been found in individuals with PTSD (Marshall, Spitzer, & Liebowitz, 1999), even though dissociation is not part of PTSD diagnosis. This has led to criticism surrounding the relevance of dissociative symptoms to ASD diagnosis. There is also a concern that ASD diagnosis may create pathology around a normal transient reaction to a traumatic event (Marshall, et al., 1999).

ASD diagnosis has created a resurgence of research within the acute period of a traumatic event that has provided strong evidence that acute stress responses are common and typically transient in nature (Bryant, 2003). Research has focused on a wide variety of traumatic events, such as rape, terrorist attacks, assault, motor vehicle accidents, cancer diagnosis, burn injury, and intensive care hospitalization. Additional research is necessary to elucidate the distinction between a normal reaction to trauma and psychopathology (Marshall, et al., 1999).

Studies conducted to specifically measure the incidence of ASD, using the Acute Stress Disorder Interview (ASDI), have been performed by Harvey and Bryant (2002). Measurement of ASD post–motor vehicle accident yielded an incidence of 13% and 21% of the individuals presented with subclinical ASD (having all symptom clusters except dissociation) two days posttrauma to one month posttrauma. Motor vehicle accident survivors with a mild traumatic brain injury yielded a 14% incident rate with a 5% subclinical diagnosis. The incidence of ASD across a wide variety of traumas (such as assault, burns, and industrial accidents) have ranged from 12 to 16%, with subclinical ASD ranging from 19 to 10%. The incidence of ASD symptoms in parents from a variety of traumas, such as pediatric intensive care unit (PICU) admission, NICU admission, pediatric cancer, and pediatric traffic injury, range from 4.7 to 32%, depending on which scale was used and the timing of measurement. A study on children newly diagnosed with pediatric cancer showed incidence rates of 51% in mothers and 40% in fathers (Patino-Fernandez, et al., 2007).

Symptoms of ASD are evident within past research studies of parental stress and the NICU experience. Parental responses to the NICU experience involve intense fear, helplessness, or horror (Affonso, et al., 1992; Jackson, et al., 2003; Jamsa & Jamsa, 1998; Miles, et al., 1991). The identification of the birth of the premature infant as a traumatic event meets Criterion A. Dissociative and avoidance symptoms (Criteria B and D), such as numbing, detachment, avoidance, and feelings of unreality, have been described as reactions of parents to the birth of the premature infant (DeMier, et al., 1996; Feldman Reichman, et al., 2000; Holditch-Davis, et al., 2003; Hughes, McCollum, Sheftel, & Sanchez, 1994; Hynan, 2005; Jackson, et al., 2003). Dissociative symptoms may be underrepresented within the literature because many studies use specific tools that measure anxiety, depressive symptoms, and symptoms of posttraumatic stress and not dissociative symptoms. Also, it is plausible that parents in a state of denial or avoidance (Criterion D) may not be actively visiting the NICU or willing to give consent to participate in a research study. Studies where dissociative symptoms are described by parents are often qualitative in nature (Holditch-Davis, et al., 2003). Different times of data collection evident within research studies on parental stress in the NICU provide evidence that the disturbance and symptoms last for a minimum of two days and a maximum of four weeks after the traumatic event (Criterion G). Parental reexperience of premature birth (Criterion C) is apparent in qualitative studies but not as evident in studies that use tools to measure parental stress. Unless a specific tool is used to measure ASD symptoms among parents of premature infants, evidence for parental reexperience of the trauma may be lost. There is a need for ASD symptoms to be studied specifically using a reliable tool of measurement.

Measurement of ASD

Measurement of ASD has been problematic because the diagnosis was published in *DSM-IV* without standardized and validated tools used to measure symptoms (Harvey & Bryant, 2002). The diagnosis has driven research on the acute reactions after a traumatic stressor and has led to the development of measures designed specifically to measure ASD symptoms. Measurement tools need to be sensitive with proven specificity to limit false positive or false negative results to result in credible research findings. There are currently four tools available to measure all symptoms of ASD (Harvey & Bryant, 2002). Each will be reviewed and compared for sensitivity, reliability, validity, specificity, and ease of use.

The Structured Clinical Interview for DSM-IV Dissociative Disorders (SCID-D) is an interview that specifically explores dissociative pathology; however, it is limited in assessment for other symptoms of ASD, such as intrusive, avoidance, and arousal symptoms. It indexes symptoms for presence, absence, or subthreshold presence, which limits its use as a measurement of severity of symptoms (Bryant & Harvey, 2000). Another limitation of this tool is the nonavailability of validity or reliability data relevant to ASD diagnosis.

The Acute Stress Disorder Interview (ASDI) was designed by Bryant, Moulds, and Guthrie (2000) to evaluate ASD. The interview was based on specific *DSM-IV* criteria and has been tested in a number of samples, including victims of motor vehicle accidents, nonsexual assaults, and industrial accidents. It has excellent internal consistency ($r = 0.90$ for the entire scale), good concurrent validity (compared with independent clinical interview), and good test–retest reliability ($r = 0.88$). This scale is scored dichotomously and has specific guidelines for ASD diagnosis. The need for a self-report measure based on the ASDI led to the development of the Acute Stress Disorder Scale (ASDS) (Bryant, et al., 2000). This scale has demonstrated reasonable internal consistency, convergent validity, and test–retest reliability. It has the ability to identify 95% of the individuals who were diagnosed with ASD on the ASDI and 83% who were not diagnosed with ASD, but it has limited ability to predict PTSD (Bryant, et al., 2000).

The Stanford Acute Stress Reaction Questionnaire (SASRQ) was developed and revised by Cardena, Koopman, Classen, Waelde, and Spiegel (2000) to evaluate *DSM-IV* criteria for ASD by evaluating anxiety and dissociative symptoms after a traumatic event. It is a 30-item self-report instrument that assesses each of the criteria of ASD diagnosis specifically: dissociation (ten items), reexperiencing the trauma (six items), avoidance (six items), anxiety and hyperarousal (six items), and impairment in functioning (two items). The presence of each symptom is scored either as a Likert-type scale (0 to 5) or dichotomously (0–2 is scored as 0; 3–5 is scored as 1). This tool began as a 98-item scale, was modified to a 67-item scale, and finally revised to the current 30-item format. It possesses high internal consistency (Cronbach's alpha 0.8 to 0.95), good concurrent validity with tools measuring PTSD, good to excellent reliability, and has proven to be predictive of subsequent PTSD severity (Cardena, et al.,

2000; Harvey, 2003; Harvey & Bryant, 2002). The psychometric properties of this tool are comparable to the ASDI with practical advantages, such as ease and efficiency of administration and scoring (Cardena, et al., 2000). Although it has been used in a diverse number of studies and samples to measure ASD symptoms and has the ability to identify symptoms of ASD, it should be compared to clinical interviews that diagnose ASD and the ASDI to substantiate its use as a diagnostic tool for ASD.

Research tools that assess individuals during a traumatic experience may be regarded as a potential risk to the study participant by study questions eliciting memories or causing distress. Kassam-Adams and Newman (2005) investigated child and parent reactions to participation in clinical research and specifically assessed reactions after completing the SASRQ. Self-reported distress from study participation was uncommon (5% of parents), with positive appraisals of the research process being more common (90% of parents). This study shows that participation has minimal risks of participation and supports the feasibility of using standardized assessment tools.

Tools to measure specific symptoms of ASD, such as dissociative symptoms, anxiety, and symptoms of avoidance, are also available (Bryant & Harvey, 2000). Examples of scales that measure dissociation are the Dissociative Experiences Scale (DES), Clinician-Administered Dissociative States Scale (CADSS), and Peritraumatic Dissociative Experiences Questionnaire (PDEQ). These scales have the ability to identify dissociative symptoms but were not designed to evaluate other parameters required for ASD diagnosis and often require a trained interviewer (Cardena, et al., 2000). One of the most commonly used scales to measure anxiety is Spielberger State-Trait Anxiety Inventory (STAI). The Impact of Event Scale (IES) has also been developed to measure intrusive and avoidance symptoms. These tools are useful to use as comparisons when determining the convergent validity of the aforementioned ASD measurement tools.

Studies of Acute Stress Disorder Symptoms in Parents

The literature was reviewed to provide a comprehensive overview of studies on ASD in parents within various sample settings and the scales that were used to measure symptoms. The timing of measurement of parental ASD symptoms and scoring methods were also compared. Eight studies specifically measured parental ASD symptoms (Balluffi, et al., 2004; Bryant, Mayou, Wiggs, Ehlers, & Stores, 2004; Daviss, et al., 2000; Kassam-Adams, Garcia-Espana, Miller, & Winston, 2006; Patino-Fernandez, et al., 2007; Shaw, et al., 2006; Winston, et al., 2002; Winston, Baxt, Kassam-Adams, Elliott, & Kallan, 2005).

Four of the eight studies used the SASRQ scale to measure parental ASD (Cronbach's alpha 0.93 and 0.90 when stated) and two used the ASD scale. One study did not use a formal scale, and one study used the Post-traumatic Stress Diagnostic Scale (as cited in Foa, Cashman, Jaycox, & Perry, 1997) to measure parental ASD. Traumatic events varied from NICU/PICU admission to pediatric injury, motor vehicle accident, traffic injury, and recent diagnosis of pediatric malignancy. In all but one study, measurement of ASD occurred within one month of the trauma. One study was retrospective and thus measurement occurred two to four weeks after discharge. Studies generally occurred within the hospital setting or outpatient clinic, except one that used telephone interviews. The percentage of ASD varied between studies and ranged between 4.7 and 51%. The reason for the varied results may be due to the variance in traumatic events studied, differences in defining symptom criteria for ASD, and the use of divergent measurement tools. The scoring method used for determining criteria for ASD was not always explicitly stated by the researchers. Only three of the eight studies examined ASD in mothers and fathers to study the divergence of ASD symptoms present within gender. Two of those studies found the differences to be significant (Patino-Fernandez, et al., 2007; Shaw, et al., 2006). More research is needed to examine how mothers and fathers differ in the portrayal of symptoms of ASD. Gender-specific interventions may be needed if differences are found to exist.

Shaw and associates (2006) specifically studied ASD symptoms in parents of infants admitted to NICU. Using a retrospective cross-sectional design, the stress symptoms of generally well-educated parents (n = 40) were assessed two to four weeks after an NICU hospitalization experience. The focus of this study was on parents of infants hospitalized in NICU. Interestingly, the mean gestational age of infants in this study was 31.46 weeks (SD 4.91), which indicates that premature infants were of the majority. ASD symptoms were found to be significantly related to parental stress as measured by the PSS:NICU, developed and revised by M. Miles. This instrument has been shown to measure parental perception of stressors arising from the NICU environment with high reliability supported by previous research (Miles, Funk, & Carlson, 1993); however, it does not take into account other sources of stress. This study was the first to document ASD symptoms in NICU parents, although the small sample makes these findings preliminary in nature. In all, 28% of the parents met all symptom criteria of ASD (of the 28%, all were women). Specific determinants of meeting symptom criteria considered to be diagnostic of ASD as measured by the SASRQ were not implicitly stated. The severity of the neonates' medical conditions failed to be associated with ASD symptoms as previous studies on PTSD have revealed (Shaw, et al., 2006). Data collection occurred two to four weeks after discharge from NICU; thus measurement of ASD symptoms occurred long after the birth of the premature infant, and the association with the infants' severity of illness may have been weakened. ASD symptoms were found to be related to concerns with parental role alteration. Increased stress from parental role alteration, supported by findings in this study, is congruent with previous research (Miles, et al., 1991). Concerns with parental role alteration may have been from the home or from the NICU experience; nonetheless, ASD symptoms were significantly related to parental stress. The retrospective design may have prevented the NICU environment from having a direct effect on the parents while the data was collected. It is debatable if the acute stress disorder symptoms being measured were from the NICU environment or from the transition to home, which has also been described as a stressful time. The timing of data collection at two to four weeks after NICU hospitalization, where the mean length of stay in NICU was 58 days (SD 36), makes it undetermined if this study was measuring ASD and not PTSD because ASD is diagnosable only within one month posttrauma. Assessment for symptoms of ASD should occur within one month posttrauma (Bryant & Harvey, 2003). Although the results support the importance of preparing parents for the psychological reactions that naturally occur during this experience, weaknesses in the design support the need for future research.

Research into ASD symptoms in parents of infants in NICU is limited, but its relevance and significance should not be disregarded. ASD symptoms have been reported in parents of children admitted to PICU, a similar intensive care environment with similar parental psychological reactions as NICU. Balluffi and associates (2004) used a prospective cohort study to measure the prevalence of parental ASD and PTSD using the ASD scale and PTSD scale (n = 272, 82% mothers, 16% fathers, 2% other female guardians). Data collection occurred at Time 1, the second day after admission to PICU (to measure ASD symptoms), and Time 2, which was two months after discharge from PICU (to measure PTSD symptoms). Of the parents studied, 32% met symptom criteria for ASD (dissociation, reexperiencing, avoidance, and hyperarousal). The severity of ASD symptoms was associated with unexpected admission and parents' degree of worry that the child might die. ASD symptom presence or severity was not associated with severity of illness, demographic factors, or number of days in PICU, as was found by Shaw et al. (2006) in NICU. Symptom criteria of PTSD were met by 21% of parents and were also associated with degree of worry that the child might die (assessed at Time 1). Parental ASD symptom severity assessed at Time 1 predicted PTSD severity at Time 2. If ASD diagnostic criteria were met, parents were more likely to meet diagnostic criteria for PTSD (of the 58% diagnosed with ASD, 42% went on to be diagnosed with PTSD). These findings have clinical implications in regard to follow-up and are actually lower than other studies showing the relationship between ASD and PTSD. In a study of motor vehicle accident survivors by Harvey and Bryant (2003), it was found that 92% of females and 57% of males diagnosed with ASD met criteria for PTSD at a follow-up assessment. Birmes and associates (2003) also confirmed the predictive power of peritraumatic dissociation and ASD to later development of PTSD in a study of assault victims. Balluffi et al. (2004) also found ASD symptoms to be common in parents with a child admitted to PICU. One or more ASD symptoms were experienced by most parents; 90% reported hyperarousal, 75% reported dissociation or reexperiencing symptoms, and 67% reported symptoms of avoidance. This study revealed higher levels of ASD symptoms compared to other studies, possibly due to early data collection at median of two days postadmission (Balluffi, et al., 2004).

In this study, mothers were more likely than fathers to develop PTSD; however, this finding was weakened by the small number of fathers studied compared to mothers. Previous literature examining gender differences in PTSD and ASD support this finding. Bryant and Harvey (2003) studied motor vehicle accident survivors and found that full criteria of ASD and PTSD were met by more females than males. Females also reported higher depression scores than males, and it appeared that the diagnosis of ASD was a more accurate predictor of PTSD for females than for males. Males and females appear to have a different incident rate of ASD; however, continued research is needed in this area. Results from this study support the potential for screening parents after PICU admission to identify families at higher risk for developing later PTSD symptoms. Screening should be done with consideration of the usual initial stress reactions of parents with the potential to persist and evolve into ASD. Research involving parents with a child admitted into PICU gives support for further research regarding ASD in parents within the NICU because both units are comparable in nature and ascertained to be a potential traumatic stressor for families (Peebles-Kleiger, 2000).

Summary

The results of this literature review support the depiction of premature birth as a traumatic event. The subsequent admission into NICU adds further trauma, and stress creates an environment where ASD symptoms may emerge. Infant prematurity has been associated with higher levels of stress, anxiety, and depression in both mothers and fathers. Limited information is available about ASD symptoms among parents within the experience of preterm birth. ASD symptoms among parents of premature infants as a focus have not been studied. There is a need to examine the incidence of ASD symptoms along with possible confounding variables to gain a further understanding of stress reactions of parents after the birth of a premature infant. Information about parental stress responses to premature birth will enable healthcare professionals to reassure parents on the normal reactions to premature birth and to grasp an awareness of the depth to which parents are affected. This knowledge can be used to identify factors that may place parents most at risk and may assist in further development of intervention strategies not only to support parents but also to assist in the prevention of psychological distress in parents of premature infants.

Theoretical Framework

In family theory the premise that a family needs to be supported as it moves into a new phase of functioning, such as the birth of a premature infant, is reinforced. The Resiliency Model of Stress, Adjustment & Adaptation (evolved from Hill's ABCX model) has been used as a framework to understand and to predict family stress (DeMarco, Ford-Gilboe, Friedemann, McCubbin, & McCubbin, 2000). ASD may be conceptualized within this model to understand and predict family stress and adaptation to the traumatic stressor of preterm birth. Stressor (A) is a life event that creates a maturational developmental crisis (i.e., preterm birth, labor and delivery, and adaptation to parenthood) and can be regarded as a traumatic event as defined in the criteria for ASD. The experience of high-risk pregnancy magnifies tensions and fears with the increased possibility of the unexpected occurring during labor (Zwelling, 2000). There are two distinct crises: the normal developmental crisis of childbirth; and the recognition that the pregnancy is not following the expected patterns, culminating with the birth of the premature infant, and admission of the infant into an intensive care environment. The appraisal of the stressor (C) (the traumatic event) is how the family defines the stressor (planned versus unplanned, normal versus high risk, expected versus unexpected). Family appraisal of the stressor may also be influenced by many factors, including fear of impending death or a previous infant who was admitted into NICU. Parental stress and the NICU environment would likely have an impact on the pileup of stressors (AA) and lead to vulnerability (V), which would influence patterns of functioning and may result in symptoms of ASD. In the proposed study, parents will be assessed for ASD symptoms seven to ten days after birth to determine degree of vulnerability. After the traumatic initial period after premature birth, parents begin to adapt to the stressor by entering the circle of situational appraisal. Resources within the family assist the family in problem solving and coping and lead to patterns of functioning. The family members' perception of the degree to which situations in one's life are appraised as stressful may also affect this process. The family may prove to be resilient and show signs of bonadaptation, or family adaptation may result in maladjustment. The parents will be assessed a second time for ASD symptoms one month after birth to determine if symptoms of ASD persist. This conceptualization of ASD within the context of the Resiliency Model of Family Stress, Adjustment, and Adaptation exemplifies the importance of assessing parents for ASD and symptom severity. It is also important to recognize that the assessment of ASD symptoms will provide just a snapshot of symptoms and feelings within this experience for the mothers and fathers of these premature infants and that a complex interaction of factors all play a role in this process. However, in the attempt to understand the experience, healthcare professionals will be better able to provide appropriate support to families. An improved understanding of the process of family stress and adaptation may assist in the development of appropriate strategies to increase adaptive resources, which may facilitate families in dealing with stressors more effectively. Adaptive resources, such as effective coping strategies, flexibility–resiliency, family connectedness, family support, communication and problem-solving process, and social and economic resources, can assist families in dealing with adversity (Walsh, 2003). Adaptive resources have been found to be a predictor of resilient outcomes and to increase coping and adaptation within a family (DeMarco, et al., 2000).

The development of appropriate strategies to assist families is contingent upon an understanding of family reactions to the traumatic event of preterm birth. Findings from the proposed study will increase understanding of the feelings and symptoms parents experience after the birth of a premature infant. Gaining a greater understanding of the incidence of ASD and severity of symptoms in parents of premature infants is important to increase knowledge of the parental experience and reactions to the birth of a premature infant. This knowledge may aid in the development of appropriate screening and intervention strategies to assist parents with symptoms of ASD.

Design

A prospective cohort study using a within–subjects research design will be used to determine the incidence of ASD in parents of premature infants.

Study Objectives

The specific objectives of this study are (1) to measure the incidence rate of ASD among parents of premature infants admitted to the NICU; (2) to describe the symptom profiles of acute stress in mothers and fathers of premature infants; (3) to examine the number and severity of ASD symptoms from each of the following categories: intrusion, avoidance, hyperarousal, and dissociation; (4) to determine if the number of ASD symptoms reported in the first seven to ten days after birth (Time 1) diminish or persist one month following birth (Time 2); (5) to determine which factors are independently associated with the total SASRQ score; and (6) to determine the factors that may increase the risk of ASD among parents of premature infants admitted to the NICU.

Study Setting

This study will be conducted within the clinical setting of the NICU at the Royal Alexandra Hospital (RAH) in Edmonton, Alberta, Canada. The RAH NICU provides Level III neonatal care to infants and their respective families within the Capital Health region, northern Alberta, parts of Northwest Territories, British Columbia, and Saskatchewan.

Study Population

The population chosen for this study will include parents of premature infants admitted to the NICU over a three-month period between January 28, 2008 and April 28, 2008. All infants will have an admitting diagnosis of premature birth. The inclusion criteria include English-speaking parents of infants less than 33 weeks completed gestational age. Either parent or both parents will be included in the study depending on consent. Exclusion criteria are a known fetal anomaly, compassionate care being offered for the infant after birth due to poor prognosis, and maternal illness that precludes NICU visitation and administration of the scale in the first seven to ten days after birth.

The decision to limit the study population to parents of infants born less than 33 weeks completed gestational age was due to lack of resources and time constraints. There is no evidence that this population will be more at risk for ASD or that a lesser gestational age predicts severity of ASD symptoms.

Study Variables

The outcome (dependent variable) to be studied is the diagnosis of ASD and the number and severity of symptoms of ASD in mothers and fathers. Other factors and covariates (independent variables) are included to examine the potential confounders that may influence the risk of developing ASD symptoms. These factors are outlined in Table C-1 and include maternal, infant, parental, obstetric, and demographic factors, with a specific focus on infant illness severity; parental worry that the infant may die; feelings of depression; feelings of support from family, friends, and spouse; perception of stressful events; history of previous infant admission into NICU; history of infertility, miscarriage, or problems conceiving; and history of infant death.

The factors and covariates chosen for this study should be considered preliminary in nature because there is potential for many complex relationships among multiple factors to exist before and after the event of premature birth. The limited number of studies of ASD in parents of infants admitted to NICU precludes the establishment of a predictive model and lends only to an examination of associative risk factors.

Study Procedure

After delivery, premature infants are admitted to the NICU at the Royal Alexandra Hospital. To determine incidence an attempt will be made to recruit as many parents of infants who fit the study criteria as possible within a three-month period. This three-month period was calculated by examining monthly statistics for inborn admissions to the NICU within the study criteria. This study is projected to take place from January 28, 2008 to April 28, 2008. According to 2006 NICU admission statistics from January to March 2006, there will be a predicted 92 potential families that meet the study criteria. For the purposes of this study, parents will be defined as the biological parents who are the primary caregivers for these infants. No guardians, relatives, or foster parents will be asked to participate.

TABLE C-1
Potential Confounders That May Influence the Risk of Developing ASD Symptoms

Demographic factors

❑ Parental age

❑ Gender

Obstetric factors

❑ Method of delivery

❑ Multiple birth versus singleton

❑ Assisted conception

Infant factors

❑ Infant illness severity

❑ Birth weight

❑ Gestational age

❑ Apgar score

Parental factors

❑ Symptoms of depression

❑ Perception of stressful life events

❑ History of infertility, infant death, difficulty conceiving

❑ Premature birth expected versus unexpected

❑ Degree of worry that the infant may die prior to discharge from NICU

❑ NICU consult and/or NICU tour prior to birth of the infant

❑ Perception of support from family, friends, and/or spouse

❑ Residence out of the city where the infant was born

❑ Other children in the family

❑ Previous history of infant admission into NICU

Maternal factors

❑ Gravity and parity

❑ History of premature birth, high risk pregnancies, miscarriage, and/or stillbirth

❑ Length of hospitalization prior to the birth of the premature infant

Study participants meeting the study inclusion criteria will be recruited by the primary investigator. Posters will be placed in the parent room outside of the NICU describing the study. A study information letter will also be provided to parents at a weekly parent support meeting. The primary investigator will obtain the parental consent and will be involved in all data collection. The primary investigator is a neonatal nurse practitioner intern who is a part of the clinical management team within the NICU. She has indirect involvement with the parents in NICU approximately 20 hours per week. She is a part of a collaborative multidisciplinary team that is responsible for developing plans of care for the infants in NICU. She does not provide daily nursing care to the infants; however, she may perform advanced skills as required.

When the infant is five to seven days old, parents of premature infants who fit the study criteria will be approached for consent to be in this study. Parents will not be approached for consent while their infant is unstable, defined as requiring above the expected intensive care support (i.e., high-frequency oscillation and inhaled nitric oxide treatment), or if the parents are in considerable distress as defined by the bedside nurse caring for the infant and/or the social worker involved. If it is deemed ethically contingent to do so, the parents will be approached for consent (five to seven days after birth). The researcher will explain the study risks and benefits to the parents and obtain informed consent. Each parent will independently sign their own consent. A letter explaining the study and a copy of the consent will be given to the parents (see Exhibits C-1 and C-2). The letter has been written in language that is comprehensible and has been assessed at a grade 8.8 by the Flesch-Kincaid Grade Level score. This is a voluntary consent, which means that parents are free to refuse consent or to discontinue participation in this study at any time without jeopardizing their infant's continuing care at the Royal Alexandra Hospital NICU. It will be reiterated that participating in the study will not affect the standards of care their infant receives in NICU.

Those parents who consent to be in the study will be given a unique ID number to protect their identity and confidentiality. Care will be taken to approach parents at a time that is most convenient and nonintrusive as possible for them. Each parent will independently sign their own consent to participate in the study. Parents will then be asked to complete the demographic form, self-report SASRQ, Edinburgh Postpartum Depression Scale, and the Perceived Stress Scale. The Acute Stress Disorder Interview will be done by the primary investigator with supervision by Dr. Kathy

Hegadoren, Canada Research Chair in Stress Disorders in Women. The parents will be asked to complete the same measures at Time 2.

Data Collection

Data collection will occur during two periods of time, and the timing will be specifically recorded. Time 1 is defined as seven to ten days postbirth. Time 1 will give information about the parents' reactions during the initial period after the birth of the preterm infant. Time 2 is defined as 28 to 30 days after birth. By collecting data at two time periods, knowledge will be gained regarding the change in nature and severity of ASD symptoms over the course of the first month of the NICU stay.

Evidence-based support for the timing of data collection is lacking. The only study on ASD symptoms in parents of infants in NICU was retrospective and completed two to four weeks after NICU hospitalization (Shaw, et al., 2006). However, in a prospective study on the prevalence of ASD and PTSD in parents of children in PICU, Balluffi and associates (2004) also used two data collection points: two days after admission (to measure ASD) and two months after discharge (to measure PTSD). The diagnosis of ASD stipulates the presence of ASD symptoms during the period after 48 hours and within four weeks posttrauma (Bryant & Harvey, 2000). This supports measuring ASD symptoms within the period of time chosen for this study. Measurement of ASD during the initial adjustment period (48 hours to one week postbirth) carries the risk of overestimation of the incidence of ASD in this population. To reduce the chance of medicalizing a normal stress reaction to premature birth, the time period of seven to ten days was chosen for this proposed study. If ASD symptoms remain high in parents at Time 2, there may be a greater chance that the symptoms will carry on longer than one month after birth, or in the diagnostic time of PTSD.

Information about support resources will be provided to all participants. Assistance in accessing those resources will be offered. There are no agreements or stated guidelines regarding the treatment of ASD in the early stages. Bryant & Harvey (2000) suggest that treatment does not need to occur within the acute phase of ASD. A supportive approach in the early stages of ASD often leads to better outcomes as individuals are able to be more involved with therapy later in the course of ASD. Parents with significant symptoms of ASD during the final data collection will be mailed or given a list of resources compiled by the primary investigator with assistance from Dr. Kathy Hegadoren. Assistance in accessing the resources will once again be offered. If ASD symptoms persist in Time 2 data collection, this would indicate the need for further study of PTSD in this population.

The Instruments

Score of Neonatal Acute Physiology (SNAP-II)

The Score of Neonatal Acute Physiology measurement tool was developed and validated prospectively on 1643 admissions in three NICUs. It was revised to include six physiologic items (lowest mean blood pressure, lowest temperature, oxygenation status, lowest serum pH, seizures, and urine output) to create the SNAP-II (Richardson, Corcoran, Escobar, & Lee, 2001). SNAP-II was recently revalidated in a SNAP Pilot Project in a large cohort of infants from various NICUs (Zupancic, et al., 2007). SNAP scores are highly predictive of neonatal mortality, and SNAP is identified as an important tool for NICU research (Richardson, Gray, McCormick, Workman, & Goldmann, 1993; Sutton, Bajuk, Berry, Eagles, et al., 2002; Sutton, Bajuk, Berry, Sayer, et al., 2002). The score parallels physician estimates of mortality risk and directly predicts in-hospital mortality. It has been used in numerous studies in NICU to measure severity of illness in premature and term infants. The SNAP-II score quantifies severity of illness among infants by using six commonly measured laboratory and clinical parameters. A score of zero is assigned if the parameter is within normal limits or if the parameter has not been measured. Lack of measurement assumes that the infant was not ill enough to induce laboratory or clinical investigation. SNAP-II scoring requires baseline data from the first 12 hours of life, found in the NICU flow sheet, to be analyzed and a scoring form to be completed. An example of an electronic version of the scoring form can be found at www.sfar.org/scores2/snap22.html. In this study, SNAP-II scoring will enable infant illness severity to be compared with the number and severity of ASD symptoms in parents. The greater the scoring on the SNAP-II scale, the greater the illness severity.

Stanford Acute Stress Reaction Questionnaire (SASRQ)

The SASRQ is a 30-item instrument with six subscales that measures symptoms of peritraumatic anxiety, dissociation, and acute stress disorder. The specific subscales measured are traumatic event, dissociative symptoms (ten items: numbing, detachment, and emotional unresponsiveness, reduced awareness of surroundings, derealization, depersonalization, and dissociative amnesia), reexperiencing of traumatic event (six items), avoidance of stimuli that arouse memories of the trauma (six items), anxiety–hyperarousal (six items), and impaired functioning (two items) (Cardena, et al., 2000). Scoring is through a 5-point Likert-type scale questionnaire, where 0 is not experienced, 1 is very rarely experienced, 2 is rarely experienced, 3 is sometimes experienced, 4 is often experienced, and 5 is very often experienced. Higher total scores reflect higher parental acute stress symptoms (the range of possible scores is 0–150). Introductory instructions can be rephrased by the researcher to refer to a specific event or certain period of time. Questions regarding the description of the event, how disturbing the event was, and how many days the individual experienced the worst symptoms are also included. The SASRQ is written in simple language, is comprehensible, can be quickly administered with minimal instruction, and can be easily scored as either a dichotomous or Likert-type measure (Cardena, et al., 2000). The scoring method for the questionnaire is as follows: total sum of raw scores for the entire scale and/or subscales or for "caseness," which is defined in the psychiatric world as whether or not the subject has the symptoms or the condition being studied or assessed for (Burger & Neeleman, 2007). The developers of SASRQ score the symptom as present (caseness) only if the respondent indicates 3 or higher (occurring at least sometimes). A total score of greater than 37 has also been found to be a good estimate of the symptom by symptom estimation of caseness (E. Cardena, personal communication, August 24, 2007).

The SASRQ was selected for this study due to the quick and easy scoring and administration and proven reliability to measure symptoms of acute stress reactions. Due to the self-report nature of this questionnaire, it provides a greater sense of anonymity for the parent participant. Although it was not designed specifically for parents within the NICU environment, it was created to be used in various traumatic events. It has been tested in a diverse number of studies involving various traumatic events to determine reliability (Cardena, et al., 2000). The major advantages of using the SASRQ questionnaire are the provision of ordinal ratings along with frequency indexes for each symptom, it involves a wide coverage of various ASD symptoms, and it has a reasonable ability to predict subsequent posttraumatic stress in acutely traumatized individuals (Bryant & Harvey, 2000). It has been used in diverse studies and samples with very good reliability, construct validity, discriminate and convergent validity, and predictive validity (Cardena, et al., 2000).

The SASRQ has been used to assess symptoms of stress in parents in four previous studies (see Table C-1). Personal communication with E. Cardena (January 17, 2008) revealed that the SASRQ and the ASD scale were well accepted by parents in previous studies. Recent use of the tool by Shaw et al. (2006) to measure the prevalence of ASD in parents of infants in NICU and in others studies on parental ASD symptoms made it appealing to the researcher. This study will provide an opportunity to calculate Cronbach's alpha to determine interitem reliability of the instrument. This tool will be used to measure the pattern and severity of symptoms, not to diagnose ASD.

Acute Stress Disorder Interview (ASDI)

The ASDI is specially validated against *DSM-IV* criteria for ASD and therefore can be used as a diagnostic tool for ASD (Bryant & Harvey, 2000). Psychometric properties are outlined in Bryant, Harvey, Dang, and Sackville (1998). It is a 19-item scale, scored dichotomously for items related to the following symptoms: five dissociative criteria, four reexperiencing criteria, four avoidance criteria, and six arousal criteria. It includes questions to assess the stressor and the impairment to functioning arising from symptoms, the trauma–assessment interval, and use of drugs or medication. This tool has been compared to independent clinician diagnostic assessment for ASD by Bryant and Harvey (2000). The sensitivity of the tool was found to be 91%, with a rate of false positives of 7%. Specificity of the tool, defined as the number not diagnosed by the ASDI as well as by the clinician was 93%, with a rate of false negatives of 9%. It has the weakest sensitivity for dissociation (79%); however, it will only be used to diagnose ASD, and the SASRQ will be used to measure severity and frequency index of each symptom. Internal consistency of the 19 items was high in previous studies of trauma survivors ($r = 0.90$). Test–retest reliability was performed by readministering the tool between two and five days after initial completion. There was strong agreement in presence or absence of symptoms (at least 80%) with strong correlations of each criterion score (at least 0.80).

The Edinburgh Postnatal Depression Scale (EPDS)

The EPDS is a ten-item self-report scale used to screen for postnatal depression. The sensitivity of the scale was found to be 86% identified as true positives for depression, with 78% identified as true negatives. It has been recognized that the sensitivity and specificity of this scale may increase when family members are not present (Cox, Holden & Sagovsky, 1987). As with all scales used within this study, the EPDS will be scored independently.

The Perceived Stressor Scale (PSS)

The PSS is a 14-item tool used to measure the degree to which situations in one's life are perceived to be stressful. Scores are obtained by reversing the scores on seven positive items (Items 4, 5, 6, 7, 9, 10, and 13) and then summing all 14 items. It contains items that are easy to understand and can be used with participants with at least junior high school education. According to Cohen, Kamarck, and Mermelstein (1983) the PSS has adequate internal and test–retest reliability and has been correlated with life-event scores, depressive and physical symptoms, social anxiety, and others. It will be used as an outcome measure of the perceived levels of general stress that parents experienced one month prior to completing the tool.

The ASDI, EPDS, PSS, and SASRQ will be given to parents during Time 1 (seven to ten days after birth) and Time 2 (28 to 30 days after birth). Every effort will be made to ensure comfort during data collection. The interview and questionnaires will be completed in a quiet room away from the bedside at a convenient time for the participant. Both parents will answer the scales separately. All data will be kept confidential. Completion of the SASRQ instrument should take approximately five minutes (Cardena, et al., 2000). Previous studies do not identify this tool as being complicated or problematic to complete. The instrument is considered to be comprehensible and easy to use (Cardena, et al., 2000). The PSS contains only ten items to rate on a scale of 0 to 4, which should take about five minutes to complete. The EPDS also contains only ten items, is a well-known, well-used scale to measure signs of postnatal depression, and should also take five minutes to complete (Cox, et al., 1987). The ASDI contains 19 items scored dichotomously, it has been defined as user friendly, and can be administered quickly (Bryant & Harvey, 2000).

Demographic data will be collected from the infant's chart by the primary investigator and from the mother and/or father. Demographic data will be used to determine specific demographic factors associated with number and severity of ASD symptoms. The primary investigator will also obtain necessary information from the chart to complete SNAP-II scoring form to measure infant illness severity. Data collection and scoring of the SNAP-II will be done only by the primary investigator.

To determine the reliability and validity of the data in a study of this nature, it is necessary to examine the instruments that measure the variables within the study (Wood & Ross-Kerr, 2006). The reliability of the SASRQ was recently supported for use within the NICU by Shaw and associates (2006), who calculated Cronbach's alpha of 0.90 for the sample of NICU parents, indicating good internal consistency. The SASRQ has possessed high internal consistency in various studies with diverse traumas (Cronbach's alpha 0.80 to 0.95), shows good to excellent reliability, and has proven to be predictive of subsequent PTSD severity (Cardena, et al., 2000; Harvey, 2003; Harvey & Bryant, 2002). The ASDI has been validated against clinician-based diagnoses of ASD (Bryant, Dang, & Sackville, 1998). It has possessed high internal consistency ($r = 0.90$), sensitivity (91%), and specificity (93%) in trauma survivors assessed within one and three weeks posttrauma. Test–retest reliability was also strong ($r = 0.88$). Diagnostic agreement was high; it has identified 91% of participants who were clinically diagnosed with ASD and 93% of those who were not diagnosed (Bryant & Harvey, 2000). The other measurement tool to be used in this study is the SNAP-II physiologic severity index. It was chosen by the researcher due to proven usefulness and validity in measuring illness severity in preterm infants (Richardson et al., 1993; Sutton, Bajuk, Berry, Sayer, et al., 2002). The internal consistency reliability coefficient (Cronbach's alpha) will be calculated for all scales used to determine the reliability of measurement for this study. The SASRQ scores will be correlated to ASD diagnosis by ASDI to provide further evidence of the futility of the scales in measuring ASD.

The cohort population was chosen because the parents have the common experience of premature birth. The results may not be generalized to all parents of premature infants but specifically to parents of premature infants born less than 33 weeks gestation. There is a chance of overestimation or underestimation of symptoms due to knowledge of the variable being studied. Within this study design there are attempts to control for extraneous variables through the use of parents without previous experience in the NICU environment and through the detection of postnatal depression, which could lead to symptoms similar to ASD.

Data Analysis

Data entry and analysis will be conducted using SPSS for Windows Version 16.0 (SPSS Inc., Chicago, Illinois). The nonparticipation rate and reasons for parents' refusal to participate will be estimated and reported. The characteristics of the study population will be described using descriptive statistics. For continuous variables means and standard deviation will be calculated; for continuous nonnormally distributed variables, median and interquartile ranges will be estimated. Frequencies and percentages will be calculated and reported for categorical and discrete variables. Graphic displays will be used to illustrate differences in the distribution of SASRQ symptoms by parental status (mothers versus fathers).

The following section describes the proposed methods of data analysis to attain each study objective. Parametric tests will be used unless normal distribution of the data cannot be assumed, then nonparametric analyses will be computed.

Objective 1: To measure the incidence rate of ASD among parents of premature infants admitted to the NICU. The following equation will be used: [(1) number of mothers with ASD; (2) number of fathers with ASD; or (3) number of parent participants with ASD)] ÷ [(1) number of maternal participants; (2) number of paternal participants; or (3) number of parent participants)] × 100. An incident rate will be reported for mothers, fathers, and for the overall study participants.

Objectives 2 and 3: To describe the symptom profiles of acute stress in mothers and in fathers of premature infants and to examine the number and severity of ASD symptoms from each of the following categories: intrusion, avoidance, hyperarousal, and dissociation. Symptom score distributions within the five SASRQ categories will be compared by parental status. For each of the symptom categories (intrusion, avoidance, hyperarousal, and dissociation) contained in the SASRQ, raw scores will be summed in accordance with the SASRQ Scoring Guide. A new variable will be created to identify study participants with scores ≥ 3 in each category. The proportion of subjects who have caseness or significant symptoms of ASD (defined as an SASRQ symptom score of ≥ 3) will be summed and reported as a percentage by parental status (i.e., mothers, fathers, and both parents). Graphic displays will be used to illustrate differences in scores in each category by parental status.

Objective 4: To determine if the number of ASD symptoms reported in the first seven to ten days after birth (Time 1) diminish or persist one month following birth (Time 2). A dependent pairs t-test will be conducted. A P-value < 0.05 will be used to establish if any of the compared differences between Time 1 and Time 2 are statistically significant.

Objective 5: To determine which factors are independently associated with the total SASRQ scores, multiple linear regression will be used with the stepwise procedure for selection of variables.

Objective 6: To determine the factors that may increase the risk of ASD among parents of premature infants admitted to the NICU. To address this study objective, bivariate logistic regression will be employed to determine which risk factors are significantly associated with the occurrence of ASD among parents of preterm infants in the NICU. Unadjusted odds ratios (OR) and 95% confidence intervals (CI) will be estimated and reported to indicate the magnitude and direction of the affect of each independent variable on the likelihood of parents reporting significant symptoms of ASD. A significant OR (greater than 1.0) will indicate that parents exposed to the risk factor had a higher risk of reporting significant symptoms of ASD than parents who were not exposed to the risk factor. All significant risk factors and covariates from the bivariate analysis will be included in a multivariate logistic regression (MLR) analysis to determine the factors that are independently associated with significant symptoms of ASD after controlling for the impact of all other variables and confounders.

Identification and the selection of potential confounding variables was based on the results of previous studies. For example, in a sample of parents of children admitted to PICU, Balluffi et al. (2004) identified that the presence of ASD was associated with parents' degree of worry that their child might die. The severity of ASD symptoms were also associated with the degree of worry that the child may die. Severity of illness was not associated with ASD presence in the PICU population. In a study by Shaw et al. (2006) in the NICU parent population, ASD symptoms were not found to be related to birth weight, gestational age, and Apgar scores. Infant illness severity was not measured in this study. These possible relationships among risk factors provided some direction as to what confounding and interaction effects should be assessed in the present study. Due to the limited research of ASD in the NICU population, some risk factors, such as birth weight, gestational age, and Apgar score, previously reported as not significantly related to ASD symptoms will be replicated in this study.

Ethical Considerations

This proposal was submitted for ethical review by the Health Research Ethics Board (HREB) at the University of Alberta. The main ethical issues within this proposal are confidentiality, anonymity, informed consent, data storage, and helping parents identified as having persistent symptoms obtain appropriate service. The primary investigator has obtained approval from the Royal Alexandra Hospital NICU research committee prior to submitting this proposal. Site approval from the Royal Alexandra Hospital has also been obtained.

Informed participant consent will be obtained according to ethical guidelines outlined by the HREB of the University of Alberta. The primary investigator will be responsible for obtaining consent. All participants will receive an information letter outlining the study and an informed consent form. The researcher will be responsible for ensuring that the participants understand the implications of being in the study. Confidentiality and anonymity will be maintained by the use of ID numbers on admission to the study to prevent any personal or identifying information from being on the questionnaires. Because infants may be discharged to home or transferred to another nursery, contact information will be obtained from each parent. Computerized data will not include personal identifying information, only anonymous data identifiers to maintain subject confidentiality. Only the primary investigator and research committee will have access to the data. All data collected will be stored in a locked filing cabinet when not in use. Computerized data stored on CD or memory stick will also be locked up when not in use. After completion of the study, data will be kept in a locked, secure place at all times and destroyed appropriately after seven years.

Every attempt has been made by the researcher to make the research process as minimally distressing as possible. Parents will not be approached for consent if their infant is unstable or if they are currently experiencing distress. This study excludes those infants being offered compassionate care. This sensitivity is a necessary part of this type of research.

There is a risk that some of the questions within SASRQ and ASDI may cause parents to remember a significantly stressful period with their infant or to recall intense feelings. The study explanation letter (Exhibit C-1) includes a clause stating that they can leave a question blank or refuse to participate at any time. Information about support resources and assistance in accessing those resources will be provided to all participants during both stages of data collection. The list of resources was compiled by the primary investigator with assistance from Dr. Kathy Hegadoren. The NICU offers parents support through parent groups, and social workers are involved in the care of the NICU families. Social workers will be on the list of resources for parents but are not a part of the research team and so will not be privy to any confidential information involved in this study.

Conclusion

Knowledge gained from this study will provide evidence on the nature of the parental stress response to premature birth, gender differences of the parental stress response, and determine the incidence of ASD symptoms within this population. Substantiation of the practicability and reliability of using the SASRQ instrument to measure parental ASD symptoms within the NICU environment is an important outcome of this study. A contribution will be made to nursing knowledge by enabling nurses and other healthcare professionals to gain insight and awareness into the extent to which parents of premature infants are affected by premature birth and subsequent admission to NICU. This is critical to understanding the dynamics of the parental experience. It will also facilitate the ability of healthcare professionals to reassure parents on the various symptoms and reactions to premature birth. The conclusions made from this study may be used to identify parents most at increased risk for ASD and assist in future development of intervention strategies to provide support and assistance for parents of premature infants.

References

Affleck, G., & Tennen, H. (1991). The effect of newborn intensive care on parents' psychological well-being. *Children's Health Care Journal, 20*(1), 6–14.

Affonso, D. D., Hurst, I., Mayberry, L. J., Haller, L., Yost, K., & Lynch, M. E. (1992). Stressors reported by mothers of hospitalized premature infants. *Neonatal Network, 11*(6), 63–70.

American Psychiatric Association. (2000). *Diagnostic and statistical manual of mental disorders* (4th ed.). Washington, DC: Author.

Ayers, S., Wright, D. B., & Wells, N. (2007). Symptoms of post-traumatic stress disorder in couples after birth: Association with the couple's relationship and parent–baby bond. *Journal of Reproductive and Infant Psychology, 25*(1), 40–50.

Bailham, D., & Joseph, S. (2003). Post-traumatic stress following childbirth: A review of the emerging literature and directions for research and practice. *Psychology, Health & Medicine, 8*(2), 159–168.

Balluffi, A., Kassam-Adams, N., Kazak, A., Tucker, M., Dominguez, T., & Helfaer, M. (2004). Traumatic stress in parents of children admitted to the pediatric intensive care unit. *Pediatric Critical Care Medicine, 5*(5), 547–553.

Beck, C. (2001). Predictors of postpartum depression. *Nursing Research, 50*(5), 275–285.

Birmes, P., Brunet, A., Carreras, D., Ducasse, J., Charlet, J., Lauque, D. H., et al. (2003). The predictive power of peritraumatic dissociation and acute stress symptoms for posttraumatic stress symptoms: A three-month prospective study. *American Journal of Psychiatry, 160*, 1337–1339.

Brooten, D., Gennaro, S., Brown, L. P., Gibbons, A. L., Bakewell-Sachs, S., & Kumar, S. P. (1988). Anxiety, depression, and hostility in mothers of preterm infants. *Nursing Research, 37*(4), 213–216.

Bryant, R. A. (2003). Acute stress disorder: Is it a useful diagnosis? *Clinical Psychologist, 7*(2), 67–79.

Bryant, R. A., & Harvey, A. G. (2000). *ASD: A handbook of theory, assessment, and treatment.* Washington, DC: American Psychological Association.

Bryant, R. A., & Harvey, A. G. (2003). Gender differences in the relationship between acute stress disorder and posttraumatic stress disorder following motor vehicle accidents. *Australian and New Zealand Journal of Psychiatry, 37*, 226–229.

Bryant, R. A., Harvey, A. G., Dang, S. T., & Sackville, T. (1998). Assessing acute stress disorder: Psychometric properties of a structured clinical interview. *Psychological Assessment, 10*(3), 215–220.

Bryant, B., Mayou, R., Wiggs, L., Ehlers, A., & Stores, G. (2004). Psychological consequences of road traffic accidents for children and their mothers. *Psychological Medicine, 34*, 335–346.

Bryant, R. A., Moulds, M. L., & Guthrie, R. M. (2000). Acute stress disorder scale: A self-report measure of acute stress disorder. *Psychological Assessment, 12*(1), 61–68.

Burger, H., & Neeleman, J. (2007). A glossary on psychiatric epidemiology. *Journal of Epidemiology and Community Health, 61*(3), 185–189.

Cardena, E., Koopman, C., Classen, C., Waelde, L. C., & Spiegel, D. (2000). Psychometric properties of the Stanford Acute Stress Reaction Questionnaire (SASRQ): A valid and reliable measure of acute stress. *Journal of Traumatic Stress, 13*(4), 719–734.

Carter, J. D., Mulder, R. T., Bartram, A. F., & Darlow, B. A. (2005). Infants in neonatal intensive care unit: Parental response [Special edition]. *Archives of Disease in Childhood, 90*, F109–F113.

Classen, C., Koopman, C., Hales, R., & Spiegel, D. (1998). Acute stress disorder as a predictor of posttraumatic stress symptoms. *American Journal of Psychiatry, 155*(5), 620–624.

Cohen, S., Kamarck, T., & Mermelstein, R. (1983). A global measure of perceived stress. *Journal of Health and Social Behavior, 24*, 385–396.

Cohen, S., Kessler, R. C., & Gordon, L. U. (1997). *Measuring stress: A guide for health and social scientists.* New York: Oxford University Press.

Cox, J., Holden, M., & Sagovsky, R. (1987). Detection of postnatal depression: Development of the 10-item Edinburgh Postnatal Depression Scale. *British Journal of Psychiatry, 150*, 782–786.

Creamer, M., O'Donnell, M., & Pattison, P. (2004). The relationship between acute stress disorder and post traumatic stress disorder in severely injured trauma survivors. *Behavior Research & Therapy, 42*, 315–328.

Creedy, D., Shochet, I., & Horsfall, J. (2000). Childbirth and the development of acute trauma symptoms: Incidence and contributing factors. *Birth, 27*(2), 104–111.

Davis, L., Edwards, H., Mohay, H., & Wollin, J. (2003). The impact of very premature birth on the psychological health of mothers. *Early Human Development, 73*, 61–70.

Daviss, B. W., Racusin, R., Fleischer, A., Mooney, D., Ford, J., & McHugo, G. (2000). Acute stress disorder symptomatology during hospitalization for pediatric injury. *Journal of the American Academy of Child & Adolescent Psychiatry, 39*(5), 569–575.

DeMarco, R., Ford-Gilboe, M., Friedemann, M., McCubbin, H., & McCubbin, M. (2000). Stress, coping and family health. In V. Hill Rice (Ed.), *Handbook of stress, coping, and health—implications for nursing research, theory, and practice* (pp. 295–332). London: Sage.

DeMier, R. L., Hynan, M. T., Harris, H. B., & Manniello, R. L. (1996). Perinatal stressors as predictors of symptoms of posttraumatic stress in mothers of infants at high risk. *Journal of Perinatology, 16*(4), 276–280.

DeMier, R., Hynan, M. T., Hatfield, R. F., Varner, M. W., Harris, H. B., & Manniello, R. L. (2000). A measurement model of perinatal stressors: Identifying risk for postnatal emotional distress in mothers of high-risk infants. *Journal of Clinical Psychology, 56*(1), 89–100.

Diefe, J., Patacek, J., Roberts, J., Barocas, D., Rives, W., Appeldorf, W., et al. (2002). Acute stress disorder after burn injury: A predictor of PTSD? *Psychosomatic Medicine, 64*, 826–834.

Doering, L. V., Dracup, K., & Moser, D. (1999). Comparison of psychosocial adjustment of mothers and fathers of high-risk infants in the neonatal intensive care unit. *Journal of Perinatology, 19*(2), 132–137.

Doering, L.V., Moser, D. K., & Dracup, K. (2000). Correlates of anxiety, hostility, depression, and psychosocial adjustment in parents of NICU infants. *Neonatal Network, 19*(5), 15–23.

Elklit, A., & Brink, O. (2004). Acute stress disorder as a predictor of posttraumatic stress disorder in physical assault victims. *Journal of Interpersonal Violence, 19*(6), 709–726.

Feldman Reichman, S. R., Miller, C. A., Gordon, R. M., & Hendricks-Munoz, K. D. (2000). Stress appraisal and coping in mothers of NICU infants. *Children's Health Care, 29*(4), 279–293.

Foa, E. B., Cashman, L., Jaycox, L., Perry, K. (1997). The validation of a self-report measure of posttraumatic stress disorder: The Posttraumatic Diagnostic Scale. *Psychological Assessment,* (9), 445–451.

Franck, L. S., Cox, S., Allen, A., & Winter, I. (2005). Measuring neonatal intensive care unit-related parental stress. *Journal of Advanced Nursing, 49*(6), 608–615.

Garel, M., Dardennes, M., & Blondel, B. (2006). Mothers' psychological distress 1 year after very preterm childbirth. Results of the epipage qualitative study. *Child: Care, Health, and Development, 33*(2), 137–143.

Grace, S. L., Evindar, A., & Stewart, D. E. (2003). The effect of postpartum depression on child cognitive development and behavior: A review and critical analysis of the literature. *Archives of Women's Mental Health, 6,* 262–274.

Hack, M., & Fanaroff, A. A. (2000). Outcomes of children of extremely low birthweight and gestational age in the 1990s. *Seminars in Neonatology, 5,* 89–106.

Harvey, A. G., & Bryant, R. A. (2002). Acute stress disorder: A synthesis and critique. *Psychological Bulletin, 128*(6), 886–902.

Holditch-Davis, D., Bartlett, T. R., Blickman, A. L., & Miles, M. S. (2003). Posttraumatic stress symptoms in mothers of premature infants. *Journal of Obstetric, Gynecologic, and Neonatal Nursing, 32*(2), 161–171.

Hughes, M., McCollum, J., Sheftel, D., & Sanchez, G. (1994). How parents cope with the experience of neonatal intensive care. *Children's Health Care, 23*(1), 1–14.

Hynan, M. T. (2005). Supporting fathers during stressful times in the nursery: An evidence-based review. *Newborn and Infant Nursing Reviews, 5*(2), 87–92.

Jackson, K., Ternestedt, B., & Schollin, J. (2003). From alienation to familiarity: Experiences of mothers and fathers of preterm infants. *Journal of Advanced Nursing, 43*(2), 120–129.

Jamsa, K., & Jamsa, T. (1998). Technology in neonatal intensive care—a study on parents' experiences. *Technology and Health Care, 6,* 225–230.

Kassam-Adams, N., Garcia-Espana, F., Miller, V. A., & Winston, F. (2006). Parent–child agreement regarding children's acute stress: The role of parent acute stress reactions. *Journal of American Academy of Child and Adolescent Psychiatry, 45*(12), 1485–1493.

Kassam-Adams, N., & Newman, E. (2005). Child and parent reactions to participation in clinical research. *General Hospital Psychiatry, 27*(1), 29–35.

Kersting, A., Dorsch, M., Wesselmann, U., Ludorff, K., Witthaut, J., Ohrmann, P., et al. (2004). Maternal posttraumatic stress response after the birth of a very low birth weight infant. *Journal of Psychosomatic Research, 57,* 473–476.

Marshall, R. D., Spitzer, R., & Liebowitz, M. R. (1999). Review and critique of the new *DSM-IV* diagnosis of acute stress disorder. *American Journal of Psychiatry, 156*(11), 1677–1685.

Miles, M. S., Carlson, J., & Funk, S. G. (1996). Sources of support reported by mothers and fathers of infants hospitalized in a neonatal intensive care unit. *Neonatal Network, 15*(3), 45–52.

Miles, M. S., Funk, S. G., & Carlson, J. (1993). Parental stressor scale: Neonatal intensive care unit. *Nursing Research, 42*(3), 148–153.

Miles, M. S., Funk, S. G., & Kasper, M. A. (1991). The neonatal intensive care unit environment: Sources of stress for parents. *AACN Clinical Issues in Critical Care Nursing, 2*(2), 346–354.

Miles, M. S., Funk, S. G., & Kasper, M. A. (1992). The stress response of mothers and fathers of preterm infants. *Research in Nursing & Health, 15*, 261–269.

Miles, M., Holditch-Davis, D., Schwartz, T., & Sher, M. (2007). Depressive symptoms in mothers of prematurely born infants. *Journal of Developmental & Behavioral Pediatrics, 28*(1), 36–44.

Nystrom, K., & Axelsson, K. (2002). Mothers' experience of being separated from their newborns. *Journal of Obstetric, Gynecologic & Neonatal Nursing, 31*, 275–282.

O'Brien, M., Heron Asay, J., & McCluskey-Fawcett, K. (1999). Family functioning and maternal depression following premature birth. *Journal of Reproductive and Infant Psychology, 17*(2), 175–188.

Padden, T., & Glenn, S. (1997). Maternal experiences of preterm birth and neonatal intensive care. *Journal of Reproductive & Infant Psychology, 15*(2), 121–139.

Patino-Fernandez, A. M., Pai, A. L. H., Alderfer, M., Hwang, W., Reilly, A., & Kazak, A. E. (2007). Acute stress in parents of children newly diagnosed with cancer. *Pediatric Blood Cancer, 50*(2), 289–292.

Peebles-Kleiger, M. (2000). Pediatric and neonatal intensive care hospitalization as traumatic stressor: Implications for intervention. *Bulletin of the Menninger Clinic, 64*(2), 257–280.

Perehudoff, B. (1990). Parents' perceptions of environmental stressors in the special care nursery. *Neonatal Network, 9*(2), 39–44.

Pierrehumbert, B., Nicole, A., Muller-Nix, C., Forcada-Guex, M., & Ansermet, F. (2003). Parental post-traumatic reactions after premature birth: Implications for sleeping and eating problems in the infant [Special edition]. *Archives of Disease in Childhood, 88*, F400–F404.

Pinelli, J. (2000). Effects of family coping and resources on family adjustment and parental stress in the acute phase of the NICU experience. *Neonatal Network, 19*(6), 27–37.

Reid, T., & Bramwell, R. (2003). Using the parental stressor scale: NICU with a British sample of mothers of moderate risk preterm infants. *Journal of Reproductive and Infant Psychology, 21*(4), 279–291.

Richardson, D. K., Corcoran, J. D., Escobar, G. J., & Lee, S. K. (2001). SNAP-II and SNAPPE-II: Simplified newborn illness severity and mortality risk scores. *Journal of Pediatrics, 138*, 92–100.

Richardson, D. K., Gray, J. E., McCormick, M. C., Workman, K., & Goldmann, D. A. (1993). Score for neonatal acute physiology: A physiologic severity index for neonatal intensive care. *Pediatrics, 91*, 617–623.

Shaw, R. J., Deblois, T., Ikuta, L., Ginzburg, K., Fleisher, B., & Koopman, C. (2006). Acute stress disorder among parents of infants in neonatal intensive care nursery. *Psychosomatics, 47*(3), 206–212.

Shields-Poe, D., & Pinelli, J. (1997). Variables associated with parental stress in neonatal intensive care units. *Neonatal Network, 16*(1), 29–37.

Singer, L. T., Davillier, M., Bruening, P., Hawkins, S., & Yamashita, T. S. (1996). Social support, psychological distress, and parenting strains in mothers of very low birthweight infants. *Family Relations, 45*(3), 343–350.

Singer, L. T., Salvator, A., Guo, S., Collin, M., Lilien, L., & Baley, J. (1999). Maternal psychological distress and parenting stress after the birth of a very low-birth-weight infant. *Journal of the American Medical Association, 281*(9), 799–805.

Spear, M. L., Leef, K., Epps, S., & Locke, R. (2002). Family reactions during infants' hospitalization in the neonatal intensive care unit. *American Journal of Perinatology, 19*(4), 205–213.

Statistics Canada. (2004). Retrieved October 4, 1007, from http://www.statcan.ca/English/freepub/84F0210XIE/84F0210XIE2004001.pdf

Statistics Canada. (2007). *Births and birth rate, by province and territory.* Retrieved October 4, 2007, from http://www40.statcan.ca/l01/cst01/demo04a.htm?sdi=birth%20rates

Sutton, L., Bajuk, B., Berry, G., Eagles, B. L., & Henderson-Smart, D. J. (2002). Reliability of SNAP (score of neonatal acute physiology) data collection in mechanically ventilated term babies in New South Wales, Australia. *Acta Pediatrica, 91*, 424–429.

Sutton, L., Bajuk, B., Berry, G., Sayer, G. B., Richardson, V., & Henderson-Smart, D. J. (2002). Score of neonatal acute physiology as a measure of illness severity in mechanically ventilated term babies. *Acta Paediatrica, 91*, 415–423.

Thomas, K. A., Renaud, M. T., & DePaul, D. (2004). Use of parenting stress index in mothers of preterm infants. *Advances in Neonatal Care, 4*(1), 33–41.

Thompson, R. J., Oehler, J. M., Catlett, A. T., & Johndrow, D. A. (1993). Maternal psychological adjustment to the birth of an infant weighing 1500 grams or less. *Infant Behavior and Development, 16*, 471–485.

Walsh, F. (2003). Family resilience: Framework for clinical practice. *Family Process, 42*(1), 1–18.

Wigert, H., Johansson, R., Berg, M., & Hellstrom, A. L. (2006). Mothers' experiences of having their newborn child in a neonatal intensive care unit. *Scandinavian Journal of Caring Sciences, 20*, 35–41.

Winston, F. K., Baxt, C., Kassam-Adams, N. L., Elliott, M. R., & Kallan, M. J. (2005). Acute traumatic stress symptoms in child occupants and their parent drivers after crash involvement. *Archives of Pediatric Adolescent Medicine, 159,* 1074–1079.

Winston, F. K., Kassam-Adams, N., Vivarelli-O'Neil, C., Ford, J., Newman, E., Baxt, C., et al. (2002). Acute stress disorder symptoms in children and their parents after pediatric traffic injury. *Pediatrics, 109*(6), e90. Retrieved September 18, 2007, from http://www.pediatrics.org/cgi/content/full/109/6/e90

Wood, M. J., & Ross-Kerr, J. C. (2006). *Basic steps in planning nursing research* (6th ed.). Sudbury, MA: Jones and Bartlett.

Young Seideman, R., Watson, M., Corff, K. E., Odle, P., Haase, J., & Bowerman, J. L. (1997). Parent stress and coping in NICU and PICU. *Journal of Pediatric Nursing, 12*(3), 169–177.

Zupancic, J. A., Richardson, D. K., Horbar, J. D., Carpenter, J. H., Lee, S. K., Escobar, G. J., et al. (2007). Revalidation of the score for neonatal acute physiology in the Vermont Oxford Network. *Pediatrics, 119*, e156–e163.

Zwelling, E. (2000). The unexpected childbirth experience. In F. H. Nichols & S. Humenick (Eds.), *Childbirth education—practice, research and theory* (pp. 399–416). Toronto, Canada: WB Saunders.

EXHIBIT C-1
Information Letter

Title of Research Study

The incidence of acute stress disorder among parents of premature infants in the neonatal intensive care unit

Investigator

Jodi Jubinville, BScN, MN(c)

Graduate Student, Faculty of Nursing, University of Alberta

Pager Number: 445-2380

Jodi.Jubinville@capitalhealth.ca

Supervisors

Dr. C. Newburn-Cook, RN, PhD

Associate Dean of Research & Associate Professor

Faculty of Nursing, University of Alberta

Office Phone Number (780) 492-6764

christine.newburn-cook@ualberta.ca

Dr. K. Hegadoren, RN, PhD

Professor & Canada Research Chair

Faculty of Nursing, University of Alberta

Office Phone Number (780) 492-4591

kathy.hegadoren@ualberta.ca

Purpose

This research study is about reactions parents may have after their child is born premature. Moms and dads can have different reactions, so we are inviting both parents to describe their reactions separately.

Research Process

If you agree to be in this study, you will fill out three short surveys. The surveys will take about 15 minutes to finish. An interview will also be done in private. This will take about 30 minutes. The surveys also include questions to let us know more about you (for example, age, education level, job status, and income). The surveys will be given to you twice: when you decide to take part in this study and again in about two weeks. It is important to us that you choose times that suit your needs. We would also like your okay to get information from your baby's medical records. We will need to find out more about the pregnancy and delivery of your baby and the care received while in the neonatal intensive care unit. You will be given a special number so that all study information will remain private.

Possible Risks

Some of the questions we ask you may cause you to remember a very stressful time with your baby. If you feel that any of these questions are too hard to answer or if they upset you, please leave the question blank. You can withdraw from the study at any time. A social worker is available if you would like to speak to someone about feelings that may have come up while answering these questions.

EXHIBIT C-1   **373**

Possible Benefits

There is no direct benefit to you for taking part in this study. However, your answers will provide useful information to families, nurses, doctors, and social workers regarding how parents feel about having a baby in the neonatal intensive care unit. It may help us in knowing which parents are at higher risk for developing signs of stress. It may also help us in developing plans of care to assist these families.

Privacy

The research team will collect the results of surveys and information from your baby's medical record. We will only collect information that is needed for the research. All information collected in this study will be kept private, as required or permitted by law. If results from this study are published, you or your infant will not be named. You will be given a special number to keep your privacy. Your information will be kept in a locked cabinet at all times. Only the research team will be able to look at your information. This is a voluntary consent, which means you are free to refuse your consent to participation or to stop taking part in this study at any time without changing your baby's care at the Royal Alexandra Hospital.

Costs

There will be no cost for taking part in this study. At each time point a small token of thanks will be given to you.

Contact Names

If at any time you have questions about this study, you may contact me, Jodi (pager 445-2380), or my supervisors, Drs. Christine Newburn-Cook (492-6764) and Kathy Hegadoren (492-4591). The study has been approved by the Health Research Ethics Board at the University of Alberta. If you have any concerns about any aspect of this study, you may contact the Nursing Research Office at (780) 492-6832. This office is not involved with the research project.

EXHIBIT C-2
Consent Form

Project Title: The incidence of acute stress disorder among parents of premature infants in the neonatal intensive care unit

Investigator:
Jodi Jubinville, BScN, MN(c)
Master of Nursing Graduate Student
Faculty of Nursing, University of Alberta
Pager Number: 445-2380

Supervisors

Dr. C. Newburn-Cook, RN, PhD
Associate Dean of Research & Associate Professor
Faculty of Nursing, University of Alberta
Office Phone Number (780) 492-6764
christine.newburn-cook@ualberta.ca

Dr. K. Hegadoren, RN, PhD
Professor & Canada Research Chair
Faculty of Nursing, University of Alberta
Office Phone Number (780) 492-4591
kathy.hegadoren@ualberta.ca

Consent of Parent Participant

Do you understand that you have been asked to be in a research study?	Yes	No
Have you read and received a copy of the attached information sheet?	Yes	No
Do you understand the benefits and risks involved in taking part in this research study?	Yes	No
Have you had the opportunity to ask questions and discuss the study?	Yes	No
Do you understand that you are free to refuse to participate or withdraw from the study at any time? You do not have to give a reason, and it will not affect the care your infant receives while in the neonatal intensive care unit.	Yes	No
Has the issue of confidentiality been explained to you?	Yes	No
Do you understand that the findings may be published or presented at conferences, but your name or any material that may identify you will not be used?	Yes	No
Do you understand that the research team will have access to your baby's medical records?	Yes	No
Do you understand who will have access to your study records?	Yes	No

Would you like a report of the research findings? If so, address:

_____

_____

This consent was explained to me by: _____   Date: _____

I agree to take part in this study

_____   _____
Signature of Research Participant   Printed Name

I believe that the person signing this form understands what is involved in the study and voluntarily agrees to participate.

_____   _____
Signature of Investigator   Printed Name

Nausea and Vomiting Following Posterior Fossa Surgery: Determination of Incidence, Risk, and Protective Factors in Children

By Susan M. Neufeld

Introduction

The successful management of nausea and vomiting is a fundamental part of nursing care of children after neurosurgery. Several risk factors have been examined as contributing to postoperative nausea and vomiting (PONV) in other surgical populations. These risk factors include a prior history of motion sickness or PONV, the age of the child, type of anesthetic, length and/or location of surgery, use of opioids, experience of pain, and exposure to other noxious stimuli (Gan, 2006). Ineffective management of PONV may result in pressure on surgical incisions, pulmonary aspiration, increased intracranial pressure, delay in recovery, increased length of hospital stay, and significant distress for the child and family (Macario, Weinger, Carney, & Kim, 1999; Scuderi & Conlay, 2003). For children who require cancer treatment after their surgery, their experience of even mild PONV could have an effect on future nausea and vomiting with their chemotherapy and/or radiation therapy protocols causing more deleterious effects (American Society of Health Systems Pharmacists, 1999). Although estimates of cumulative incidence of PONV in other populations of children are more than 40% (Rose &

Watcha, 1999; Rowley & Brown, 1982), little attention has been paid to PONV in children following neurosurgery.

From clinical observation, children who have undergone posterior fossa surgery (surgery for brain tumors or malformations that occur in the back bottom part of the brain, below the tentorium, where the brainstem and cerebellum reside) appear to be at highest risk for long-lasting, severe, and unremitting PONV (Neufeld, 2002). However, this observation has not yet been substantiated by any research. Even the adult neurosurgery literature that has examined the contribution of location of neurosurgery to PONV is inconclusive (Fabling, et al., 1997; Irefin, et al., 2003). Even more troublesome is the lack of investigation into the kind of severe intractable PONV that is occasionally observed clinically after posterior fossa surgery.

The development of protocols for preventing and treating adverse outcomes, such as PONV, requires that the characteristics of those in the population who do and do not experience the outcome be determined. The identification of these risk and protective factors for PONV in neurosurgery is limited to studies in adults (Fabling, et al., 1997; Flynn & Nemergut, 2006; Irefin, et al., 2003; Meng & Quinlan, 2006; Stieglitz, et al., 2005). Multivariable models of PONV developed for adults to delineate significant risk factors for prognosis show limited validity for use for children (Eberhart, Morin, et al., 2004). The only multivariable model of PONV developed for children (Eberhart, Geldner, et al., 2004) did not examine risk factors that are unique to pediatric neurosurgical populations because it excluded these children in their sample.

The purpose of this study is to determine the epidemiology of PONV in children after posterior fossa surgery. A five-year retrospective chart review of all children who had posterior fossa surgery will be conducted at participating children's hospital sites across Canada. First, the cumulative incidence of nausea and vomiting and retching at specific time periods after surgery will be determined. Second, the number of children with severe PONV will be determined. Third, risk and protective factors for the occurrence of vomiting, retching, and severe PONV will be explored. Fourth, the relationship among these two outcomes and other adverse events will be examined.

Following neurosurgery, the care of children requires a comprehensive approach to the prevention and management of PONV, including careful assessment; the use of an efficacious PONV protocol; and implementation of nonpharmacological strategies, such as appropriate delay of oral intake, assuring slow movements, and providing a low stimulation environment that limits noise, activity, motion, and light. Reliable and valid preventive intervention programs must target those at highest risk to prevent unnecessary related risk, burden to the child and family, and expense to the healthcare system. The results of this study will advance our knowledge of PONV in a vulnerable group of children by establishing risk and protective factors to help clinical decision making and will provide the foundation for further studies.

Background

The term "postoperative nausea and vomiting (PONV)" covers one or more of three symptoms: nausea, retching, and vomiting (Gan, 2006). Nausea is the unpleasant sensation of the urge to vomit that occurs along with neurological changes, such as excessive salivation and swallowing (Apfel, Roewer, & Korttila, 2002). Retching is the first phase of vomiting (Hornby, 2001) and is commonly defined as an unproductive attempt to vomit (Apfel, et al., 2002). Vomiting is the forceful expulsion of stomach contents through the mouth that involves coordinated autonomic processes in the brain and gut (Hornby, 2001). Occurring alone or in combination, these symptoms may cause discomfort and distress for the individual, put pressure on surgical incisions, increase intracranial pressure, cause dehydration and electrolyte imbalance, delay recovery, and prolong hospitalization (Macario, et al., 1999; Scuderi & Conlay, 2003).

PONV is common in children following craniotomy (Furst, et al., 1996). Although its incidence has not been described, severe refractory PONV has been reported as a clinical concern for children after posterior fossa surgery (Neufeld, 2002). Clinical experience and the proximity of neurological processes associated with nausea and vomiting to the location of the surgical procedure makes the exploration of PONV in children after posterior fossa surgery an important area of research. In this paper, the rationale for research that is focused on PONV in children after posterior fossa surgery will be developed. A literature review of critical aspects of PONV in children and adults will follow to establish the rationale for further study. Finally, the research design of a multisite retrospective study to determine the incidence of PONV and its risk and protective factors for children after posterior fossa surgery will be presented.

Why Focus on PONV in Children After Posterior Fossa Surgery?

Children who require neurosurgery form a heterogeneous group that ranges from healthy children to children with severe disabilities. Surgical treatment spans from one-hour shunt operations to brain tumor operations that last more than 12 hours. One approach to addressing the heterogeneity in pediatric neurosurgery in the study of PONV is to limit the sample to a particular area of neurosurgery and build on knowledge from there. By specifically studying children after posterior fossa surgery, the research questions can also be focused on the determination of incidence and the unique risk and protective factors for PONV for this group of children. This approach has shown success in determining risk and protective factors specific to the location of the neurosurgery in three adult studies (Flynn & Nemergut, 2006; Meng & Quinlan, 2006; Stieglitz, et al., 2005).

Neurosurgeons have determined by experience that certain specific areas of the brain are frequently associated with protracted postoperative vomiting. Along with vomiting usually comes varying degrees of nausea but also sometimes hiccups, bradycardia episodes, or apnea spells. Sudden or dramatic changes in intracranial pressure alone, especially low intracranial pressure, can be associated with intractable vomiting, but the most serious vomiting seems to be associated with posterior fossa surgery.

Posterior fossa surgery takes place below the tentorium cerebelli in the posterior cranial fossa. The posterior cranial fossa houses the back bottom part of the brain, including the cerebellum, brainstem, and cranial nerves III–XII. Complex physical, chemical, and emotional processes are involved in nausea, retching, and vomiting. Although the reticulospinal tracts, diencephalon, limbic system, and discrete areas of the cerebral hemispheres may all be involved in nausea and vomiting (Ganong, 1987), the coordination of the autonomic changes associated with retching and vomiting occurs at the level of the medulla oblongata in the posterior fossa (Hornby, 2001; Miller, 1999). Areas of the medulla oblongata that are involved in retching and vomiting include the area postrema in the lower lateral wall of the fourth ventricle, which has cells that are more sensitive to circulating emetic substances than the underlying medulla; the nucleus tractus solitarius (NTS), which receives input from the area postrema, vestibular apparatus, and abdominal vagal afferents; as well as groups of neurons that are scattered throughout the medulla that may be activated in sequence by a central pattern generator (CPG), which receives input from the NTS.

Biologically and clinically, children after posterior fossa surgery appear to be at highest risk for PONV, especially severe refractory PONV. Lesions anywhere in the posterior fossa can be associated with intractable vomiting, both preoperatively and postoperatively. The worst cases of PONV seem to occur with surgery near the dorsal surface of the brainstem (floor of fourth ventricle). The lower in the brainstem, the worse the vomiting, with the worst areas being close to the midline below the striae medullares (vagal trigone) or near the lateral recesses (vestibular area). Intractable vomiting is such a problem with surgery in and around the medulla oblongata that plans for tracheostomy tube airway management and gastrostomy tube feeding are usually discussed with the family before proposed midline posterior fossa surgery.

Literature Review

The incidence, risk and protective factors, prevention, and treatment of PONV in children after posterior fossa surgery have not been identified in the literature. The purpose of this review is to bring together relevant literature from studies of PONV in other patient groups to provide insight and direction for this research project. First, the incidence of PONV in children after craniotomy is discussed. Second, risk and protective factors for PONV will be identified along with a discussion of the applicability of adult studies to children. Third, the applicability of the only pediatric study of children after neurosurgery is reviewed. Finally, the literature on strategies for prevention and treatment of PONV and severe refractory PONV in neurosurgery is reviewed.

Incidence of PONV in Children After Craniotomy

Although PONV has been identified as frequent following craniotomy in adults (Du Pen, et al., 1992; Irefin, et al., 2003; Manninin, Raman, Boyle, & el-Beheiry, 1999; Wong, O'Regan, & Irwin, 2006), studies aimed at determining its incidence in children have not been published. One small randomized controlled trial provides some insight into the incidence of PONV in children after craniotomy. Furst and colleagues (1996) examined postoperative vomiting (POV) to determine the efficacy of ondansetron in the first 24 hours after either supratentorial or infratentorial craniotomy in children. In this study of 60 children aged 2–16 years, 57% of children experienced at least one episode of vomiting within 24 hours of craniotomy despite prophylactic treatment with antiemetics. This result is higher than the estimated 40% of children in other surgical populations who experience POV (Rose & Watcha, 1999; Rowley & Brown, 1982). Finally, even in the overall pediatric literature, little work has been done to look at postoperative nausea (PON) in children (Fisher, 1997), and no one has looked at severe refractory PONV, even though Rowley and Brown called for such studies in 1982 (Rowley & Brown, 1982).

Risk and Protective Factors for PONV

Knowledge about risk and protective factors helps guide clinical decision making and furthers research into mechanisms of disease, prognosis, and efficacy of new interventions (Concato, Feinstein, & Holford, 1993; Gan, 2006; Harrell, Lee, & Mark, 1996). Currently, there are no studies of risk and protective factors for PONV in children after neurosurgery. Overall, there are numerous published studies of risk and protective factors for PONV and a few studies of PONV in adults after neurosurgery. The application of these results to children may be appealing, but multivariable models of risk and protective factors for PONV in adults do not appear to generalize to children (Eberhart, Morin, et al., 2004). Furthermore, the one published study of risk factors for PONV in children (Eberhart, Geldner, et al., 2004) has limitations for use in children after posterior fossa surgery.

Overall Risk and Protective Factors for PONV

In his recent systematic review of more than 20 multivariable models of risk and protective factors for PONV (including one developed with a pediatric sample) and dozens of univariable studies and clinical trials, Gan (2006) identified established, possible, and disproved risk factors. Established risk factors included female gender postpuberty; nonsmoking status; history of PONV or motion sickness; childhood after infancy and younger adulthood; increasing duration of surgery; and the use of volatile anesthetics, nitrous oxide, a large dose of neostigmine, and intraoperative or postoperative opioids. Possible, but not confirmed, risk factors included better American Society of Anesthesiologists (ASA) physical status; history of migraine (nausea only); preoperative anxiety; ethnicity; history of PONV or motion sickness in a parent or sibling; certain surgery types (among them neurosurgery); less intraoperative fluid administration; increasing duration of anesthesia; general anesthesia versus other forms; and use of longer-acting opioids. The short list of disproved risk factors included early phase menstruation; obesity; and lack of supplemental oxygen.

Risk and Protective Factors for PONV in Neurosurgery

There are five published studies that focus on risk and protective factors for PONV in neurosurgery—all are limited to surgery in adults. First, Fabling and colleagues (1997), in a multivariable analysis of retrospective data from 199 adults after craniotomy, found that posterior fossa surgery, female gender, and younger age were predictors of PONV by 24 hours. Duration of anesthetic, fentanyl dose, and postoperative opioid use were removed from their model as insignificant. Irefin et al. (2003) conducted a prospective study of PON and pain in 128 patients following craniotomy and did not find a relationship between craniotomy location (supratentorial versus posterior fossa) and nausea (vomiting was not examined).

Stieglitz and colleagues (2005) conducted a retrospective analysis of the preoperative symptoms and conditions that contributed to nausea and dizziness in 115 patients after vestibular schwannoma surgery. This study was the only one that attempted to quantify postoperative symptoms by describing the number of days that the patients experienced symptoms. The mean number of days that patients suffered from nausea was 2.3 (range of 0–16 days), and 32% had symptoms longer than three days. Of preoperative vertigo symptoms, examination findings, gender, tumor size, tumor grade, side of tumor, body mass index, and positive stepping test, univariate analysis (Student's t-tests) showed significant differences for gender and tumor grade. Interestingly, those with tumor classes 4a (compression of the brainstem) and 4b (severe dislocation of the brainstem and compression of the fourth ventricle) showed less nausea than those with early tumor classes 1 (localized intrameatal), 2 (has an extrameatal part), 3a (fills the cerebellopontine cistern), and 3b (reaches the brainstem). The authors hypothesized that patients with later tumor grades were accustomed to vestibular dysfunction and better able to compensate postoperatively than those with early tumor grades. The greater degree of retraction on the cerebellum and vestibular nerves required to expose smaller tumors was another proposed explanation for this unexpected finding.

Flynn and Nemergut (2006), in a retrospective analysis of 877 adults after transsphenoidal surgery, found an incidence of postoperative vomiting of 7.5% in this patient population during the period of their postanesthesia care unit stay. A higher incidence of vomiting was reported in patients who required a lumbar intrathecal catheter (11.4%), those who experienced a cerebral spinal fluid leak and subsequent fat grafting (17.1%), and those who presented with craniopharyngiomas (18%). Antiemetic prophylaxis was related to a lower incidence of nausea but was not related to vomiting. In this study, nausea was measured by the documented use of an antiemetic drug after complaining of nausea, so the reliability of the researchers' measure for nausea could explain this result (i.e., nurses were less likely to give a second dose of an antiemetic for nausea if an intraoperative dose was already given).

Most recently, Meng and Quinlan (2006) conducted a five-year retrospective analysis of PONV in 185 patients following retromastoid craniectomy with microvascular decompression of cranial nerves. Sixty percent of the patients experienced nausea, vomiting, or both, even though 99% of them received prophylactic ondansetron. These authors developed a multivariable model that included the risk factors of decompressive surgery for cranial nerve V (versus cranial nerves VII, IX, and X), use of desflurane (versus sevoflurane), and female gender, and the protective factor of the use of a transdermal scopolamine (TDS) patch to account for PONV in this population. Anesthetic time, muscle relaxants, reversal drugs, intraoperative propofol, use of fentanyl, and use of postoperative opioids were excluded in their model.

The literature on neurosurgery and PONV shows two different approaches to the identification of risk and protective factors for PONV: general and specific. Studies that focus on a specific neurosurgical approach (transsphenoidal, retromastoid) or type of tumor (vestibular schwannoma, craniopharyngioma) allow for the delineation of risk factors specific to those patients. These factors may be missed in studies that take a broader focus with a more heterogeneous population if a similar number of participants were included.

Applicability of Adult Studies to Children

Because there are studies of risk and protective factors for adults after neurosurgery and refined prognostic models for adults, there may be a temptation to apply these findings to children. To determine the applicability of adult multivariable risk models of PONV to children, Eberhart, Morin, and colleagues (2004) selected five models (Apfel, et al., 1998; Apfel, et al., 1999; Koivuranta & Laara, 1998; Palazzo & Evans, 1993; Sinclair, Chung, & Mezei, 1999) that allowed for the calculation of risk during the first 24 hours after surgery and showed content validity for a pediatric population. To validate these models, Eberhart and colleagues measured POV in the first 24 hours in 1150 children aged 0–12 years. The study took place over 22 months and included a university hospital, a community hospital, and an outpatient surgical center. There were no children with neurosurgery in the sample. The majority of children had ear, nose, and throat surgery (42%), urological surgery (24%), ophthalmic surgery (16%), or abdominal procedures (10%). Anesthetic protocols were not standardized, but 128 children who were given prophylactic antiemetics or dexamethasone had their data withdrawn. Thirty-nine patients were also lost to follow-up. Of the 983 children remaining, 326 experienced at least one episode of POV in 24 hours. As shown in Table D-1, the models were not well calibrated. Even more disappointing was the limited ability of any of

TABLE D-1
Validation of Adult Models of PONV in Children

First author	Formula	Calibration curve (Eberhart, Morin, et al., 2004)	Area under the ROC curve* (95% CI) (Eberhart, Morin, et al., 2004)
Palazzo (1993)	Risk of PONV = $1/1 + e^{-logit(p)}$ P = 5.03 + 2.24 (postoperative opioids) + 3.97 (history PONV) + 2.4 (female gender) + 0.78 (motion sickness) − 3.2 (female gender × motion sickness)	$y = 0.55x + 30$	0.56 (0.52–0.60)
Koivuranta (1998)	Risk of POV = 7, 17, 25, 38, and 61% when 0–5 factors are present: Female gender, previous PONV, duration of surgery >60 min, nonsmoking, motion sickness	$y = 1.18x + 8$	0.61 (0.58–0.65)
Apfel (1998)	Risk of POV = $1/1 + e^{-logit(p)}$ P = −1.92 + 1.28 (female gender) − 0.029 (age) − 0.74 (smoking) + 0.63 (history of POV or motion sickness) + 0.26 (duration of surgery)	$y = 0.51x + 18$	0.59 (0.56–0.63)
Sinclair (1999)	Risk of PONV = $1/1 + e^{-logit(p)}$ P = 2.36 + 0.014 (age) − 1.03 (male gender) − 0.42 (smoking) + 1.14 (history PONV) + 0.46 (duration of surgery/30) + 1.48 (ENT) + 1.9 (plastics) + 1.2 (gynecological non-D&C) + 1.04 (orthopedic knee) + 1.78 (orthopedic shoulder) + 0.94 (orthopedic other) − 5.97	$y = 0.64x + 13$	0.65 (0.61–0.69)
Apfel (1999)	Risk of PONV = 10, 21, 39, 61, and 79% when 0–4 factors are present: Female gender, postoperative opioids, previous PONV or motion sickness, nonsmoking	$y = 0.64x + 14$	0.58 (0.54–0.62)

*0.50 = No discrimination; 0.60 = Poor; 0.70 = Acceptable; 0.80 = Good; 0.90 = Excellent

the models to discriminate among children who developed POV and those who did not. These authors concluded that prognostic models for children needed development.

Risk Factors for PONV in Children

After testing models of PONV from the adult literature, Eberhart, Geldner, and colleagues (2004) developed a multivariable model followed by a risk scoring system specifically for pediatric patients. Again, the outcome was an episode of POV within 24 hours. A total of 1401 children aged 0–14 years were prospectively enrolled, with 88 excluded for receiving a prophylactic antiemetic or dexamethasone and 56 lost to follow-up, leaving 1257 children in the final sample. A split sample technique was used for internal validation with 657 in the evaluation data set and 600 in the validation data set. Similar types of surgery were performed as in their initial study; again, there were no neurosurgical patients.

The final model included four predictor variables: (1) strabismus surgery; (2) age ≤ 3 or > 3 years; (3) duration of surgery >30 minutes; (4) history of POV in the child and/or history of PONV in father, mother, or siblings. The factors excluded from the model due to lack of statistical significance were female gender, administration of local or regional anesthesia, and the use of intraoperative and postoperative opioids. There was no testing for interaction effects or confounders. From their final multivariable model, Eberhart, Geldner, and colleagues created a clinical prediction rule: 0, 1, 2, 3, and 4 of the risk factors translated into a 9%, 10%, 30%, 55%, and 70% incidence of POV.

The results of the study by Eberhart, Geldner, and colleagues (2004) may help guide the development of a multivariable model of the risk and protective factors for PONV in children after neurosurgery, but the applicability of their prognostic model and the simplified risk score is limited. Any attempt to validate the prognostic model would likely show underfitting because important predictive factors for children after neurosurgery are missing. Furthermore, two of the factors in the simplified risk score do not apply to this group of children. Strabismus surgery is not a variable for neurosurgical patients and likely reflects the idiosyncrasies of the sample, that is, the predominantly day surgery population. A second limitation is that even the shortest neurosurgical procedures last longer than 30 minutes. Using their simplified risk score, children after neurosurgery could only score from 1–3 and would therefore never be considered at low or very high risk for PONV.

The exclusion of children who received antiemetics and dexamethasone is also a concern because these drugs are often used as a standard of care for brain tumor operations. The administration of dexamethasone and/or antiemetics could better be examined within a multivariable model as protective factors. Finally, Eberhart, Geldner, and colleagues' (2004) failure to examine interaction effects may explain why gender was excluded from the model. Gender is a confirmed risk factor in adult studies (Gan, 2006); therefore, females after menarche may be at greater risk in a pediatric study.

Prevention and Treatment Strategies for PONV After Neurosurgery

The literature on treatment strategies for PONV after neurosurgery has no reports of nonpharmacologic prophylactic or treatment strategies for adults or children. Nonpharmacologic strategies encompass acupuncture, acupoint stimulation, and acupressure (Lee & Done, 1999), delaying oral intake (Kearney, Mack, & Entwistle, 1998), and environmental changes. In the few reports on the use of pharmacologic strategies that have been published, it remains uncertain whether or not the current strategies have much of an impact on the incidence of PONV after craniotomy (Flynn & Nemergut, 2006; Furst, et al., 1996; Neufeld & Newburn-Cook, 2007). Finally, treatment for severe, refractory PONV is limited to a single case report.

Pharmacologic Prevention Strategies

That Furst and colleagues (1996) found no effect for ondansetron in preventing POV after craniotomy in children concurs with the few studies of protective interventions for adults that have been conducted in neurosurgery. Studies of total intravenous anesthesia (TIVA) (Wong, et al., 2006) and prophylactic $5HT_3$ receptor antagonists (Neufeld & Newburn-Cook, 2007) suggest that the rates of PONV remain high even with interventions that have shown efficacy in other surgical populations. Awake supratentorial craniotomy versus general anesthetic showed a decrease in PONV only in the first four hours after surgery (Manninen & Tan, 2002). Because the risk for PONV may depend on what areas of the brain are manipulated (Fabling, et al., 1997; Flynn & Nemergut, 2006; Meng & Quinlan, 2006), effective strategies for prevention and treatment may need to depend more on the area and type of surgery than on individual risk factors and anesthetic techniques.

In their retrospective analysis of PONV in adults after microvascular decompression of the cranial nerves, Meng and Quinlan (2006) found a lower incidence of PONV with the preoperative use of a transdermal scopolamine (TDS) patch. The TDS patch has shown limited efficacy for prevention of PONV in other surgical populations (Kranke, Morin, Roewer, Wulf, & Eberhart, 2002), and its role for neurosurgical patients has not been well studied. Scopolamine is an anticholinergic that acts on all five subtypes of muscarinic receptors (Yates, Miller, & Lucot, 1998), whose proposed antiemetic mechanism of action is in the central nervous system through inhibition of vestibular impulses to the vestibular nuclei, the cerebellum, and the brainstem reticular areas (Murray, 1997). This centrally mediated mechanism of action on vestibular impulses may be the reason for its proposed effectiveness with this type of surgery.

Other prevention strategies that have been investigated with limited success in the adult neurosurgical population include droperidol (Fabling, Gan, El-Moalem, Warner, & Borel, 2000) and metoclopramide (Cremonesi, Tenuto, & Bairao, 1967; Kuwabara & Amano, 1966; Pugh, Jones, & Barsoum, 1996). Dimenhydrinate has commonly been given in neurosurgery but has not been researched in this population. A systematic review and meta-analysis of dimenhydrinate shows some efficacy in preventing PONV for other surgical populations (Kranke, Morin, Roewer, & Eberhart, 2002). Dexamethasone, which is commonly used by neurosurgeons perioperatively to control cerebral edema (Hartsell, Long, & Kirsch, 2005), has antiemetic properties as well and may work best when used in combination with other classes of antiemetics (Henzi, Walder, & Tramer, 2000).

Treatment for Severe Refractory PONV

The literature on treatment for severe, refractory, and/or cyclic vomiting after posterior fossa surgery is limited to a single adult case study. Guttuso, Vitticore and Holloway (2005) describe a 58-year-old man who underwent a resection for a 6.5 cm posterior fossa cholesteatoma that was compressing his left cerebellar hemisphere. This individual went on to experience PONV, which resolved in three days. He was then discharged home only to return two days later with a resumption of his nausea and vomiting. His symptoms continued despite a polypharmaceutical attempt at symptom control: trimethobenzamide, a promethazine suppository, metoclopramide, lorazepam, and a one-week trial of ondansetron and dexamethasone. Four weeks later, his symptoms remained, he had a 40 pound weight loss, and he was readmitted for life-threatening nausea and vomiting. A lateral decubitus and flexed position in bed was the only thing that appeared to relieve his symptoms. At the time of his second postoperative admission, he was also experiencing frequent hiccups, which would culminate in an emetic episode. There was no evidence of hydrocephalus on diagnostic imaging, and a lumbar puncture showed an opening pressure of 21 cm H_2O. He did not experience vertigo; however, he did have bilateral end gaze lateral nystagmus. Further treatment with ondansetron, dexamethasone, and famotidine showed no improvement, nor did treatment with granisetron or chlorpromazine. Finally, all antiemetics were discontinued and a dose of gabapentin and a TDS patch were tried. Within 14 hours of administering gabapentin and applying the TDS patch, the symptoms improved. A regimen of these two drugs proved successful for long-term therapy and were discontinued after six months (missing a single dose of gabapentin resulted in retching, as did an attempt to reduce the TDS patch at two months postdischarge).

This case study is important in a number of ways. Primarily, it highlights the effect that severe, unremitting PONV can have on individuals. It also points to the need for studies of PONV that go beyond the first few days after surgery. The case study highlights the frustrations of using an uncoordinated and underresearched polypharmaceutical approach to PONV. Finally, it points to a need for research into combined regimens, such as the use of a TDS patch and gabapentin. Gabapentin is a gamma-aminobutyric acid analog whose mechanism of action in chemotherapy-induced nausea has been suggested to be the mitigation of central tachykinin neurotransmitter activity (Guttuso, Roscoe, & Griggs, 2003). Currently, the use of gabapentin in neurosurgery is limited to treatment of neuralgia; however, given its central mechanism of action, it holds promise for future research in PONV, especially for those who are at risk for experiencing severe unremitting and/or cyclic vomiting. Before comprehensive prevention and treatment strategies can be developed and tested, however, the magnitude of the problem of PONV in specific neurosurgical populations needs to be elucidated and risk and protective factors need to be identified.

Research Study of Nausea and Vomiting Following Posterior Fossa Surgery: Determination of Incidence, Risk, and Protective Factors in Children

Clearly, there is a need to identify the incidence of PONV and the risk and protective factors for PONV in children after neurosurgery to improve their postoperative care. Childhood and neurosurgery are risk factors that have not been examined together. Previous research has identified important risk factors for children and adults that may be investigated in children after neurosurgery. For example, age, length of surgery, and history of PONV are important general risk factors for children. Female after menarche is an established risk factor in adult studies and may have an important affect on older girls. Adult neurosurgical studies that focus on a particular craniotomy site delineate specific risk and protective factors for that area. Posterior fossa surgery may pose unique risks for PONV due to the proximity of the surgery to key neurocircuits for vomiting. Posterior fossa surgery is also an area of clinical concern for PONV and severe refractory PONV. Focusing research on this vulnerable group of children will allow for the examination of factors, such as type of surgery, location of surgery (midline versus hemispheric), and histopathology, that have not been examined before.

Measurement of PONV is also an issue for neurosurgery. As was highlighted by the case report (Guttuso, et al., 2005) and the study of vestibular schwannoma surgery (Stieglitz, et al., 2005), the risk period for nausea and vomiting after posterior fossa surgery may extend well past 24 hours. By looking at the distribution of PONV over the entire length of the postoperative neurosurgical admission, critical time periods can be further delineated. The severity of PONV is also important to describe because the risk factors and choice of interventions for this population may be different for those with brief self-limited PONV than for children experiencing severe refractory PONV. When the incidence of PONV in children after posterior fossa surgery is described and risk and protective factors are delineated, further research into the development of prognostic models and on determining the efficacy of interventions that are targeted to those at greatest risk can be conducted.

Research Goal

The goal of this research project is to describe PONV in children after posterior fossa surgery. Strategies to achieve this goal include determining the cumulative incidence of nausea and vomiting/retching at specified time periods over the course of the children's neurosurgical postoperative hospital admissions; quantifying the severity of PONV; identifying documented prevention and treatment strategies; determining significant risk and protective factors; and exploring the relationship of PONV to adverse outcomes.

Design

The study design will be a multisite retrospective study. The accurate estimation of the incidence, risk, and protective factors of PONV requires a sample size that would otherwise take years to collect prospectively. A retrospective study design is therefore an efficient way to get initial estimates of cumulative incidence and risk and protective factors and to guide the design of future studies.

Research Questions

1. What is the cumulative incidence of nausea in children after posterior fossa surgery by 4, 8, 12, 24, and subsequent 24-hour periods until discharge from neurosurgical postoperative hospital care?

2. What is the cumulative incidence of vomiting/retching in children after posterior fossa surgery by 4, 8, 12, 24, and subsequent 24-hour periods until discharge from neurosurgical postoperative hospital care?

3. What is the frequency distribution of the number of vomiting/retching events experienced in children after posterior fossa surgery over the course of the neurosurgical postoperative hospital care?

4. What is the frequency distribution of the number of days that vomiting/retching and nausea were experienced in children after posterior fossa surgery over the course of the neurosurgical postoperative hospital care?

5. What are the major risk and protective factors for vomiting/retching over the course of the children's postoperative neurosurgical stay?

6. What comorbidities do children with vomiting/retching experience after posterior fossa surgery?

Sample Selection and Sample Size Estimation

Children aged 0–16 years who had posterior fossa surgery between March 2002 and March 2007 at the Stollery Children's Hospital in Edmonton, SickKids in Toronto, and other children's hospital sites (pending approval) will be included in the study. Children with infratentorial tumors and Chiari I malformations will make up the majority of the sample. Fourth ventricular shunt procedures, operations without dural and arachnoid openings (outside the brain), surgery for traumatic brain injury, and children requiring prolonged intubation (greater than 48 hours) will be excluded. If the child required a second posterior fossa surgery during the course of the data collection period, data will be collected separately for each surgery with the same participant identification number. Data from any second and subsequent procedures will not be included in the initial analysis but may be considered for a secondary within-subjects analysis and will be collected only when other data collection is complete.

By collecting data in a number of sites, there will be data from approximately 300 children. This will also allow for an estimation of incidence and 95% confidence interval within a 6% margin of error (Piface & Lenth, 2006) and for a multivariable analysis of 10–15 variables for an outcome incidence ranging from 30–70% (Peduzzi, Concato, Kemper, & Holford, 1996).

Data Collection Procedures

A case report developed specifically for the study by the author, in collaboration with a pediatric educator in children's surgery, a neurosurgeon at the Stollery Children's Hospital, and two clinical nurse specialists/advanced nurse practitioners in children's neurosurgery at SickKids (Exhibit D-1), will be used for data collection. Data will be collected by review of the child's medical history, previous surgery (for any history of PONV), anesthesia records, operative reports, recovery room records, in and out flowcharts, nursing records, and medication administration records (Exhibit D-2). The data collection period extends over the course of a child's neurosurgical postoperative hospital stay. This time period is defined as the duration of the child's hospital stay that is related to his or her surgery. Thus, data collection will end when the child goes home, is transferred from neurosurgical care to rehabilitation care (i.e., to a rehabilitation hospital or rehabilitation unit), or is transferred from neurosurgery care to oncology care for further treatments. The reason for any readmission to the hospital or neurosurgical care, if not discharged within 30 days of discharge from neurosurgical postoperative care, will also be noted.

Data will be collected at each site by nurses with extensive pediatric neurosurgical experience. To ensure reliability, all those involved in data collection will train on five charts, and the case report form will be revised as needed. Each person will then review the same five randomly selected charts to establish interrater reliability. Discrepancies will be resolved through discussion. If necessary, the procedure will be repeated until 90% interrater reliability is achieved for the overall case report form and 100% interrater reliability is achieved for the cumulative incidence of retching/vomiting over the course of the children's neurosurgical postoperative hospital care and cumulative incidence of nausea over the course of the children's neurosurgical postoperative hospital care.

Measurement

Table D-2 contains a review of the definition and measurement of the outcome measures of PONV for this study. It is widely accepted that PON and POV data be collected separately (Apfel, et al., 2002; Gan, 2006; Korttila, 1992). Because of their similar physiology, retching and vomiting should be considered together in the data analysis (Korttila, 1992) but again can be collected separately. It is likely that retching will only be documented when it occurs repeatedly without vomiting; therefore, estimates of retching will not be accurate enough to analyze this variable on its own. Nausea may also not be well documented unless it occurs over a prolonged period without vomiting. For these reasons, multivariable modeling for this study will be limited to the measures of vomiting/retching taken at 48 hours and over the course of the child's postoperative neurosurgical admission and combined for the outcome of severe, refractory PONV.

Other variables that will be collected include demographic information, presenting symptoms, use of steroids, use of preventive antiemetics, anesthetic procedures, surgery details, and use of pain medications. For brain tumors, location, size, degree of resection, and pathology will be noted.

Data Analysis

Data analysis will be conducted using SPSS Version 14.0 software. Demographic and study variables will be summarized using descriptive statistics that are appropriate to their level of measurement. The primary outcome of cumulative incidence of vomiting/retching (number of individuals experiencing at least one event ÷ total number of individuals in the sample) will be calculated at 0–4, 0–8, 0–12, and 0–24 hours and subsequent 24-hour periods until discharge, as will the cumulative incidence of nausea.

To examine important risk and protective factors, multivariable logistic regression models will be developed (Hosmer & Lemeshow, 2000; Kleinbaum, Kupper, Muller, & Nizam, 1998). The multivariable models will be used to quantify the level of risk or protection that individual variables have on PONV while accounting for other main effect variables, interactions, and confounders (Concato, et al., 1993). A purposeful method of model development will be used to incorporate what is currently known about PONV in children and adults with the variables that are specific to children after posterior fossa surgery (Exhibit D-3). The cumulative incidence of vomiting/retching over the course of the child's hospital stay will be used as the outcome for the multivariable model. Variables that will initially be examined will include age; length of surgery; documented history of PONV or motion sickness; postmenarche; presenting with nausea,

TABLE D-2
Study Outcome Measures

Outcome	Definition	Measurement
Primary outcomes		
Nausea	Subjective sensation of the urge to vomit or retch	Any charting in the nursing notes or flow sheets that nausea was experienced at 4, 8, 12, and 24 hours and subsequent 24-hour periods until discharge from neurosurgical postoperative hospital care. Documented children's statements, parental concerns, or behaviors that refer to nausea, such as "states that he feels like throwing up" or "feels like puking" will be included. Judgement statements like "appears nauseous" will also be included.
Vomiting	Forceful expulsion of gastric contents through the mouth	Each time vomiting is noted on the in and out flowchart at 4, 8, 12, and 24 hours and subsequent 24-hour periods until discharge from neurosurgical postoperative hospital care. If no vomiting is noted on the flowchart in a time period, the nursing notes for that time period will be reviewed to confirm that there were no episodes.
Retching	Attempts to vomit without expulsion of gastric contents through the mouth	Any charting in the nursing notes that indicates retching or gagging in an attempt to vomit.
Secondary outcomes		
Severe refractory PONV	Nausea, retching, and/or vomiting that continues despite treatment and interferes with the child's recovery	The severity of nausea and vomiting/retching will first be determined by the data collector based on the overall chart review using a four-point scale (none, mild, moderate, severe). A content analysis of the data for nausea, retching, and vomiting will also be conducted to determine levels of severity by two independent reviewers with discrepancies resolved through discussion and a third-party review if necessary.
Use of rescue antiemetics	Administration of an antiemetic "as needed" (prn) in response to a child's nausea, vomiting, or retching	The medication administration records will indicate when these drugs were administered. The data collector will indicate if the drugs were given after the first episode occurred.
Adverse events	Other outcomes that may impede the child's recovery	Cerebral spinal fluid leak, wound infection, cerebellar mutism, ataxia, and cranial nerve deficits that are documented in the progress notes and/or discharge summary.

retching, or vomiting; use of prophylactic antiemetics; use of dexamethasone; type of surgery; surgical site; histopathology; and development of hydrocephalus. Finally, chi-square tests of association among cumulative PONV over the course of the child's hospital stay, severe PONV, and adverse events will be examined.

Limitations

The primary limitation of this study is its retrospective nature because it limits the researchers' control over the data that can be collected. For the outcomes of nausea, vomiting, and retching, the quality of the charting by healthcare professionals is paramount. The exact count of vomiting episodes will likely be underestimated, but the cumulative incidence of vomiting at the specified time period should be accurate. Retching may be charted if it occurs without vomiting; however, it may be unobserved by the healthcare team. Because of their similar physiology, the cumulative incidence will be of combined vomiting and retching. I am confident that severe vomiting will be reflected in the charting and flow sheets. The subjective nature of nausea will not be measurable; only the presence or absence of nausea as charted will be available for analysis. Young children and children with disabilities may not have the capacity to express nausea, and nausea, as perceived by the child, may not be indicated at all. Should I be unable to capture nausea through the chart review, the study will be limited to an examination of vomiting/retching, which is still an important area for investigation.

There are also challenges in the multisite aspects of the study. Differences in the way that postoperative neurosurgical care is provided and the timing of transfer of the child to home, for rehabilitation, or for oncology treatment may vary among institutions. A clear definition of the postoperative care time period has been developed in collaboration with the participating researchers at SickKids, and if other sites are also involved, this definition may need to be further refined. Differences in documentation styles and charting practices among the participating sites will also affect data collection. Many of the challenges in defining the data collection period will be determined when training and establishing interrater reliability, with issues resolved through discussion.

Due to the retrospective nature of the data collection, the multivariable models that are developed in this study will be used to identify risk and protective factors for PONV in children after posterior fossa surgery. They will not be developed for prognosis or risk scoring at the individual level.

The study will also not determine the efficacy of treatments, only their contribution as protective factors. Finally, it is well recognized that the analysis of adverse events and PONV will not establish a causal direction but merely reflect whether there is a relationship between them.

Ethical Considerations

Application for ethical approval will first be sought through the Capital Health Institutional Ethical Review Board (Panel A). When approved, each participating site will apply to their appropriate internal review board prior to any data collection. There are no individual risks to being included in the study. The study does involve a sample from a vulnerable population; however, as shown in the proposal, children have unique needs that must be studied separately from adults.

Because it is a retrospective study, there will be no contact with any children or families in the process of data collection. There will be no identifying information collected on the case report form. All names, birth dates, and addresses will be kept confidential and will not appear on the case report form or any research document. The children's age will be determined at the time of surgery in years and months so that their birth dates will not appear on the case report form or any research document. Each site will identify the child by subject number on the case report form. For audit purposes, the subject number as it appears on the case report form and child's unique hospital identification number will be kept on paper in a locked clinic file cabinet that is separate from the case report forms and is accessible only to the researchers at that particular site. This link will be destroyed at the time indicated by the policies of the participating site or at two years after completion of the study if no policy is in place. Completed case report forms will be kept in a locked file cabinet at each site, and when complete they will be confidentially couriered to Susan Neufeld at the Stollery Children's Hospital for data entry. Each site will keep copies of their case report forms according to institutional policies or two years after completion of the study if no policy is in place. The original case report forms will be kept in a locked cabinet at the University of Alberta, Faculty of Nursing for seven years following completion of the study. Any computer files will be password protected and accessible only to the research team. These will also be kept for seven years following completion of the study. Findings will be presented in aggregate form so that no single child's data will be used or identified. Any secondary data analysis will require further ethical approval from the appropriate institutional review board.

References

American Society of Health Systems Pharmacists. (1999). ASHP therapeutic guidelines on the pharmacologic management of nausea and vomiting in adult and pediatric patients receiving chemotherapy or radiation therapy or undergoing surgery. *American Journal of Health-System Pharmacy, 56*, 729–764.

Apfel, C. C., Greim, C. A., Haubitz, I., Grundt, D., Goepfert, C., Sefrin, P., et al. (1998). A risk score to predict the probability of postoperative vomiting in adults. *Acta Anaesthesiologica Scandinavica, 42*, 495–501.

Apfel, C. C., Laara, E., Koivuranta, M., Greim, C. A., & Roewer, N. (1999). A simplified risk score for predicting postoperative nausea and vomiting: Conclusions from cross-validations between two centers. *Anesthesiology, 91*, 693–700.

Apfel, C. C., Roewer, N., & Korttila, K. (2002). How to study postoperative nausea and vomiting. *Acta Anaesthesiologica Scandinavica, 46*, 921–928.

Concato, J., Feinstein, A. R., & Holford, T. R. (1993). The risk of determining risk with multivariable models. *Annals of Internal Medicine, 118*, 201–210.

Cremonesi, E., Tenuto, R. A., & Bairao, G. S. (1967). Methochlopramide in the prevention of post-operative vomiting. Results in neurosurgery. *Revista Brasileira de Anestesiologica, 17*, 44–47.

Du Pen, S., Scuderi, P., Wetchler, B., Sung, Y. F., Mingus, M., Clayborn, L., et al. (1992). Ondansetron in the treatment of postoperative nausea and vomiting in ambulatory outpatients: A dose-comparative, stratified, multicentre study. *European Journal of Anaesthesiology, 6*(Suppl.), 55–62.

Eberhart, L. H., Geldner, G., Kranke, P., Morin, A. M., Schauffelen, A., Treiber, H., et al. (2004). The development and validation of a risk score to predict the probability of postoperative vomiting in pediatric patients. *Anesthesia and Analgesia, 99*, 1630–1637.

Eberhart, L. H., Morin, A. M., Guber, D., Kretz, F. J., Schauffelen, A., Treiber, H., et al. (2004). Applicability of risk scores for postoperative nausea and vomiting in adults to paediatric patients. *British Journal of Anaesthesia, 93*, 386–392.

Fabling, J. M., Gan, T. J., El-Moalem, H. E., Warner, D. S., & Borel, C. O. (2000). A randomized, double-blinded comparison of ondansetron, droperidol, and placebo for prevention of postoperative nausea and vomiting after supratentorial craniotomy. *Anesthesia and Analgesia, 91*, 358–361.

Fabling, J. M., Gan, T. J., Guy, J., Borel, C. O., el-Moalem, H. E., & Warner, D. S. (1997). Postoperative nausea and vomiting. A retrospective analysis in patients undergoing elective craniotomy. *Journal of Neurosurgical Anesthesiology, 9*, 308–312.

Fisher, D. M. (1997). The "big little problem" of postoperative nausea and vomiting: Do we know the answer yet? *Anesthesiology, 87*, 1271–1273.

Flynn, B. C., & Nemergut, E. C. (2006). Postoperative nausea and vomiting and pain after transsphenoidal surgery: A review of 877 patients. *Anesthesia and Analgesia, 103*, 162–167.

Furst, S. R., Sullivan, L. J., Soriano, S. G., McDermott, J. S., Adelson, P. D., & Rockoff, M. A. (1996). Effects of ondansetron on emesis in the first 24 hours after craniotomy in children. *Anesthesia and Analgesia, 83*, 325–328.

Gan, T. J. (2006). Risk factors for postoperative nausea and vomiting. *Anesthesia and Analgesia, 102*, 1884–1898.

Ganong, W. F. (1987). Central regulation of visceral control. In W. F. Ganong (Ed.), *Review of medical physiology* (pp. 235–254). Norwalk, CT: Appleton and Lange.

Guttuso, T., Jr., Roscoe, J., & Griggs, J. (2003). Effect of gabapentin on nausea induced by chemotherapy in patients with breast cancer. *Lancet, 361*, 1703–1705.

Guttuso, T., Jr., Vitticore, P., & Holloway, R. G. (2005). Responsiveness of life-threatening refractory emesis to gabapentin–scopolamine therapy following posterior fossa surgery. Case report. *Journal of Neurosurgery, 102*, 547–549.

Harrell, F. E., Jr., Lee, K. L., & Mark, D. B. (1996). Multivariable prognostic models: Issues in developing models, evaluating assumptions and adequacy, and measuring and reducing errors. *Statistics in Medicine, 15*, 361–387.

Hartsell, T., Long, D., & Kirsch, J. R. (2005). The efficacy of postoperative ondansetron (Zofran) orally disintegrating tablets for preventing nausea and vomiting after acoustic neuroma surgery. *Anesthesia and Analgesia, 101*, 1492–1496.

Henzi, I., Walder, B., & Tramer, M. R. (2000). Dexamethasone for the prevention of postoperative nausea and vomiting: A quantitative systematic review. *Anesthesia and Analgesia, 90*, 186–194.

Hornby, P. J. (2001). Central neurocircuitry associated with emesis. *American Journal of Medicine, 111*(Suppl. 8A), 106S–112S.

Hosmer, D. W., & Lemeshow, S. (2000). *Applied logistic regression.* Hoboken, NJ: John Wiley and Sons.

Irefin, S. A., Schubert, A., Bloomfield, E. L., DeBoer, G. E., Mascha, E. J., & Ebrahim, Z. Y. (2003). The effect of craniotomy location on postoperative pain and nausea. *Journal of Anesthesia, 17*, 227–231.

Kearney, R., Mack, C., & Entwistle, L. (1998). Withholding oral fluids from children undergoing day surgery reduces vomiting. *Paediatric Anaesthesia, 8*, 331–336.

Kleinbaum, D. G., Kupper, L. L., Muller, K. E., & Nizam, A. (1998). *Applied regression analysis and other multivariable methods*. Pacific Grove, CA: Duxbury Press.

Koivuranta, M., & Laara, E. (1998). A survey of postoperative nausea and vomiting. *Anaesthesia, 53*, 413–414.

Korttila, K. (1992). The study of postoperative nausea and vomiting. *British Journal of Anaesthesia, 69*, 20S–23S.

Kranke, P., Morin, A. M., Roewer, N., & Eberhart, L. H. (2002). Dimenhydrinate for prophylaxis of postoperative nausea and vomiting: A meta-analysis of randomized controlled trials. *Acta Anaesthesiologica Scandinavica, 46*, 238–244.

Kranke, P., Morin, A. M., Roewer, N., Wulf, H., & Eberhart, L. H. (2002). The efficacy and safety of transdermal scopolamine for the prevention of postoperative nausea and vomiting: A quantitative systematic review. *Anesthesia and Analgesia, 95*, 133–143.

Kuwabara, T., & Amano, K. (1966). Experience in the use of metoclopramide in the field of neurosurgery. *No To Shinkei, 18*, 943–948.

Lee, A., & Done, M. L. (1999). The use of nonpharmacologic techniques to prevent postoperative nausea and vomiting: A meta-analysis. *Anesthesia and Analgesia, 88*, 1362–1369.

Macario, A., Weinger, M., Carney, S., & Kim, A. (1999). Which clinical anesthesia outcomes are important to avoid? The perspective of patients. *Anesthesia and Analgesia, 89*, 652–658.

Manninen, P. H., Raman, S. K., Boyle, K., & el-Beheiry, H. (1999). Early postoperative complications following neurosurgical procedures. *Canadian Journal of Anaesthesia, 46*, 7–14.

Manninen, P. H., & Tan, T. K. (2002). Postoperative nausea and vomiting after craniotomy for tumor surgery: A comparison between awake craniotomy and general anesthesia. *Journal of Clinical Anesthesia, 14*, 279–283.

Meng, L., & Quinlan, J. J. (2006). Assessing risk factors for postoperative nausea and vomiting: A retrospective study in patients undergoing retromastoid craniectomy with microvascular decompression of cranial nerves. *Journal of Neurosurgical Anesthesiology, 18*, 235–239.

Miller, A. D. (1999). Central mechanisms of vomiting. *Digestive Diseases and Sciences, 44*, 39S–43S.

Murray, J. B. (1997). Psychophysiological aspects of motion sickness. *Perceptual and Motor Skills, 85*, 1163–1167.

Neufeld, S. (2002). Pharmacology review: The role of ondansetron in the management of children's nausea and vomiting following posterior fossa neurosurgical procedures. *Axone, 23*, 24–29.

Neufeld, S. M., & Newburn-Cook, C. (2007). Post-operative nausea and vomiting in craniotomy: A systematic review of the literature and meta-analysis. *Journal of Neurosurgical Anesthesiology, 19*, 10–17.

Palazzo, M., & Evans, R. (1993). Logistic regression analysis of fixed patient factors for postoperative sickness: A model for risk assessment. *British Journal of Anaesthesia, 70*, 135–140.

Peduzzi, P., Concato, J., Kemper, E., Holford, T. R., & Feinstein, A. R. (1996). A simulation study of the number of events per variable in logistic regression analysis. *Journal of Clinical Epidemiology, 49*, 1373–1379.

Lenth, R. V. (2006). Java applets for power and sample size [Computer software]. Retrieved September 18, 2006, from http://www.cs.uiowa.edu/~rlenth/Power/

Pugh, S. C., Jones, N. C., & Barsoum, L. Z. (1996). A comparison of prophylactic ondansetron and metoclopramide administration in patients undergoing major neurosurgical procedures. *Anaesthesia, 51*, 1162–1164.

Rose, J. B., & Watcha, M. F. (1999). Postoperative nausea and vomiting in paediatric patients. *British Journal of Anaesthesia, 83*, 104–117.

Rowley, M. P., & Brown, T. C. (1982). Postoperative vomiting in children. *Anaesthesia Intensive Care, 10*, 309–313.

Scuderi, P. E., & Conlay, L. A. (2003). Postoperative nausea and vomiting and outcome. *International Anesthesiology Clinics, 41*, 165–174.

Sinclair, D. R., Chung, F., & Mezei, G. (1999). Can postoperative nausea and vomiting be predicted? *Anesthesiology, 91*, 109–118.

Stieglitz, L. H., Samii, A., Kaminsky, J., Gharabaghi, A., Samii, M., & Ludemann, W. O. (2005). Nausea and dizziness after vestibular schwannoma surgery: A multivariate analysis of preoperative symptoms. *Neurosurgery, 57*, 887–890.

Wong, A. Y., O'Regan, A. M., & Irwin, M. G. (2006). Total intravenous anaesthesia with propofol and remifentanil for elective neurosurgical procedures: An audit of early postoperative complications. *European Journal of Anaesthesiology, 23*, 586–590.

Yates, B. J., Miller, A. D., & Lucot, J. B. (1998). Physiological basis and pharmacology of motion sickness: An update. *Brain Research Bulletin, 47*, 395–406.

EXHIBIT D-1
Nausea and Vomiting After Posterior Fossa Surgery
Case Report Form

Child Demographics

Age at surgery: _____ years _____ months   Gender: M   F   Started menses: Y   N   Unknown   N/A

Other health issues: _____   Weight: _____

Surgery Summary

Surgery: _____

Surgery date: ____/____/____   Discharge (from surgery) date: ____/____/____

Discharge location: Home   Oncology unit   Rehabilitation unit   Other: _____

Hospital discharge date: ____/____/____

Pathology/final diagnosis: _____

Preoperative

History:

Yes   No

____ ____   Other surgery (specify) _____

____ ____   Postoperative nausea

____ ____   Postoperative vomiting

Presenting signs and symptoms:

Yes   No

____ ____   Nausea (Describe:) _____

____ ____   Vomiting (Describe:) _____

____ ____   Hydrocephalus

____ ____   Syringomyelia/scoliosis

____ ____   Headache

____ ____   Ataxia

____ ____   Cranial nerve deficits (Specify:) _____

____ ____   Other (Specify:) _____

Antiemetics in 24 hours before surgery:

Yes   No

____ ____   Dimenhydrinate (Gravol)

____ ____   Granisetron (Kytril)

____ ____   Metoclopramide (Maxeran)

____ ____   Ondansetron (Zofran)

____ ____   Scopolamine

____ ____   Other (Specify:_____)

Steroids in 24 hours before surgery:

Yes   No

____ ____   Dexamethasone

____ ____   Other steroid (Specify:_____)

CSF Management

Yes	No			Date inserted	Date D/C
____	____	EVD	Pre/intra/post	__/__/__	__/__/__
____	____	Lumbar drain	Pre/intra/post	__/__/__	__/__/__
____	____	Other (Specify: _____)	Pre/intra/post	__/__/__	__/__/__
____	____	Third ventriculostomy	Pre/intra/post	__/__/__	__/__/__
____	____	VP shunt	Pre/intra/post	__/__/__	__/__/__

Intraoperative

ASA status: I II III IV

Anesthetic start time: __ __:__ __   Anesthetic finish time: __ __:__ __

Surgery start time: __ __:__ __   Surgery finish time: __ __:__ __

Anesthesia:

    Induction: Thiopenta   Propofol N_2O Rocuronium   Other _____

    Maintenance: Isoflurane   Desflurane   Sevoflurane N_2O Other _____

    Reversal: Neostigmine Atropine   Glycopyrrolate

    Opioid: Fentanyl   Morphine   Remifentanil

    Antiemetic: _____ Time: __ __:__ __

    Steroids: _____ Time: __ __:__ __

    Mannitol: _____ Time: __ __:__ __

Estimated size of lesion: Preoperative/intraoperative MRI _____

Location of lesion:

    ❏ Cerebellar vermis

    ❏ Cerebellar hemisphere: Right   Left

    ❏ Intraventricular

    ❏ Outside of fourth ventricle and cerebellum (i.e., cerebellopontine angle, undersurface of cerebellar hemisphere)

    ❏ Other: _____

Degree of resection: _____

Evidence of: Extensive bleeding   Cranial nerve damage   Other _____

Notes on surgery:

_____

_____

_____

Postoperative

	PARR	___–4 hr	4–8 hr	8–24 hr	24–48 hr	48–72 hr
Location	_____	_____	_____	_____	_____	_____
Nausea	Y N	Y N	Y N	Y N	Y N	Y N
Vomiting (counts)	_____	_____	_____	_____	_____	_____
Retching	Y N	Y N	Y N	Y N	Y N	Y N
Pain	❑ None noted ❑ Headache ❑ Neck ❑ Other	❑ None noted ❑ Headache ❑ Neck ❑ Other	❑ None noted ❑ Headache ❑ Neck ❑ Other	❑ None noted ❑ Headache ❑ Neck ❑ Other	❑ None noted ❑ Headache ❑ Neck ❑ Other	❑ None noted ❑ Headache ❑ Neck ❑ Other
Antiemetics ordered	_____	_____	_____	_____	_____	_____
Antiemetics given	_____	_____	_____	_____	_____	_____
Dexa-methasone/ steroid	_____	_____	_____	_____	_____	_____
Nonpharm strategies	_____	_____	_____	_____	_____	_____
Activity	❑ Bed rest ❑ Mobilizing	❑ Bed rest ❑ Mobilizing	❑ Bed rest ❑ Mobilizing	❑ Bed rest ❑ Mobilizing	❑ Bed rest ❑ Mobilizing	❑ Bed rest ❑ Mobilizing
Opioids given	_____	_____	_____	_____	_____	_____
Intake type	❑ NPO ❑ Sips/CF ❑ FF/DAT ❑ NG/NJ	❑ NPO ❑ Sips/CF ❑ FF/DAT ❑ NG/NJ	❑ NPO ❑ Sips/CF ❑ FF/DAT ❑ NG/NJ	❑ NPO ❑ Sips/CF ❑ FF/DAT ❑ NG/NJ	❑ NPO ❑ Sips/CF ❑ FF/DAT ❑ NG/NJ	❑ NPO ❑ Sips/CF ❑ FF/DAT ❑ NG/NJ
EVD	❑ Open @___ ❑ Clamped ❑ D/C ❑ N/A	❑ Open @___ ❑ Clamped ❑ D/C ❑ N/A	❑ Open @___ ❑ Clamped ❑ D/C ❑ N/A	❑ Open @___ ❑ Clamped ❑ D/C ❑ N/A	❑ Open @___ ❑ Clamped ❑ D/C ❑ N/A	❑ Open @___ ❑ Clamped ❑ D/C ❑ N/A
Evidence of hydro-cephalus	Y N CT MRI	Y N CT MRI	Y N CT MRI	Y N CT MRI	Y N CT MRI	Y N CT MRI

Notes:

_____

_____

First postoperative antiemetic given:

❏ Before first emetic episode   ❏ After first emetic episode   ❏ None given

First recorded oral/gastric intake _____ hours postoperative

Nausea and Vomiting After Posterior Fossa Surgery
Case Report Form
Additional Inpatient Days

Postoperative

	72–96	96–120	120–144	144–168	168–192	192–216	216–240
Location	_____	_____	_____	_____	_____	_____	_____
Nausea	Y N	Y N	Y N	Y N	Y N	Y N	Y N
Vomiting (counts)	___	___	___	___	___	___	___
Retching	Y N	Y N	Y N	Y N	Y N	Y N	Y N
Pain	❏ None noted	❏ None noted	❏ None noted	❏ None noted	❏ None noted	❏ None noted	❏ None noted
	❏ Headache	❏ Headache	❏ Headache	❏ Headache	❏ Headache	❏ Headache	❏ Headache
	❏ Neck	❏ Neck	❏ Neck	❏ Neck	❏ Neck	❏ Neck	❏ Neck
	❏ Other	❏ Other	❏ Other	❏ Other	❏ Other	❏ Other	❏ Other
Antiemetics ordered	_____	_____	_____	_____	_____	_____	_____
Antiemetics given	_____	_____	_____	_____	_____	_____	_____
Dexamethasone/ steroid	_____	_____	_____	_____	_____	_____	_____
Nonpharm strategies	_____	_____	_____	_____	_____	_____	_____
Activity	❏ Bed rest	❏ Bed rest	❏ Bed rest	❏ Bed rest	❏ Bed rest	❏ Bed rest	❏ Bed rest
	❏ Mobilizing	❏ Mobilizing	❏ Mobilizing	❏ Mobilizing	❏ Mobilizing	❏ Mobilizing	❏ Mobilizing
Opioids given	_____	_____	_____	_____	_____	_____	_____
Intake type	❏ NPO	❏ NPO	❏ NPO	❏ NPO	❏ NPO	❏ NPO	❏ NPO
	❏ Sips/CF	❏ Sips/CF	❏ Sips/CF	❏ Sips/CF	❏ Sips/CF	❏ Sips/CF	❏ Sips/CF
	❏ FF/DAT	❏ FF/DAT	❏ FF/DAT	❏ FF/DAT	❏ FF/DAT	❏ FF/DAT	❏ FF/DAT
	❏ NG/NJ	❏ NG/NJ	❏ NG/NJ	❏ NG/NJ	❏ NG/NJ	❏ NG/NJ	❏ NG/NJ

EVD	❑ Open @＿	❑ Open @＿	❑ Open @＿	❑ Open @＿	❑ Open @＿	❑ Open @＿	❑ Open @＿
	❑ Clamped	❑ Clamped	❑ Clamped	❑ Clamped	❑ Clamped	❑ Clamped	❑ Clamped
	❑ D/C	❑ D/C	❑ D/C	❑ D/C	❑ D/C	❑ D/C	❑ D/C
	❑ N/A	❑ N/A	❑ N/A	❑ N/A	❑ N/A	❑ N/A	❑ D/C
Evidence of hydro-cephalus	Y N CT MRI	Y N CT MRI	Y N CT MRI	Y N CT MRI	Y N CT MRI	Y N CT MRI	Y N CT MRI

Notes:

_____

_____

_____

Outcomes

Rating of vomiting and/or retching: None   Mild   Moderate   Severe

	Self-limited or responsive to treatment	Responsive to treatment	Not responsive to treatment
	1–3 episodes	> 3 episodes	Limits activity

Rating of nausea: None   Mild   Moderate   Severe

	Responsive to treatment	Responsive to treatment	Not responsive to treatment
	≤ 48 hrs	> 48 hrs	Limits activity

Yes   No

____ ____   Wound failure

____ ____   CSF leak

____ ____   Pseudomeningocele (Clinically noted OR MRI/CT noted only)

____ ____   Infection

____ ____   Cerebellar mutism/posterior fossa syndrome

____ ____   Cranial nerve deficits (Describe:) _____

____ ____   Other: _____

____ ____   Other: _____

Readmission within 30 days? ❑ Yes   ❑ No

Reason for readmission: _____

Notes

_____

_____

_____

_____

EXHIBIT D-2
Nausea and Vomiting After Posterior Fossa Surgery
Data Collection Notes

Inclusion/Exclusion Criterion

Inclusion:

1. Children under the age of 17 years (0–16)
2. Posterior fossa surgery between March 2002 and March 2007

Exclusion:

1. Fourth ventricular shunt procedures only
2. Operations without dura/arachnoid opening (outside the brain)
3. Surgery for traumatic brain injury
4. Prolonged postoperative intubation >48 hours
5. Surgery with a supratentorial component (except placement of EVD)

If the child requires a second posterior fossa surgery during the course of the data collection period, data may be collected separately for each surgery with the same participant identification number. Data from any second and subsequent procedures will not be included in the initial analysis but may be considered for a secondary within-subjects analysis. These data should not be collected until all other data collection is complete.

Child Demographics

- History, admission record
- Menses started: Circle Y if LMP noted

Surgery Summary

- OR records and discharge summary
- Pathology report

Preoperative

History:

- Anesthesia history
- History of PONV; check charts of previous surgeries if not on anesthesia history
- Presenting symptoms; admission record, physical exam record

Antiemetics/steroid:

- Admission record
- If admitted, medication administration record

CSF Management

- OR records
- Progress notes

Intraoperative

- Anesthesia flow sheet
- Surgical summary
- Location of lesion: Preoperative MRI report and operative report. If conflicting (i.e., vermis versus fourth ventricular, use operative report). If both the vermis and cerebellar hemisphere are involved, check both locations.
- Size of lesion: Preoperative MRI. Note that we will use the largest diameter reported in the analysis.

Postoperative

Nausea

- Recovery room record
- Nurses' notes
- Note time of documentation

Vomiting

- Recovery room record
- Counts from in and out flow sheet (after reviewing flow sheet, go to nurses' notes and note each separately charted episode; if it corresponds to the flow sheet, do not count again)
- Note time of documentation

Retching

- Recovery room record
- Nurses' notes

Pain

- Nurses' notes, pain flow sheet, progress notes
- Note headache, neck/back of head/incision, and other

Activity

- Order sheets, nurses' notes
- Note mobilizing (active in crib, held, carried) or bed rest

Antiemetics ordered

- Order sheets and medication administration records

Antiemetics given*

- Medication administration records, effectiveness charted in nurses' notes

Nonpharm strategies

- Nurses' notes; directly following any charting of nausea or vomiting

Opioids given

- Medication administration records
- Note type of drug: Morphine/codeine, etc.

Intake

- In and out flow sheets, nurses' notes, order sheet, dietary records
- Note time to first oral intake (including oral meds administered)

EVD @

- EVD flow sheet, nurses' notes

Evidence of hydrocephalus

- CT/MRI report

*Note: Any significant changes as noted on progress notes or nurses' notes; for example, intubation (<48 hours), surgery for VP shunt, IV started for dehydration

Last recorded vomit or retch/nausea: If >10 days, follow nurses' notes and in and out flow sheets until resolved (may also show in progress notes and discharge summary if severe and refractory).

Outcomes

Rating of vomiting and/or retching: This rating is the subjective impression of the data collector with quantitative guidelines. When data has been collected and the initial analysis is complete, the categories may be further refined. Include the rationale for the rating in notes section.

Rating of nausea: This is also the subjective impression of the data collector with quantitative guidelines. When data has been collected and initial analysis is complete, the categories may be further refined. Include the rationale for the rating in the notes section.

Wound failure

- This is failure at the surgical site; progress notes and nurses' notes

CSF leak

- This is a CSF fluid leak through the skin
- Note location (surgical site, shunt site, EVD exit site, etc.); progress notes and nurses' notes

Pseudomeningocele

- Present if "pseudomeningocele" or "bulging" noted in clinical records or if a fluid collection is present superficial to the craniotomy flap on postoperative CT scan or MR scan (even if not clinically noted)

Infection

- Note location: CSF (progress notes), wound (progress notes, nurses' notes)

Cerebellar mutism/posterior fossa syndrome

- Progress notes, speech/language notes, nurses' notes

Cranial nerve deficits

- Progress notes, ophthalmology consults, ENT consults, physiotherapy notes, speech language notes

Other

- Any other outcomes indicated on the progress notes

EXHIBIT D-3
Purposeful Selection Methods for Multivariable Modeling

Purposeful Method to Building Main Effects Model

Step 1: Fit a univariate logistic regression model with each variable.

Step 2: Select as candidates for a multivariable model all significant variables ($p < 0.02$) and clinically important variables.

Step 3: Fit a multivariable model from significant variables identified in Step 2.

Step 4: Identify, using Wald statistic, those variables in the multivariable model that are statistically significant ($p < 0.05$).

Step 5: Assess the confounding effects of important variables that were removed. Keep changes that are greater than 15%.

Step 6: Fit a model with significant predictors from Step 4 and confounders in Step 5.

Step 7: Check linear assumptions of continuous variables. If not linear replace with categorical variables.

Step 8: Prepare a list of clinically plausible interactions.

Step 9: Examine interaction effects one at a time and use the Wald test to determine the significance of the interaction ($p < 0.05$).

Step 10: Fit a model with main effects and interactions.

Step 11: Proceed to assessing the fit of the model using goodness of fit statistics.

Adapted from:

Hosmer, D. W., & Lemeshow, S. (2000). *Applied logistic regression.* Hoboken, NJ: John Wiley and Sons.

Kleinbaum, D. G., Kupper, L. L., Muller, K. E., & Nizam, A. (1998). *Applied regression analysis and other multivariable methods.* Pacific Grove, CA: Duxbury Press.

By: Y. Yasui and A. Senthilselvan, Public Health Sciences 698, Class Notes, 2005.

The Impact of Older Maternal Age at First Birth on the Risk of Spontaneous Preterm Birth in Northern and Central Alberta

By Safina Hassan McIntyre

Introduction

Statement of the Problem

Preterm birth remains the most significant public health problem facing providers of maternal and infant care (Kramer, et al., 1998; McCormick, 1985). Despite improvements in high-risk obstetrical care and neonatal medicine, efforts to manage and to prevent preterm birth have failed to reduce its incidence. Instead, the preterm birth rate has increased steadily in many developed countries, including both Canada and the United States. Between 1991 and 2002, the Canadian preterm birth rate increased from 6.6% to 7.5%. From 1996 to 2003, the rate in the United States rose from 11% to 12.3% (Health Canada, 2003; Statistics Canada, 2005; Hamilton, Martin, & Sutton, 2004; Ventura, Martin, Curtin, & Mathews, 1999). The rise in preterm birth rates has been linked to a number of factors, including advanced maternal age at first birth, the use of assisted reproductive technology (ART) and/or ovulation induction, increasing rates of multiple births, changes in the registration of infants weighing <500 g, and improvements in obstetrical intervention that have resulted in gestational age and birth-weight-specific declines in infant mortality and a rise in the number of infants surviving at lower limits of viability (Blondel, et al., 2002; Joseph, Demissie, & Kramer, 2002; Joseph & Kramer, 1996; Joseph, et al., 1998; Kramer, et al.,1998; Tough, et al., 2002).

The increasing preterm birth rate is of great concern to healthcare professionals and policy makers due to its association with increased neonatal mortality and infant and childhood morbidity. Although preterm births account for only 5–12% of all live births in Canada, they are associated with 60–80% of infant deaths and approximately 50% of cognitive delays and learning disabilities (Health Canada, 2003; Moutquin & Papiernik, 1990). Neurodevelopmental handicaps, such as cerebral palsy, seizure disorders, mental disorders, and delays in psychomotor development, are more likely to occur in infants born preterm (Brown, 1993; Knoches & Doyle, 1993; Paneth, 1995; Stoelhorst, et al., 2003). These disorders are related to the complications of prematurity, including perinatal asphyxia, bronchopulmonary dysplasia, respiratory distress syndrome, and intraventricular hemorrhage (Brown, 1993; Knoches & Doyle, 1993).

The medical impact of preterm birth also places an enormous psychological and economic burden on caregivers and society in general (Petrou, Sach, & Davidson, 2001). In 1995, it was conservatively estimated that for every preterm low birth weight infant born in Canada, neonatal intensive care and postneonatal care up to one year of age cost approximately $48,183 per survivor (Moutquin & Lalonde, 1998). Similar findings in the United States suggest that infants born at <37 weeks gestation between 1989 and 1992 accounted for 57% of the total initial costs for neonatal care (St. John, Nelson, Cliver, Bishnoi, & Goldenberg, 2000). The mean costs associated with initial hospitalization ranged from $10,561 for infants born between 33 and 36 weeks gestational age to a mean of $239,749 for extremely preterm infants born at 26 and 28 weeks (Cuevas, Silver, Brooten, Youngblut, & Bobo, 2005). In the longer term, preterm infants are more likely to be rehospitalized within the first two years of life, experience chronic conditions requiring ongoing medical care, and need special education and social services well into later childhood (Lewit, Baker, Corman, & Shiono, 1995; Petrou, et al., 2003; Petrou, et al., 2001; Tommiska, Tuominen, & Fellman, 2003). The costs attributed to caring for preterm birth infants over a lifetime have been estimated to be more than $8 billion (Moutquin & Lalonde, 1998). Canadian researchers have suggested that healthcare costs could be reduced by $2 billion per year if the preterm birth rate could be decreased by 20% through prevention efforts (Statistics Canada, 2004b)—an important consideration in the current era of fiscal restraint and limited healthcare resources.

There have been numerous studies focusing on the etiology of preterm birth. In these studies, researchers were able to demonstrate that preterm birth is a multifactorial and heterogeneous outcome (Ananth, Joseph, Oyelese, Demissie, & Vintzileos, 2005) resulting from the interaction of demographic, biomedical, psychological, and behavioral/lifestyle risk factors. After completing extensive literature reviews, some authors were able to identify variables with well-established causal effects (Berkowitz & Papiernik, 1993; Kramer, 1987). However, much of the etiology of prematurity remains unexplained.

Unfortunately, many of the identified risk factors for preterm birth are not modifiable and therefore cannot be targeted for reduction by prevention programs. However, one potentially modifiable risk factor is maternal age at first birth. Researchers have shown that older maternal age (defined as age 35 years and older at time of delivery) is associated with subfertility, chromosomal abnormalities, and multiple gestation (Cleary-Goldman, et al., 2005; Cnattinguis, Forman, Berendes, & Isotalo, 1992; Edge & Laros, 1993; Scholz, Hass, & Petru, 1999). Furthermore, some researchers have found an association between older maternal age and preterm birth. Other researchers have challenged these findings, however (Barkan & Bracken, 1987; Beydoun, et al., 2004; Kolas, Nakling, & Salvesen, 2000; Malloy, 1999). More women are delaying childbirth into their mid-30s and later. Therefore, healthcare providers need current conclusive research findings regarding the impact of older maternal age on the risk of preterm birth for preconceptual and antenatal counseling. Women of childbearing age need this information to help inform their decisions regarding when to start a family to minimize the risk of adverse maternal and infant outcomes.

Trends in Delayed Childbearing

Older maternal age is becoming increasingly common. Since the 1970s there has been a rise in the number of Canadian women postponing the birth of their first child. Between 1974 and 1994, the proportion of first births to women aged 35–39 years rose from 13% to 25% (Ford & Nault, 1996). By 2002, this number increased to 26.5% (Statistics Canada, 2004b). Similarly, the proportion of first births to women aged 40–44 years increased from 22.6% in 1991 to 23.8% in 2002, with 2.5% of all live births being to women of this age group, up from 1.04% 10 years earlier (Health Canada, 2003; Statistics Canada, 2005). In Alberta, the mean maternal age at first birth increased steadily from 26 to 27 years of age between 1992 and 2002 (Reproductive Health Report Working Group, 2004).

Similar trends have been reported in other industrialized countries. For example, approximately 40% of all live births in the United States are first births, with women 30 years of age and older accounting for 25.8% of these births in 2003, up from 22.5% in 1997 (Hamilton, et al., 2004; Ventura, et al., 1999). The United States also reported a birth rate increase of 31% for women aged 35–39 years and 51% for women aged 40–44 years between 1990 and 2002 (Martin, et al., 2003). In 2002, the mean age of women having their first child reached an all-time high of 25.1 years, and the birth rate declined for women 15–24 years of age (Martin, et al., 2003) .

Demographic trends in Canada and the United States suggest that there are a number of socioeconomic changes contributing to women delaying childbirth. More women are now pursuing higher education and advancing their careers while postponing marriage to achieve these goals. For example, the number of Canadian women aged 24–44 years participating in the labor force with a university education increased by 35.5% between 1995 and 2003, which corresponds with an increase in the mean age of brides (from 25.3 to 31.2 years between 1979 and 2000) (Statistics Canada, 2003; Statistics Canada, 2004a). In addition, by 1994, almost half of the first births to American females were to women with 16 or more years of education (Heck, Schoendorf, Ventura, & Kiely, 1997). The availability of birth control, second marriages, the need for dual incomes, the desire for career advancement (Freeman-Wang & Beski, 2002; Newburn-Cook & Onyskiw, 2005), and a history of infertility (Kessler, Lancet, Borenstein, & Steinmetz, 1980) have also been cited as other factors contributing to the postponement of childbirth.

Unfortunately, the longer women delay starting a family, the more fertility concerns may arise. Decreasing fertility and fecundity in women older than 35 years has been well documented (Berendes & Forman, 1991; Gosden & Rutherford, 1995; Hansen, 1986). Reasons for this biological outcome include poor ovulatory function, poor oocyte quality, an increase of genetic anomalies in oocytes and embryos, and a decreased rate of embryo implantation (Bowman & Saunders, 1995; Pal & Santoro, 2003).

Difficulty conceiving has led to the increased use of ART and/or ovulation induction. As a result, an associated rise in the number of multiple gestations has been documented and linked to both older maternal age at first birth and to increased rates of preterm birth (Luke & Martin, 2004). Canadian researchers reported that Alberta women who had children at age 35 years and older (excluding in vitro fertilization pregnancies) accounted for a 23% increase in the multiple birth rate (Tough, et al., 2002). Delayed childbearing in this population was also associated with a 40% increased risk of delivering a preterm baby (Tough, et al., 2002).

Etiologic Heterogeneity of Preterm Birth

Although some researchers have shown that there is an increased risk of preterm birth with older maternal age (Astolfi & Zonta, 1999; de Sanjose & Roman, 1991; Mohsin, Wong, Bauman, & Bai, 2003; Verkerk, Zaadstra, Reerink, Herngreen, & Verloove-Vanhorick, 1994; Wen, Goldenberg, Cutter,

Hoffman, & Cliver, 1990), other researchers have demonstrated no increased risk (Arbuckle & Sherman, 1989; Barkan & Bracken, 1987; Kolas, et al., 2000; Nordentoft, et al., 1996; White, 2004). These equivocal findings may be due to a number of methodological differences and limitations present across the various studies, such as inconsistencies in defining what constitutes older maternal age, inadequate control for potential risk factors and age-dependent covariates, inadequate sample sizes (reduced study power), differences in the age category selected for reference group comparisons, the use of hospital-based versus population-based samples, and a failure to consider the heterogeneity of preterm birth itself (Berkowitz & Papiernik, 1993; Kramer, 1987; Newburn-Cook & Onyskiw, 2005). Contradictory findings have led to confusion surrounding whether older maternal age has an independent (direct) negative effect on gestational age and an increased risk of preterm birth. In addition, the majority of past researchers have treated preterm birth as a single outcome (i.e., the birth of an infant <37 weeks gestational age) and may have prevented them from "determining conclusively the relationship between older maternal age and the risk of preterm delivery" (Newburn-Cook & Onyskiw, 2005, p. 855).

Preterm births are classified into three distinct clinical presentations (or subtypes): those that arise from idiopathic preterm labor (spontaneous onset of uterine contractions with or without rupture of the chorioamniotic membranes), preterm birth following premature rupture of membranes, and medically indicated preterm birth (also referred to as iatrogenic preterm birth), which is often necessitated in the presence of fetal distress or maternal indications such as preeclampsia and other pregnancy complications (Savitz, Blackmore, & Thorp, 1991). Some authors who oppose the separation of preterm births into these subtypes make the theoretical argument that these subtypes may not reflect etiologically different entities but rather result from differences in the timing of diagnosis and access to medical care (Klebanoff, 1998; Klebanoff & Shiono, 1995). These authors suggest that there may be substantial etiologic overlap between preterm birth caused by spontaneous preterm labor or premature rupture of membranes, thereby making the separation of these categories difficult. Moreover, they argue that there is etiologic overlap between spontaneous preterm births and medically indicated preterm births, stating that in the absence of medical intervention many of these births would have occurred spontaneously due to underlying medical causes. Although some researchers have shown there is etiologic overlap among the preterm birth subtypes (Moutquin, 2003; Pickett, Abrams, & Selvin, 2000; Savitz, et al., 2005), other researchers have demonstrated that distinct causal factors leading to the different subtypes may exist (Berkowitz, Blackmore-Prince, Lapinski, & Savitz, 1998; Harlow, et al., 1996; Kristensen, Langhoff-Roos, & Kristensen, 1995; Meis, et al., 1995; Pickett, et al., 2000).

Overall, researchers suggest that relatively little attention has been given to the possibility that different causal mechanisms can lead to different prematurity outcomes (Savitz, et al., 1991). They also note that the etiology of preterm birth following spontaneous onset of labor is poorly understood even though it is a significant contributor to all preterm births (Savitz, et al., 1991). Moreover, each preterm birth subtype may not respond to the same prevention activities (Goffinet, 2005). Only a limited number of researchers have examined the determinants of spontaneous preterm birth (Table E-1). Their studies will be discussed in the literature review.

Etiologic research should consider the heterogeneity of preterm birth so that the different causal mechanisms for each subtype can be identified. In addition, researchers need to consider simultaneously multiple potential risk factors to understand how they interact and whether they act independently or indirectly (mediated through other factors) to influence gestational age at birth.

It will be difficult to reduce preterm births without acting on their causes (Goffinet, 2005). Identifying the modifiable factors early in the pregnancy, or even before pregnancy, will help to enable more effective preventive measures to be taken (Robinson, Regan, & Norwitz, 2001) and thus help to reduce the preterm birth rate.

With the increasing number of women delaying childbirth into their mid-30s and older and the concurrent rise in preterm birth rates, the question of whether older maternal age increases the risk of preterm birth needs to be addressed. Furthermore, given the heterogeneity of preterm birth, the impact of older maternal age on each preterm birth subtype must be assessed. Women need to be assured that healthcare professionals have the correct information regarding the risks associated with older maternal age and adverse birth outcomes so that they too can become aware of any potential adverse outcomes and make an informed decision about when to begin their family.

Purpose of the Study

The overall purpose of this study is to determine the impact of older maternal age on the risk of spontaneous preterm labor (defined as delivery <37 weeks gestation not associated with either ruptured membranes or iatrogenic intervention) (Ananth, et al., 2005) among nulliparous women.

TABLE E-1
Characteristics and Results of the Studies Examining the Effect of Older Maternal Age on the Risk of Spontaneous Preterm Birth

[1,2]**Aldous, M. B., Edmonson, B. (1993). Maternal age at first birth and risk of low birth weight and preterm delivery in Washington State.**

Sample:
USA; n = 16,492 white, first-born infants delivered in Washington State between 1984 and 1988

Included n = 4,403 black infants

Population-based study

Purpose: To study the effect of delayed childbearing on the risk of low birth weight (LBW; <2500g), very low birth weight (<1500g) and preterm delivery

Design: Retrospective cohort study

Methods: Used Washington State birth certificates. Gestational age (GA) was confirmed by first day of last menstrual period (LMP; 80% accurate; excluded cases with unknown gestational age)

Risk factors and covariates included: Hypertension, paternal and maternal occupation, marital status, smoking, prenatal care, prior fetal loss, and cesarean delivery. Preeclampsia, gestational diabetes, and diabetes mellitus assessed but not included in final model

Birth outcome: PT-both (adjusted for cesarean delivery in analysis)

Results:
AOR for PT-both =
1.0 (0.86, 1.3) for white women aged 25–29 years;
1.4 (1.1, 1.7) for white women aged 30–34 years;
1.6 (1.4, 2.0) for white women aged 35–39 years;
1.8 (1.3, 2.6) for white women aged ≥40 years
No statistically significant findings for black women (small sample size)
Reference age group: 20–24 years

Discussion:
Older maternal age a significant risk factor for PT-both in white, nulliparous women
Risk increases as a function of increasing maternal age (1.4 to 1.6 to 1.8 for women 30–34 years, 35–39 years, and ≥40 years, respectively, when compared with women 20–24 years of age)

Berkowitz, G. S. (1985). Clinical and obstetric risk factors for preterm delivery.

Sample:
USA; n = 488 infants (175 preterm, 313 term infants) delivered at Yale-New Haven Hospital between 1977 and 1978

Hospital-based study

Purpose: To study the clinical and obstetric risk factors of preterm delivery

Design: Case-control study

Methods: Study data obtained from a structured interview and hospital delivery records; GA was confirmed by Dubowitz score

Risk factors and covariates included: First trimester bleeding, antepartum hemorrhage, third trimester urinary tract infection, sociodemographic factors, maternal height, prepregnancy weight, weight gain, previous preterm delivery, reproductive history, and incompetent cervix

Birth outcome: PT-both (restricted to preterm births preceded by spontaneous labor or spontaneous rupture of membranes)

Results:
Crude OR for PT-both =
1.8 (1.2, 2.6) for women under 25 years of age (compared to those over 25 years of age)

Discussion:
In the multivariate analysis, maternal age was not a significant predictor of preterm birth preceded by spontaneous labor or spontaneous rupture of membranes (odds ratio estimate not reported)

(continues)

TABLE E-1 (continued)
Characteristics and Results of the Studies Examining the Effect of Older Maternal Age on the Risk of Spontaneous Preterm Birth

[2]Berkowitz, G. S., Blackmore-Prince, C., Lapinski, R. H., Savitz, D. A. (1998). Risk factors for preterm birth subtypes.

Sample:		Results:	Discussion:
USA; n = 31,107 births at Mount Sinai Hospital between 1986 and 1994 (randomly selected one pregnancy for women who had more than one eligible pregnancy) Hospital-based study	**Purpose:** To examine the epidemiologic risk factors for the preterm birth subtypes **Design:** Retrospective cohort study **Methods:** Used computerized perinatal database; GA confirmed by LMP and ultrasound; if menstrual date was missing, used best clinical judgement **Risk factors and covariates included:** Preexisting medical conditions (e.g. diabetes, hypertensive disorder); pregnancy complications; sociodemo-graphic, lifestyle, obstetric, and nutritional factors **Birth outcome:** Preterm PROM (preterm birth preceded by preterm premature rupture of membranes), preterm labor (onset of labor before rupture of membranes leading to preterm birth)	AOR for preterm PROM = 1.4 (1.2, 1.6) for women aged 30–24 years; 1.5 (1.3, 1.8) for women aged ≥35 years AOR for preterm labor = 0.95 (0.8, 1.1) for women aged 30–34 years; 0.93 (0.8, 1.1) for women aged ≥35 years Reference age group: 20–29 years	Older maternal age (30–34 years and ≥35 years) significant for preterm birth due to preterm premature rupture of membranes only

[2]Harlow, B. L., Frigoletto, F. D., Cramer, D. W., et al. (1996). Determinants of preterm delivery in low-risk pregnancies.

Sample:		Results:	Discussion:
USA; n = 14,948 low risk participants form the Routine Antenatal Diagnostic Imaging with Ultrasound Study (RADIUS) Excluded women with preexisting medical conditions (i.e., diabetes mellitus, chronic hypertension, chronic renal disease)	**Purpose:** To examine potential risk factors associated with each category of preterm birth in low-risk pregnancies (i.e., no medical indication for ultrasound at first obstetrical visit) **Design:** Randomized clinical trial that recruited subjects from 109 obstetrical and family practices **Methods:** Used personal interview and hospital and obstetrical office medical records; GA confirmed by LMP and ultrasound **Risk factors and covariates included:** Parity, prior LBW infant, race, abnormal glucose load, urine protein, smoking (past and present), serum alpha-fetoprotein, infant sex, positive urine culture, and prepregnancy weight/height **Birth outcome:** Spontaneous preterm labor (preterm birth with spontaneous labor and membranes intact), preterm PROM (preterm birth with PROM with or without spontaneous labor)	RR (relative risk) for preterm PROM = 1.25 for women >30 years of age (no confidence interval or p-value reported, but stated as an increased risk) Not adjusted for potential confounders Reference age group 20–30 years of age When adjusted for other risk factors, the RR for preterm PROM (maternal age per 5 years) = 1.3 (1.0, 1.5)	Stated in research discussion that maternal age predictive for preterm PROM only (p. 446) Not significant for spontaneous preterm labor

TABLE E-1
Characteristics and Results of the Studies Examining the Effect of Older Maternal Age on the Risk of Spontaneous Preterm Birth

Heaman, M. I., Blanchard, J. F., Gupton, A. L., Moffatt, M. E. K., Currie, R. F. (2005). Risk factors for spontaneous preterm birth among Aboriginal and non-Aboriginal women in Manitoba.

Sample:	Purpose:	Results:	Discussion:
Canada; n = 684 (226 preterm and 458 term; 82 preterm Aboriginal and 176 term Aboriginal) infants delivered at two tertiary care hospitals in Winnipeg, Manitoba between October 1999 and December 2000 Hospital-based study.	To identify risk factors for spontaneous preterm birth and to compare risk factors among Aboriginal and non-Aboriginal women **Design:** Case-control study **Methods:** Used labor and delivery log books, standardized questionnaire, and an in-person interview; GA confirmed by LMP and ultrasound **Risk factors and covariates included:** Sociodemographic, behavioral, psychosocial, and biomedical risk factors (e.g. vaginal bleeding, gestational hypertension, urinary tract infection) **Birth outcome:** PT-both (preterm delivery preceded by spontaneous labor or rupture of the membranes without induction or elective cesarean section)	Crude OR for PT-both = 1.27 (0.74, 2.19) for non-Aboriginal women aged >35 years. Crude OR for PT-both = 1.07 (0.31, 3.66) for Aboriginal women aged >35 years. Older maternal age not a significant risk factor for PT-both, so not included in the final analysis Reference age group: 19–35 years	Older maternal age does not increase the risk of PT-both in Aboriginal and non-Aboriginal women

Kramer, M. S., McLean, F. H., Eason, E. L., Usher, R. (1992). Maternal nutrition and spontaneous preterm birth.

Sample:	Purpose:	Results:	Discussion:
Canada; n = 13,102 infants born at Montreal's Royal Victoria Hospital between 1 January 1980 and 31 March 1989 (8,022 births less than 37 weeks gestation used for regression analysis; 10,358 births <34 weeks and <32 weeks gestation used for regression analysis) Hospital-based study	To investigate the impact of maternal nutrition and other determinants on delivery prior to 37 weeks, 34 weeks, and 32 weeks gestation **Design:** Retrospective cohort study **Methods:** Used McGill Obstetric and Neonatal Database; GA confirmed by LMP and ultrasound (dates required to agree within +/- 7 days) **Risk factors and covariates included:** Pregnancy-induced hypertension, prepregnancy hypertension, prior at-risk obstetrical history, diabetes, urinary tract infection, height, education, marital status, smoking, and alcohol **Birth outcome:** PT-both (includes spontaneous preterm births and preterm cesarean deliveries due to medical complications)	AOR for women aged ≥35 years and delivering an infant <37 weeks gestation = 1.13 (0.98, 1.24) AOR for women aged ≥35 years and delivering an infant <34 weeks gestation = 1.15 (0.93, 1.41), AOR for women aged ≥35 years and delivering an infant <32 weeks gestation = 1.05 (0.79, 1.40) Reference age group: 20–34 years	Older maternal age not a significant risk factor for PT-both

(continues)

TABLE E-1 *(continued)*
Characteristics and Results of the Studies Examining the Effect of Older Maternal Age on the Risk of Spontaneous Preterm Birth

Lang, J.M., Lieberman, E., Cohen, A. (1996). A comparison of risk factors for preterm labor and term small-for-gestational-age birth.

Sample:
USA; n = 11,505 women recruited into the delivery interview program conducted at the Boston Hospital for Women from August 1977 to March 1980 (n = 9, 490 for preterm analysis)
Excluded women with menstrual abnormalities for whom gestational dating was problematic and women with preexisting chronic diseases (i.e., diabetes mellitus, hypertension, epilepsy, asthma)
Hospital-based study

Purpose: To determine the effect of prematurity and fetal growth retardation in healthy women and to compare the different risk models

Design: Cohort study

Methods: Used interviews and medical records; GA confirmed by LMP

Risk factors and covariates included: Urinary tract infection; genetic and constitutional, sociodemographic, obstetrical, nutritional, and lifestyle factors; and prenatal care. Pregnancy complications treated as intermediate outcomes (no effect on AOR for maternal age adding these factors into the risk model last)

Birth outcome: PT-both (excluded women whose pregnancies were artificially interrupted before term)

Results:
AOR for PT-both = 1.1 (0.8, 1.6) for women aged ≥35 years
Reference age group: 25–34 years

Discussion:
Older maternal age (≥35 years) not a significant predictor of spontaneous preterm birth

Mercer, B. M., Das, A., Moawad, A. H., et al. (1996). The preterm prediction study: A clinical risk assessment system.

Sample:
USA; n = 2,929 women participating in the Preterm Birth Prediction Study between October 1992 and July 1994 (followed up at 10 participating centers; assessed between 23 and 24) weeks gestation
Population-based study

Purpose: To develop a risk assessment system for predicting preterm delivery preceded by spontaneous labor or preterm PROM

Design: Prospective cohort

Methods: Used structured interview, medical records, laboratory testing and medical exams; GA confirmed by LMP and/or ultrasound.

Risk factors and covariates included: Assessed numerous risk factors to develop a risk assessment model, including preexisting medical conditions and pregnancy complications

Birth outcome: PT-both (included infants delivered before 37 weeks gestation after spontaneous labor) or preterm PROM)

Results:
Crude RR for PT-both = 1.1 (0.8, 1.6) for nulliparous women >35 years of age
Crude RR for PT-both = 1.08 (0.61, 1.92) for multiparous women >35 years of age
Reference age group: 16–35 years

Discussion:
Older maternal age (>35 years) was not a significant predictor of PT-both for nulliparous or multiparous women, so it was not included in the final model

TABLE E-1
Characteristics and Results of the Studies Examining the Effect of Older Maternal Age on the Risk of Spontaneous Preterm Birth

Abbreviation	Term	Description
Preterm PROM	Preterm premature rupture of membranes	The rupture of chorioamniotic membranes anytime before the onset of labor prior to 37 weeks completed gestation (Newburn-Cook & Onyskiw, 2005).
RR	Relative risk	A "ratio of risk" estimated in cohort studies. For example, in the studies reviewed where PT-both is the outcome, it is defined as the incidence of spontaneous preterm birth in women 35 years of age and older divided by the incidence of spontaneous preterm birth in the reference age group (e.g., women under the age of 35). A relative risk greater than 1.0 and a 95% confidence interval not including 1.0 indicates that there is an increased risk of spontaneous preterm birth for women 35 years of age and older (Newburn-Cook & Onyskiw, 2005).
OR	Odds ratio	An estimate of the relative risk in case-control studies. It is the probability or likelihood of spontaneous preterm birth occurring for women 35 years of age and older when compared to women of younger maternal age. An odds ratio greater than 1.0 and a 95% confidence interval not including 1.0 indicates that the probability of having a spontaneous preterm birth is greater for women of older maternal age (Newburn-Cook & Onyskiw, 2005).
AOR	Adjusted odds ratio	Estimates the independent effect of older maternal age on spontaneous preterm birth after controlling for the effects of age-dependent (e.g. preexisting medical conditions) and other potential confounders (e.g. psychosocial, behavioral, nutritional factors) (Newburn-Cook & Onyskiw, 2005).

Notes:

Studies adjusted for maternal age or included maternal age as the independent variable; study samples included only singleton, live births, unless separate analysis provided for multiple births and/or stillbirths; in all studies preterm birth and preterm delivery defined as delivery <37 weeks gestation; all studies adjusted for preexisting medical conditions and/or pregnancy complications.

[1]The impact of maternal age is the primary focus of the study.

[2]Results show significant association between older maternal age and PT-both, spontaneous labor or preterm PROM.

Source: Adapted from Newburn-Cook & Onyskiw, 2005.

Study Objectives

The specific objectives of this study will be (1) to determine if older maternal age at first birth (≥35 years of age at time of delivery) is an independent risk factor for spontaneous preterm birth or a risk marker that exerts its influence indirectly through other age-dependent risk factors (e.g., preexisting maternal illnesses, such as chronic hypertension and diabetes mellitus or pregnancy complications such as pregnancy-induced hypertension); and (2) to establish separate risk models for healthy, low-risk nulliparous women (i.e., no preexisting illness) and high-risk nulliparous women (i.e., those with preexisting chronic health problems).

Significance of the Study

An epidemiological framework and a population health approach will guide the development and implementation of the proposed research study. These two approaches are complementary, both seeking to identify the many determinants that influence health among women of childbearing age, including the effect of older maternal age on gestational age and the occurrence of spontaneous preterm birth. This information can then be used to control or prevent preterm birth.

Originally focused on the etiological determinants of disease, the focus of epidemiology has evolved to include investigating the distribution and determinants of health and illness in individuals and populations (Brunt & Shields, 2000; Gordis, 2000; Mackenbach, 1995; Valanis, 1999). Epidemiologic methods are becoming increasingly important to healthcare providers, including nurses, because health system priorities have changed and are now focused primarily on primary prevention (upstream thinking) rather than on treatment or cure of illness (Brunt & Shields, 2000).

Factors outside of the healthcare system identified as being influential to the health of individuals and populations are known as the determinants of health. These health determinants include income and social status; social support; education; physical, social, and work environments; biology and genetics; personal health practices and coping skills; gender; culture; health services; and healthy child development (Federal, Provincial and Territorial Advisory Committee on Population Health, 1994; Health Canada, 1996). Like epidemiology, a population health approach is concerned with the determinants of health in populations, specifically the interaction among individual and collective factors and conditions contributing to the health and well-being of populations (Health Canada, 1996). To effectively influence population health, a better understanding of these health determinants and the complex interactions among them needs to be addressed (Federal, Provincial and Territorial Advisory Committee on Population Health, 1994).

Understanding the determinants of health is important for primary prevention. However, the role of nurses in the identification of these determinants is still in its infancy. Butterfield (2002) noted that "with few exceptions, nursing has not been active in efforts to understand the etiology of disease" (p. 33). She believes that nurses have an important role in advancing upstream thinking through research efforts that address the determinants of diseases impacting their clients. Nurses are in a key position to influence birth outcomes due to their contact with families before, during, and after pregnancy. Consequently, they need to understand what factors are involved and how these factors interact to influence pregnancy outcomes, including gestational duration.

The results of the proposed study will provide further insight into the determinants of spontaneous preterm birth in northern and central Alberta and, in particular, whether or not pregnancy in nulliparous women ≥35 years of age is associated with an increased risk of spontaneous preterm birth. As stated by the World Health Organization (2002), focusing on the risks to health is important to prevention and requires examining both proximal and distal causes of adverse health outcomes because risks do not occur in isolation (Misra, O'Campo, & Strobino, 2001; Myslobodsky, 2001). Examining the direct and indirect effects of biologic, genetic, lifestyle, and sociodemographic variables, including maternal age, will increase understanding of how these factors work together to influence gestational age at birth. Furthermore, identifying any modifiable risk factors, such as maternal age, and their impact on pregnancy outcomes can be used to develop interventions and/or prevention programs.

With more women delaying the birth of their first child until 35 years of age and beyond, and with the preterm birth rate on the rise, nurses need to know whether older maternal age (a potentially modifiable risk factor) has an independent–direct effect or interacts with other factors to increase the likelihood of spontaneous preterm birth. This information is needed by healthcare providers in the provision of preconceptual and antenatal counseling, as well as by women who are deciding on when to begin their families. The knowledge gained from this study will help nurses to develop effective primary prevention interventions or programs aimed at reducing modifiable risk factors that shorten gestational duration. In addition, nurses will be better equipped to work with healthcare policy makers to create and implement health-oriented public policy targeted to improving maternal, fetal, and newborn health, and hence, population health (Glass & Hicks, 2000; White, 2004). These actions will promote the health of childbearing women and possibly lead to better birth outcomes.

Literature Review

Concern about the potential risks of older maternal age on birth outcomes arose over three decades ago when the International Federation of Gynecology and Obstetrics (FIGO) classified women who delivered their first child at age 35 years or older as elderly primigravida (Cunningham & Leveno, 1995; Kirz, Dorchester, & Freeman, 1985). Since then, there have been numerous researchers who investigated the effect of older maternal age ($\geq$35 years of age at time of delivery) on various maternal and fetal outcomes, including the risk of preterm birth. Unfortunately, the results of these studies have been inconclusive and sometimes contradictory. For example, several researchers have found an association between older maternal age and the risk of preterm birth (Alexander, Baruffi, Mor, & Kieffer, 1992; Astolfi & Zonta, 1999; de Sanjose & Roman, 1991; Ekwo & Moawad, 2000; Mohsin, et al., 2003; Mor, Alexander, Kogan, Kieffer, & Ichiho, 1995; Newburn-Cook, et al., 2002; Tough, Svenson, Johnston, & Schopflocher, 2001; Verkerk, et al., 1994; Wen, Goldenberg, Cutter, Hoffman, & Cliver, 1990). However, other researchers have not supported this finding. They have concluded that older maternal age does not increase the risk of preterm birth (Arbuckle & Sherman, 1989; Barkan & Bracken, 1987; Beydoun, et al., 2004; Frisbie, Biegler, de Turk, Forbes, & Pullum, 1997; Kolas, et al., 2000; Mvula & Miller, 1998; Nordentoft, et al., 1996; Shiono & Klebanoff, 1986; Shults, Arndt, Olshan, Martin, & Royce, 1999; Virji & Cottington, 1991; White, 2004).

As discussed previously, the disparate findings among past studies may be due to methodological limitations and study differences. These include inadequate sample sizes and lack of study power; differences in the study setting and population sampled (i.e., population-based versus hospital-based studies); inadequate control of age-dependent confounders that are also associated with pregnancy outcomes; failure to consider the relationship between maternal age and preexisting chronic diseases and pregnancy complications that are associated with older maternal age; inconsistency in the definition of what constitutes older maternal age and choice of the specific reference age group for comparisons; differences in data sources used, resulting in incomplete and/or inaccurate data on risk factors; and varying definitions of birth outcomes being assessed (Berkowitz & Papiernik, 1993; Kramer, 1987; Newburn-Cook & Onyskiw, 2005). In addition, the equivocal results may be due to the fact that the majority of the researchers have treated preterm birth as a single entity or homogeneous birth outcome without acknowledging that preterm birth is a "cluster of conditions with different etiologies" or different etiological pathways (Pickett, et al., 2000, p. 305).

The impact of maternal age on the incidence of preterm birth may, in fact, vary as a function of the specific preterm birth subtype (i.e., preterm birth following spontaneous labor, preterm birth following ruptured membranes, or medically indicated preterm birth) (Savitz, et al., 1991). Failing to consider the heterogeneity of preterm birth may prevent the identification of any differential age effects for each subtype.

The purpose of this literature review is to identify, select, and examine the results of studies where researchers have estimated the impact of older maternal age on two preterm birth subtypes (i.e., preterm birth following ruptured membranes or preterm birth following spontaneous labor) or PT-both (preterm birth with or without ruptured membranes). The review will include a discussion of the methodological shortcomings and limitations of the studies selected.

Selecting the Studies for Inclusion in the Literature Review

The present literature review extends the work of Newburn-Cook and Onyskiw (2005). These researchers conducted a systematic review of the literature (1985 to 2002) to examine the impact of advancing maternal age on spontaneous preterm birth and fetal growth restriction. Studies were selected by these researchers if they met the following inclusion criteria: (1) assessed risk factors for preterm birth by subtype (i.e., idiopathic preterm labor, preterm premature rupture of membranes) and small-for-gestational age birth (fetal growth restriction); (2) used acceptable definitions of these birth outcomes; (3) were restricted to singleton live births; (4) were conducted in a developed country; and (5) were published in English. The same criteria were used in retrieving and selecting the literature included in this review.

A comprehensive search for additional published and unpublished studies for the time period from January 2003 to July 2005 was undertaken using a number of search strategies. These included a computerized search of various online databases (i.e., MEDLINE, CINAHL, EMBASE, HealthSTAR, Web of Science, ABI/INFORM, Academic Search Premier, Sociological Abstracts), abstracting services (i.e., ProQuest Dissertations & Theses), and the Cochrane Collaboration Database. The medical subject headings (MeSH) and keywords used to locate and retrieve articles were older maternal age, maternal age, maternal age 35 and over, advanced maternal age, spontaneous preterm labor, spontaneous preterm delivery, premature rupture of membranes, preterm birth subtypes, preterm delivery subtypes, preterm birth, low birth weight, risk factors, pregnancy complications, pregnancy outcome, and a combination of these terms. In addition to the online searches, reference lists of pertinent studies were examined for other potentially relevant articles.

Articles were screened for any words in the title or abstract that indicated an investigation into the risk factors for preterm birth. Studies that focused primarily on other risk factors were considered for review if the researchers provided a risk estimate of older maternal age on preterm birth. The majority of articles included in this review had risk factors other than maternal age as the primary focus (e.g., nutrition, various clinical and obstetric risk factors). For example, Berkowitz and her colleagues (1998) assessed simultaneously the effect of previously identified sociodemographic, obstetric, nutritional, and medical risk factors on preterm birth due to spontaneous labor, premature rupture of membranes, or medical indications. Because older maternal age was included in the analysis, this investigation met the inclusion criteria outlined by Newburn-Cook and Onyskiw (2005) and was included in this review, along with studies that considered maternal age as the independent variable of interest.

Approximately 50 articles were retrieved, but only one study by Heaman, Blanchard, Gupton, Moffatt, and Currie (2005) met the criteria established by Newburn-Cook and Onyskiw (2005). This study was added to the investigations previously selected by these authors. The characteristics and results of the eight studies included in this literature review are summarized in Table E-1.

Older Maternal Age and Its Association with Spontaneous Preterm Birth

All of the studies included in this review had at least two preterm birth subtypes as the dependent variable (Aldous & Edmonson, 1993; Berkowitz, 1985; Berkowitz, et al., 1998; Harlow, et al., 1996; Heaman, et al., 2005; Kramer, McLean, Eason, & Usher, 1992; Lang, Lieberman, & Cohen, 1996; Mercer, et al., 1996). In six of these studies, researchers grouped preterm birth due to spontaneous (idiopathic) labor or preterm premature rupture of membranes into the single category of spontaneous preterm birth (Aldous & Edmonson, 1993; Berkowitz, 1985; Heaman, et al., 2005; Kramer, et al., 1992; Lang, et al., 1996; Mercer, et al., 1996). For the purposes of this review, this classification of spontaneous preterm birth will be referred to as PT-both. The remaining researchers conducted separate analyses for preterm birth due to spontaneous labor, preterm premature rupture of membranes, or preterm births that were medically indicated (Berkowitz, et al., 1998; Harlow, et al., 1996).

Although the majority of the authors equated spontaneous preterm birth (PT-both) to preterm birth preceded by preterm premature rupture of membranes or spontaneous labor, Kramer et al. (1992) used a different definition that concurred with the theoretical argument of Klebanoff and Shiono (1995). Klebanoff and Shiono argued that "a non-trivial fraction of 'elective' preterm births would have been 'spontaneous' had the managing clinician not intervened" (p. 126). Based on this argument, Kramer et al. controlled for any preterm births not considered spontaneous or potentially spontaneous by including only those preterm births occurring from spontaneous labor, from inductions for preterm premature rupture of membranes or chorioamnionitis, or from cesarean sections due to maternal or fetal indications (e.g., abruptio placentae, placenta previa). Kramer et al. excluded preterm births following induced labor or a cesarean section for which there was no medical threat. These researchers acknowledged that any discrepancies between their results and the findings in other studies could be due to the inclusion of induced preterm deliveries in their analyses. Because Kramer and his colleagues defined spontaneous preterm birth (PT-both) differently, caution should be taken when comparing their results with the findings of other studies included in this review.

The studies varied with respect to study design, sample size, and data sources used to obtain the potential risk factors (including maternal age) and birth outcomes. In six studies, researchers used a cohort study design (Aldous & Edmonson, 1993; Berkowitz, et al., 1998; Harlow, et al., 1996; Kramer, et al., 1992; Lang, et al., 1996; Mercer, et al., 1996), and in the other two studies, researchers conducted case-control investigations (Berkowitz, 1985; Heaman, et al., 2005). All but three studies had hospital-based samples and included study data gathered from administrative databases, interviews, and medical records (Berkowitz, 1985; Berkowitz, et al., 1998; Heaman, et al., 2005; Kramer, et al., 1992; Lang, et al., 1996). Two of the cohort studies were prospective and were restricted to women participating in larger research projects (i.e., RADIUS and the Preterm Birth Prediction Study, respectively) (Harlow, et al., 1996; Mercer, et al., 1996). Women in these studies were followed prenatally through to delivery with data being collected prior to delivery via interview (e.g., demographic information, lifestyle choices). The remaining study by Aldous and Edmonson (1993) was the only population-based study. These investigators used birth certificates to acquire information on all white and black infants born in Washington State between 1984 and 1988.

Due to the differences in how samples and data were acquired, the number of subjects varied among the studies. Sample sizes ranged from 488 to 31,107 births. A small sample size present in three studies may have prevented an adequate examination of the impact that older maternal age had on PT-both (Berkowitz, 1985; Heaman, et al., 2005; Mercer, et al., 1996). In two of these studies, researchers excluded older maternal age from the final regression model when it proved to be insignificant in the univariate analysis (Heaman, et al., 2005; Mercer, et al., 1996). In the other study, investigators found that older maternal age was insignificant in the multivariate analysis (no odds ratio was reported) (Berkowitz, 1985). These studies may have been underpowered because of their limited sample sizes. For example, Berkowitz (1985) recruited only n = 488 participants (175 cases and 313 controls) who delivered at Yale-New Haven Hospital to assess various clinical and obstetric risk factors for PT-both. However, as Berkowitz points out, the sample size may have been insufficient to properly assess the independent effects of variables entered simultaneously into the multivariate model.

Similarly, Heaman et al. (2005) modeled several sociodemographic, behavioral, psychosocial, and biomedical risk factors for PT-both for both Aboriginal and non-Aboriginal women. The subjects in this study consisted of n = 226 preterm infants (82 Aboriginal) and n = 458 term infants (176 Aboriginal) born at two tertiary care hospitals. Through multivariate analysis, they found young maternal age (<19 years of age; AOR = 0.19, 95% CI = 0.04–0.89) to be a protective factor for Aboriginal women, a finding that was contrary to the results for non-Aboriginal women. However, these results may be questionable given the small sample size. Heaman et al. concluded that there were insufficient numbers of subjects for adequate racial–ethnic stratification. Therefore, this study was an exploratory study and, as such, did not provide definitive findings for the determinants of PT-both in Aboriginal and non-Aboriginal Canadian women.

Mercer et al. (1996) were at the same disadvantage with only 1218 nulliparous and 1711 multiparous women participating in the Preterm Birth Prediction Study to investigate the predictability of a risk assessment system for PT-both. After assessing several risk factors simultaneously, including maternal age, they established that all the risk factors had low predictive value for PT-both in both nulliparous and multiparous women. Unfortunately, the large number of risk factors assessed, along with the small sample size used, led to tentative and inconclusive results.

Although the rest of the researchers in this review used larger sample sizes, they had other methodological limitations present in their research that need to be considered before accepting the conclusions. Kramer et al. (1992) were the only researchers to develop separate risk models for PT-both at <37, <34, and <32 completed weeks gestation. Dividing PT-both in this manner enabled Kramer and his colleagues to detect any varying effects each determinant had for moderately preterm, very preterm, and extremely preterm births. Their study sample included n = 13,102 single-ton, live-born infants delivered at Montreal's Royal Victoria Hospital. Using a retrospective cohort study design, they investigated the impact of maternal nutrition and other determinants, including older maternal age, on PT-both. After controlling for age-dependent confounders (i.e., pregnancy-induced hypertension, prepregnancy hypertension, diabetes, education), Kramer et al. concluded that women aged 35 years and older were at no greater risk for delivering an infant at <37 weeks gestation (AOR = 1.13, 95% CI = 0.98–1.24), <34 weeks gestation (AOR = 1.15, 95% CI = 0.93–1.41), or <32 weeks gestation (AOR = 1.05, 95% CI = 0.79–1.40) when compared to women 20–34 years of age. However, the generalizability of the study findings is limited given the use of a hospital-based sample. Moreover, as mentioned previously, Kramer and colleagues included inductions and cesarean sections in their study, unlike the other studies in this review, which makes comparing their findings to the other study results difficult.

Aldous and Edmonson (1993) conducted the only study that specifically investigated the effects of older maternal age on various birth outcomes (i.e., low birth weight, very low birth weight, and PT-both). Using a population-based study, a total of n = 16,492 white and n = 4403 black, first-born, singleton, live-born infants were included in their investigation. Information recorded on Washington State birth certificates was used for acquiring the risk factors included in the risk modeling and PT-both. Aldous and Edmonson grouped maternal age into five-year categories, with older maternal age being separated into women aged 35–39 years and ≥40 years of age. This was the only study that provided a separate risk estimate for women ≥40 years of age. By stratifying maternal age into these categories and through adequate control for age-dependent confounders (i.e., preexisting hypertension, socioeconomic status, smoking), Aldous and Edmonson were able to establish a moderate but progressive increased risk of PT-both with advancing maternal age. The highest risk was seen in women ≥ 40 years of age (AOR = 1.8, 95% CI = 1.3–2.6) with significant risk beginning in women aged 30–34 years (AOR = 1.4, 95% CI = 1.1–1.7). Although an analysis for black infants was completed, the results showed no significant findings. However, the small number of black infants born to women 35 years and older (n = 127) and the resulting imprecise risk estimates made these findings inconclusive. Because this was the only study to demonstrate a significant association between older maternal age and PT-both, and it was the only study to have older maternal age as the independent variable, more research is needed to investigate the relationship between older maternal age and this birth outcome.

One of the methodological strengths exhibited in all the studies was the inclusion of age-dependent confounders in the analyses; these are factors associated with increasing age and have a negative impact on birth outcomes (e.g., pregnancy complications and/or preexisting medical conditions). However, the researchers varied as to what risk factors they included, making comparison of results difficult. To focus on women who were healthy at the start of their pregnancies, both Harlow et al. (1996) and Lang et al. (1996) excluded women with preexisting medical conditions, but they varied in which women they excluded with different medical conditions. Lang and associates excluded those women with epilepsy, asthma, diabetes mellitus, and hypertension, and Harlow et al. excluded those women with chronic renal disease, diabetes mellitus, and hypertension. All but two of the remaining studies (Berkowitz, 1985; Heaman, et al., 2005) had adjustments for chronic medical conditions in the analyses. In two of these studies, the researchers included a wide range of pregnancy complications (Lang, et al., 1996; Mercer, et al., 1996); the rest included as few as one to as many as three potential pregnancy complications (e.g., gestational diabetes, pregnancy-induced hypertension, proteinuria).

The studies included in this literature review also differed on how older maternal age, as well as the reference age group chosen for comparison, were defined. Despite the FIGO definition of older maternal age as being ≥ 35 years of age, only half the researchers used this definition, and when they did, they differed on the choice of reference age group. One study had women 20–29 years of age (Berkowitz, et al., 1998) and another had women 25–29 years of age (Harlow, et al., 1996) as the age groups for comparison. Kramer et al. (1992) and Lang et al. (1996) used women 20–34 years of age and 25–34 years of age, respectively, as the reference age groups for their analyses. Berkowitz (1985) defined older maternal age as 35–41 years but did not report a reference group due to the insignificant findings between older maternal age and PT-both. In two studies where older maternal age was defined as >35 years, women 19–35 years of age and 16–35 years of age, respectively, were chosen as the groups for comparison (Heaman, et al., 2005; Mercer, et al., 1996). In the study where older maternal age was stratified into 35–39 years and ≥40 years, women 20–24 years of age were included as the reference group (Aldous & Edmonson, 1993). All the differing definitions of age make comparison of results across studies a challenge.

Overall, the studies reviewed here show that the effect of older maternal age on PT-both remains inconclusive. A lack of population-based samples, along with the use of smaller samples in three studies (Berkowitz, 1985; Heaman, et al., 2005; Mercer, et al., 1996), limits the generalizability and validity of the findings. Interestingly, the only study to find a significant association between older maternal age and PT-both was also the only population-based study in this review (Aldous & Edmonson, 1993). The discrepancy in findings between this study and the others may reflect differing sample characteristics. Several confounders were included in all the studies, but the type and number of confounders varied. Furthermore, with the exception of one study (Lang, et al., 1996), there was no clear assessment of the direct or indirect effect of risk factors. More attention to the determinants of the different preterm birth subtypes that may play an intermediate role in the etiological chain is necessary for there to be clarity around the direct causes of this birth outcome. Finally, in all studies, age definition and choice of reference age group need more refinement if results are to be compared in the future.

Heterogeneity of Preterm Birth

Two groups of researchers in this review developed separate risk models for preterm birth due to spontaneous labor or preterm premature rupture of membranes using several previously identified risk factors (Berkowitz, et al., 1998; Harlow, et al., 1996). Berkowitz et al. (1998) included both high- and low-risk pregnancies in their study and used a retrospective cohort design to investigate the impact of several risk factors on each preterm birth subtype (i.e., preterm birth due to spontaneous labor, preterm birth due to preterm premature rupture of membranes, or medically indicated preterm births). A hospital-based sample of n = 31,107 births was used. After controlling for several known risk factors, Berkowitz et al. found that both women 30–34 years of age (AOR = 1.4, 95% CI = 1.2–1.6) and women ≥35 years of age (AOR = 1.5, 95% CI = 1.3–1.8) were at greater risk for preterm birth due to preterm premature rupture of membranes when compared to women 20–29 years of age. Older maternal age was not a significant predictor of preterm birth due to spontaneous labor.

Like Berkowitz et al. (1998), Harlow and his colleagues (1996) had a large hospital-based sample (n = 14,948) to conduct their analysis of potential risk factors for each preterm birth subtype. However, their study sample was restricted to low-risk pregnancies (i.e., no medical indication for ultrasound at the first visit and exclusion of women with preexisting diseases). Unlike Berkowitz et al., Harlow and his associates were not able to clearly demonstrate their maternal age result. These researchers classified maternal age as a continuous variable (maternal age per five years) and as a result could only make a conclusion about maternal age, not older maternal age. The findings showed borderline significance for maternal age and preterm premature rupture of membranes (AOR = 1.3, 95% CI = 1.0–1.5); however, these researchers concluded that maternal age "was predictive for premature rupture of membranes" (p. 446). This weak result may have been a reflection of the healthy population used to investigate their objectives. Like Berkowitz et al., Harlow and his colleagues did not find a significant association between maternal age and preterm birth due to spontaneous labor.

Both Berkowitz et al. (1998) and Harlow et al. (1996) acknowledged that distinguishing between preterm birth arising from preterm premature rupture of membranes and spontaneous labor could be problematic. However, the findings from both studies indicate that there may be differential effects for maternal age on each preterm birth subtype. The results in Berkowitz et al. show that older maternal age increases the risk of preterm birth arising from preterm premature rupture of membranes, but not spontaneous labor, and the results in Harlow et al. show the same findings for maternal age. Unfortunately, the hospital-based samples and varying definitions of older maternal age used in these studies prevent the establishment of definitive conclusions. As a result, more research is needed to examine causal factors for each preterm birth subtype. Future studies should include a population-based sample, differentiate between high- and low-risk women, and control for a wide range of potential confounders.

Age-Dependent Confounders

There are several researchers that have investigated the complications of pregnancy, particularly in older gravida. The overwhelming majority has shown that there is an increased risk of chronic medical conditions and pregnancy complications in women of older maternal age. In a recent US study, researchers found that certain maternal complications demonstrated a positive association with maternal age in a dose-dependent fashion (Salihu, Shumpert, Slay, Kirby, & Alexander, 2003). For example, the rate of chronic hypertension per 1000 deliveries in women 20–29 years of age was 5.3. This rate increased to 10.4 for women aged 30–39 years, to 23.8 for women aged 40–49 years, and to 27.8 for women aged 50 and older.

This study confirmed previous results that established older women were more likely to be at higher risk for antepartum and intrapartum complications when compared to their younger counterparts (Berkowitz, Skovron, Lapinski, & Berkowitz, 1990; Gilbert, Nesbitt, & Danielsen, 1999; Jolly, Sebire, Harris, Robinson, & Regan, 2000; Prysak, Lorenz, & Kisly, 1995). For example, in a population-based study in the United Kingdom, it was found that women >40 years of age were three times more likely to have placenta previa compared to women 18–34 years of age (AOR = 3.09, 99% CI = 2.19–4.36) (Jolly, et al., 2000). Similarly, it was determined that, after adjusting for race and underlying medical conditions, women ≥35 years of age were two times more likely to have antepartum complications than women 20–29 years of age (i.e., gestational diabetes, abruptio placentae, and placenta previa; AOR = 2.0, 95% CI = 1.6–2.5) (Berkowitz, et al., 1990). Results of these studies indicate the importance of including age-dependent confounders in an analysis of older maternal age and spontaneous preterm birth so that the presence of any independent association between older maternal age and this birth outcome can be determined.

Pregnancy complications have been identified as intermediate outcomes of preterm birth in the literature (i.e., other risk factors act indirectly through these factors) (Kramer, 1987). As a result, in one study where the mediating role of pregnancy complications was examined, the researchers first assessed the effect of 23 different risk factors on PT-both without pregnancy complications in the risk model and then assessed their effect with pregnancy complications added in (Lang, et al., 1996). By proceeding in this fashion, the indirect effects of other risk factors were determined by noting any significant changes in the risk estimates. Although there was no significant change in the odds ratio for older maternal age, Lang et al. were able to identify the direct and indirect effects of other risk factors. For example, the odds ratios for low prepregnant weight, previous preterm birth, three or more miscarriages, two or more stillbirths, in utero DES exposure, and low weekly weight gain showed significant moderate decreases after pregnancy complications were added into the model. These results indicate that these particular risk factors may act indirectly through pregnancy complications to influence PT-both. Older maternal age was a nonsignificant risk factor for PT-both (AOR = 1.1, 95% CI = 0.8–1.6) regardless of whether pregnancy complications were in the risk model. Lang et al. were unique in their assessment of pregnancy complications and, as a result, were able to provide methodological direction for future studies to specifically address the effects of older maternal age on spontaneous preterm birth.

To accurately assess the impact of older maternal age on spontaneous preterm birth, other potential confounders, along with chronic medical conditions and pregnancy complications, need to be considered in the risk modeling. Kramer (1987) and Berkowitz and Papiernik (1993) completed two comprehensive reviews of potential risk factors for preterm birth. These two reviews were used to determine which risk factors and covariates would be included, along with maternal age, in the risk modeling proposed in this study.

Summary

The results of the studies reviewed provide some evidence that there is an older maternal age effect on the incidence of spontaneous preterm birth (PT-both) and preterm birth due to preterm premature rupture of membranes. Other studies have shown that older maternal age is associated with an increased prevalence of chronic diseases, medical problems during pregnancy, as well as antepartum and labor complications (Berkowitz, et al., 1990; Gilbert, et al., 1999; Jolly, et al., 2000; Prysak, et al., 1995; Salihu, et al., 2003). However, it is not known whether older maternal age exerts an independent and direct effect on preterm birth (i.e., the different preterm birth subtypes) or if it acts indirectly through its association with age-dependent confounders, factors that affect birth outcome and are a function of increasing maternal age (e.g., preexisting maternal illness, pregnancy complications). Therefore, the aim of this study is to determine if older maternal age at first birth is an independent risk factor for spontaneous preterm birth (preterm birth not associated with either ruptured membranes or iatrogenic intervention) (Ananth, et al., 2005) or a risk marker that exerts its influence indirectly through other age-dependent risk factors.

The specific methodology used to address this inquiry is important. From the studies reviewed it has become apparent that it will be necessary to define what constitutes older maternal age, to decide on the choice of reference group based on the age associated with optimal reproduction (less risk to pregnancy outcomes), and to control for age-dependent confounders, other risk factors, and interactions among these variables.

None of the researchers of the studies reviewed provided a rationale for the age categories selected and used in their analyses. It seems that the majority based their definitions on what had been done or defined in the past; however, definitions today may be changing. Although most researchers use ≥35 years of age as the benchmark for older maternal age, some are now considering women aged 40 years and beyond as the high-risk older primigravida (Ekblad & Vilpa, 1994; Miletic, et al., 2002; Salihu, et al., 2003; Spellacy, Miller, & Winegar, 1986; Ziadeh & Yahaya, 2001).

It is unknown today at what age young ends and old begins (Blickstein, 2003). The definition of older maternal age (≥35 years) seems to be an archaic one, developed by FIGO in a time when women had lower life expectancies (Kirz, et al., 1985). Now women are leading healthier lives and may be delivering healthier babies in their mid-30s and beyond than was previously thought. Women who choose to delay childbearing are often better educated, more psychologically ready for pregnancy, and more socially advantaged, which all contribute to more positive pregnancy outcomes (Chen & Millar, 2000; Freeman-Wang & Beski, 2002; Lansac, 1995; Mansfield & McCool, 1989; Newburn-Cook & Onyskiw, 2005). A detailed analysis is warranted to determine where the older age cutoff truly lies. Only when health professionals are aware of where actual risk begins can they provide more effective counseling and treatment.

Although there have been numerous researchers who examined the etiologic factors influencing preterm birth, the majority have treated this birth outcome as a single entity. The research reviewed here indicates that preterm birth may consist of separate etiological pathways that need to be considered if this adverse birth outcome is to be fully understood. Although the results of these studies are equivocal, they are also fewer in number. Methodological limitations in previous research justify the need for more etiological research that acknowledges the heterogeneity of preterm birth and examines the causal mechanisms of each preterm birth subtype. As delineated by Berkowitz et al. (1998), investigation into the components of preterm birth must continue until the components appear to be homogeneous. Only then can preterm birth as a whole be considered. Ignoring the heterogeneity of preterm birth at this point may impede our ability to determine conclusively any differential effects that older maternal age has on the varying pathways leading to early delivery.

The proposed study will provide further insight into the relationship between older maternal age and spontaneous preterm birth. It will be the first study to have maternal age as the independent variable of interest and to be focused on determining the direct and indirect effects of various previously identified etiologic determinants of spontaneous preterm birth (i.e., preterm birth not associated with either ruptured membranes or iatrogenic intervention) (Ananth, et al., 2005). As in Lang et al. (1996), pregnancy complications will be treated as intermediate outcomes of spontaneous preterm birth and entered last into the risk modeling so that the mediating effects of these risk factors can be established. Unlike previous research, the heterogeneity of the maternal population will be taken into account by comparing two risk models, one for women who are healthy versus one for women diagnosed with preexisting medical conditions. These separate models will help to demonstrate any differences in the causal mechanisms that exist for these two groups of women.

The lack of population-based studies incorporating maternal age as the independent variable was evident from the studies reviewed. This will be the first population-based study to have older maternal age as the independent variable and one preterm birth subtype (preterm birth due to spontaneous labor) as the dependent variable. Finally, this study will have smaller age groupings of maternal age to more clearly establish where the at risk age for spontaneous preterm birth begins and to determine if there is a differential risk effect. Establishing the direct or indirect effect of older maternal age at first birth on spontaneous preterm birth in both low-risk and high-risk women will help to improve counseling and preterm birth prevention efforts for women of childbearing age.

Design

A retrospective population-based cohort study will be used to determine the impact of older maternal age at first birth on the risk of spontaneous preterm birth in northern and central Alberta.

Study Objectives

The specific study objectives are (1) to determine if older maternal age at first birth (≥35 years of age at time of delivery) is an independent risk factor for spontaneous preterm labor (preterm birth not associated with ruptured membranes or iatrogenic intervention) or a risk marker that exerts its influence indirectly through other age-dependent confounders (e.g., preexisting maternal illnesses, such as chronic hypertension and diabetes mellitus, or pregnancy complications, such as pregnancy-induced hypertension); and (2) to establish separate risk models for healthy, low-risk nulliparous women (i.e., no preexisting illness) and high-risk nulliparous women (i.e., those with preexisting chronic health problems). For the development of all risk models, older maternal age will be stratified into two age groups, consisting of women 35–39 years of age and women 40 years of age and older.

Study Subjects

The study population will consist of n = 193,575 women who were residents of, and gave birth in, northern and central Alberta between January 1, 1996 and December 31, 2004. Subjects will include all Alberta women who delivered a live born, singleton infant. Cases will be composed of nulliparous women 35 years of age and older who delivered a live born, singleton infant at less than 37 completed weeks gestational age and for whom the delivery was spontaneous (not associated with either ruptured membranes or iatrogenic intervention) (Ananth, et al., 2005). Controls will be composed of nulliparous women aged 20–24 years of age (considered the optimal age for childbearing) who delivered a live born, singleton infant between 37 and 41 completed weeks gestation and for whom the delivery was spontaneous (not associated with either ruptured membranes or iatrogenic intervention).

The study focus will be restricted to singleton births because preterm birth rates and causal mechanisms differ between singleton and multiple births (Demissie, et al., 2001; Joseph, et al., 1998). Medically indicated preterm births, defined as births that follow iatrogenic intervention (i.e., labor induction or a primary or repeat cesarean delivery) (Ananth, et al., 2005), will be excluded for both cases and controls.

Data Source

This study will use maternal and newborn data recorded in the Alberta Perinatal Health Program (APHP) North Perinatal Database. This is one of two regional perinatal databases maintained by the APHP. Data are collected from healthcare facilities that provide maternal and newborn care in Health Regions 4 through 9. This computerized population-based perinatal database contains pregnancy and birth data recorded on the provincial delivery records (parts 1 and 2) by hospital staff at the time of delivery. These provincial delivery records are completed for all deliveries. The database also includes information on home births supervised by registered midwives.

Perinatal data are recorded based on the place of delivery, and this information is forwarded to the APHP for data entry. Data collected by participating hospitals are forwarded to the APHP using one of three methods: (1) photocopies of the provincial delivery records; (2) a log book that is transcribed from the provincial delivery records; or (3) electronic transfer of the data from the provincial delivery records.

A number of precautions are taken to ensure both completeness and accuracy of the data entered into the APHP databases. After the data are entered, a data validation procedure is implemented. This consists of a monthly cross check of the manual tabulation of key variables with an electronic tabulation of these same variables. A minimum of one in 20 records is verified with the actual data entry to check its accuracy. Participating hospitals are provided with guidelines for validating electronic data so that validation of hospital data can occur before it is sent to the APHP. In addition, the APHP completes a validation process for electronically submitted data. This consists of electronic tabulation and comparison of results with the Monthly Statistical Report that is supplied with the data.

The APHP North Perinatal Database includes information on genetic and constitutional factors, maternal age at time of delivery, lifestyle factors, obstetrical history, medical problems in the current pregnancy, pregnancy complications, birth outcomes, and limited information about the infant. This database also contains information on maternal health status, including the presence of any preexisting chronic diseases.

Study Variables

The outcome (dependent variable) in this study is spontaneous preterm labor. It is defined as the delivery of a live born, singleton infant prior to 37 completed weeks gestational age that is not associated with either ruptured membranes or iatrogenic intervention (i.e., labor induction or a primary or repeat cesarean delivery) (Ananth, et al., 2005). Of particular interest in the proposed study is the impact of older maternal age (independent variable) on the risk of spontaneous preterm birth. Older maternal age will be defined as women who deliver their first child at 35 years of age or older.

There is some controversy in the literature regarding what constitutes older maternal age. Are women aged 35–39 years at increased risk for preterm birth if they are in good health? Does the risk increase among older nulliparous women ≥40 years of age regardless of health status? Or does the risk for adverse birth outcomes start earlier for women at the age of 30 years as opposed to later, as some researchers suggest (Aldous & Edmonson, 1993; Berkowitz, et al., 1998)? Therefore, to assess the impact of maternal age on the risk of spontaneous preterm birth, maternal age will be stratified into the following age categories: 20–24 years (reference group), 25–29 years, 30–34 years, 35–39 years, and ≥40 years. By stratifying maternal age in this manner, there will be a clearer indication of where the older at risk maternal age begins for preterm birth, and the occurrence of any differential age effects will be established.

Other risk factors and age-dependent covariates (independent variables) will be included in the risk models to examine the impact of older maternal age on the risk of spontaneous preterm birth for low-risk and high-risk women. These factors are outlined in Table E-2 and include maternal and newborn factors, obstetric and medical factors, lifestyle behaviors, medical problems arising during pregnancy, and pregnancy complications. The variables selected for inclusion in this study were based on two reviews of the published literature that focused on the etiology of preterm birth. In particular, the systematic review and meta-analysis completed by Kramer (1987) and the review of the epidemiology of preterm birth (risk factors causally related to decreased gestational age) by Berkowitz and Papiernik (1993) guided the selection of other independent variables to be included in the risk models (see Table E-2).

The risk modeling will be limited to maternal and clinical variables recorded in the APHP North Perinatal Database and the way in which these potential risk factors were measured or aggregated. Consequently, only a partial risk model can be provided. A full explanatory model would require further research and consideration of other potential determinants not recorded in the data source (perinatal database) to be used in this study. This is a limitation of using administrative data in the conduct of etiological research.

Data Analysis

The APHP data will be cleaned and analyzed using SPSS for Windows Version 13.0 (SPSS Inc., Chicago, Illinois). Each study variable will be examined for outliers (implausible values) and coding errors that will be corrected, if feasible, or coded as missing values. New variables will be created as required from existing variables in the database using the transform recode command in the SPSS data analysis program.

The prevalence and distribution of the study variables will be summarized by group (i.e., spontaneous preterm births or cases versus term controls) using descriptive statistics. Means and standard deviations (SD) will be reported for continuous variables, and frequencies and percentages will be used to summarize categorical variables. To determine if the prevalence and distribution of variables across the study groups are different, a Student's t-test to compare means and a chi-square test for

TABLE E-2
Risk Factors to Be Included in the Proposed Study

Demographic
- Maternal age (≥20 years stratified into five age categories: 20–24 years, 25–29 years, 30–34 years, 35–39 years, and 40 years and older)

Genetic and constitutional
- Maternal height (<152 cm or ≥152 cm)
- Prepregnancy weight (≤45 kg, 46–90 kg, ≥91kg)

Lifestyle factors
- Smoker (smoked anytime during pregnancy)
- Alcohol consumption (defined as any alcohol consumed during pregnancy)
- Drug dependent (inappropriate/excessive drug use of any substance that may adversely affect pregnancy outcome)

Preexisting medical diseases (for model 2 only; see Figure E-2)
- Diabetes (insulin dependent or diet controlled)
- Hypertension (defined as a blood pressure of 140/90 mmHg or greater with or without the use of antihypertensive drugs)
- Chronic renal disease
- Heart disease (symptomatic or asymptomatic)
- Other medical disorders (e.g., epilepsy, asthma, lupus, Crohn disease)

Nutritional problems during pregnancy
- Poor gestational weight gain (<0.5 kg/week or weight loss between 26 and 36 weeks)
- Anemia (hemoglobin <100 g/l)

Medical problems during current pregnancy
- Gestational diabetes
- Poly- or oligohydramnios
- Presence of blood antibodies (Rh, anti-C, anti-K, etc.)
- Acute medical disorder (e.g., urinary tract infection, acute asthma, thyrotoxicosis)

Current pregnancy status
- Diagnosis of an SGA infant (<10th percentile)
- Diagnosis of an LGA infant (>90th percentile)
- Presence of a fetal anomaly
- Fetal malpresentation

Pregnancy complications
- Bleeding <20 weeks
- Placenta previa
- Bleeding ≥20 weeks
- Pregnancy-induced hypertension (PIH)
- Preeclampsia (defined as the presence of PIH with proteinuria (≥+1))
- Eclampsia/toxemia (defined as PIH with proteinuria and seizures)

proportions will be calculated. A two-sided P-value ≤ 0.05 will be used to establish if any of the compared differences between cases and controls are statistically significant.

Univariate logistic regression will be used to determine the contribution of every predictor (independent) variable and interaction on the incidence of spontaneous preterm labor, without controlling for the influence of other risk factors and potential covariates. Unadjusted odds ratios (OR) and 95% confidence intervals (CI) will be estimated and reported to indicate the magnitude and direction of the effect of each variable on the outcome (dependent) variable—spontaneous preterm labor.

Unconditional multivariate logistic regression (MLR) will then be used to determine the independent effect of each study variable (including maternal age) on the occurrence of spontaneous preterm labor while simultaneously controlling for the other study variables and covariates. Adjusted odds ratios (AOR) and 95% CIs will be reported.

Separate risk models will be developed to examine the impact of older maternal age on the risk of spontaneous preterm labor for low-risk nulliparous healthy women (no preexisting maternal illnesses or chronic conditions) and high-risk nulliparous women (presence of preexisting maternal illness or chronic conditions). The study variables will be entered in a stepwise fashion in blocks as outlined in Figures E-1 and E-2. This will be done to determine if older maternal age has a direct (independent) or indirect effect (mediated through other factors, including age-dependent variables) on the dependent variable (i.e., spontaneous preterm birth). The hypothetical models (see Figures E-1 and E-2) were based on the risk model used by White (2004) to determine the direct and indirect effects of previously identified risk factors on birth weight and gestational age.

A number of factors guided the development of these models and the order in which the individual study variables and interaction terms will be entered. These included (1) consideration of the risk factors that were present prior to the current pregnancy (e.g., maternal age, height, prepregnancy maternal weight); (2) reflection on the proximal and distal causes and the pathways leading to preterm birth; (3) examination of the relationships among the different study variables (e.g., maternal age may influence the incidence of preexisting maternal illness and chronic conditions, as well as the development of pregnancy complications that necessitate preterm delivery); and (4) consideration of the interaction among different variables and their differential impact on the risk of preterm birth (White, 2004). The risk factors outlined in Figures E-1 and E-2 and their order of entry into the logistic regression models reflects the distal

Block 1 Demographic (maternal age)

Block 2 Genetic and constitutional (maternal height and prepregnancy weight)

Block 3 Lifestyle factors (smoking status, alcohol consumption during pregnancy, drug dependency)

Block 4 Interaction: Age by smoking

Block 5 Interaction: Smoking by alcohol consumption during pregnancy

Block 6 Interaction: Smoking by drug dependency

Block 7 Interaction: Smoking by drug dependency by alcohol consumption during pregnancy

Block 8 Nutritional problems during pregnancy (poor gestational weight gain, anemia)

Block 9 Medical problems during current pregnancy (gestational diabetes, poly- or oligohydramnios, presence of blood antibodies, acute medical disorder)

Block 10 Interaction: Age by gestational diabetes

Block 11 Current pregnancy status (diagnosis of an SGA infant, diagnosis of an LGA infant, presence of a fetal anomaly, fetal malpresentation)

Block 12 Pregnancy complication (bleeding <20 weeks)

Block 13 Pregnancy complication (placenta previa)

Block 14 Interaction: Age by placenta previa

Block 15 Pregnancy complication (bleeding ≥20 weeks)

Block 16 Pregnancy complication (pregnancy-induced hypertension, i.e., PIH)

Block 17 Interaction: Age by PIH

Block 18 Pregnancy complication (preeclampsia—PIH + proteinuria ≥+1)

Block 19 Interaction: Age by preeclampsia

Block 20 Pregnancy complication (eclampsia/toxemia)

Block 21 Interaction: Age by eclampsia/toxemia

Spontaneous preterm birth

FIGURE E-1   Model 1 (nulliparous women with no preexisting medical diseases or pregnancy complications): Order of entry of variables into the logistic regression model

Block 1 Demographic (maternal age)
▼
Block 2 Genetic and constitutional (maternal height and prepregnancy weight)
▼
Block 3 Lifestyle factors (smoking status, alcohol consumption during pregnancy, drug dependency)
▼
Block 4 Interaction: Age by smoking
▼
Block 5 Interaction: Smoking by alcohol consumption during pregnancy
▼
Block 6 Interaction: Smoking by drug dependency
▼
Block 7 Interaction: Smoking by drug dependency by alcohol consumption during pregnancy
▼
Block 8 Preexisting medical diseases (diabetes, hypertension, chronic renal disease, heart disease, other medical disorders)
▼
Block 9 Nutritional problems during pregnancy (poor gestational weight gain, anemia)
▼
Block 10 Medical problems during current pregnancy (gestational diabetes, poly- or oligohydramnios, presence of blood antibodies, acute medical disorder)
▼
Block 11 Interaction: Age by gestational diabetes
▼
Block 12 Current pregnancy status (diagnosis of an SGA infant, diagnosis of an LGA infant, presence of a fetal anomaly, fetal malpresentation)
▼
Block 13 Pregnancy complication (bleeding <20 weeks)
▼
Block 14 Pregnancy complication (placenta previa)
▼
Block 15 Interaction: Age by placenta previa
▼
Block 16 Pregnancy complication (bleeding ≥20 weeks)
▼
Block 17 Pregnancy complication (pregnancy-induced hypertension, i.e., PIH)
▼
Block 18 Interaction: Age by PIH
▼
Block 19 Pregnancy complication (preeclampsia—PIH + proteinuria ≥+1)
▼
Block 20 Interaction: Age by preeclampsia
▼
Block 21 Pregnancy complication (eclampsia/toxemia)
▼
Block 22 Interaction: Age by eclampsia/toxemia
▼
Spontaneous preterm birth

FIGURE E-2   Model 2 (nulliparous women with no preexisting medical problems): Order of entry of variables into the logistic regression model and proximal relationship of each risk factor to the dependent variable. For example, maternal age is considered the most distal risk factor in the proposed models because it was assumed that subsequent risk factors were a function of maternal age (e.g., problems in the index pregnancy, the development of one or more pregnancy complications). These figures do not distinguish between indirect and direct effects of the risk factors on spontaneous preterm labor.

Pregnancy complications are assumed to be intermediate (intervening) pregnancy outcomes and hence will be entered last into the regression analysis. If pregnancy complications are entered earlier into the risk models it could lead to an underestimation or elimination of the effect of maternal age on spontaneous preterm birth whose impact may be mediated through pregnancy complications (Kramer, 1987; Lang, et al., 1996). Each pregnancy complication will be entered separately to assess both the direct and indirect effect of each complication on spontaneous preterm labor.

Interaction terms will also be included in the risk models. The selection of the interaction terms was based on the results of previous studies. For example, the literature suggests that the incidence of gestational diabetes and pregnancy complications increases as maternal age increases (Jacobsson, Ladfors, & Milsom, 2004; Jolly, et al., 2000; Joseph, et al., 2005; Salihu, et al., 2003). Furthermore, it has been demonstrated that the effect of smoking on preterm birth is greater as maternal age advances (Cnattinguis, Forman, Berendes, Graubard, & Isotalo, 1993; Wen, Goldenberg, Cutter, Hoffman, Cliver, et al., 1990) and that a person who smokes is more likely to use illicit drugs and alcohol (Visscher, Feder, Burns, Brady, & Bray, 2003). These interactions will be entered into the risk model following the entry of the individual variables (see Figures E-1 and E-2).

Ethical Considerations

The proposal was submitted to the University of Alberta Health Research Ethics Board (Panel B) for expedited review and approval. The Alberta Perinatal Health Program (APHP), as part of its audit program, has already collected the data for the proposed study. A data request was submitted to the APHP for data access and the use of the APHP database for this study. Approval by the Alberta Health Research Ethics Board and the APHP for this proposed study was received.

The data file provided for this study does not contain any personal identifiers, only anonymous subject ID numbers, to maintain subject confidentiality. Data will be stored on an external hard drive and will be securely locked up when not in use. Only members of the thesis supervisory committee will have access to the data to assist with data management and analysis. All data will be kept in a locked filing cabinet for seven years.

References

Aldous, M. B., & Edmonson, M. B. (1993). Maternal age at first childbirth and risk of low birth weight and preterm delivery in Washington state. *Journal of the American Medical Association, 270*(21), 2574–2577.

Alexander, G. R., Baruffi, G., Mor, J., & Kieffer, E. (1992). Maternal nativity status and pregnancy outcome among U.S.-born Filipinos. *Social Biology, 39*(3–4), 278–284.

Ananth, C. V., Joseph, K. S., Oyelese, Y., Demissie, K., & Vintzileos, A. M. (2005). Trends in preterm birth and perinatal mortality among singletons: United States, 1989 through 2000. *Obstetrics and Gynecology, 105*(5), 1084–1091.

Arbuckle, T. E., & Sherman, G. J. (1989). Comparison of the risk factors for pre-term delivery and intrauterine growth retardation. *Paediatric and Perinatal Epidemiology, 3*, 115–129.

Astolfi, P., & Zonta, L. A. (1999). Risks of preterm delivery and association with maternal age, birth order, and fetal gender. *Human Reproduction, 14*(11), 2891–2894.

Barkan, S. E., & Bracken, M. B. (1987). Delayed childbearing: No evidence for increased risk of low birth weight and preterm delivery. *American Journal of Epidemiology, 125*(1), 101–109.

Berendes, H. W., & Forman, M. R. (1991). Delayed childbearing: Trends and consequences. In M. Kiely (Ed.), *Reproductive and perinatal epidemiology* (pp. 27–41). Boca Raton, FL: CRC Press.

Berkowitz, G. S. (1985). Clinical and obstetric risk factors for preterm delivery. *Mount Sinai Journal of Medicine, 52*(4), 239–247.

Berkowitz, G. S., Blackmore-Prince, C., Lapinski, R. H., & Savitz, D. A. (1998). Risk factors for preterm birth subtypes. *Epidemiology, 9*, 279–285.

Berkowitz, G. S., & Papiernik, E. (1993). Epidemiology of preterm birth. *Epidemiologic Reviews, 15*(2), 414–443.

Berkowitz, G. S., Skovron, M. L., Lapinski, R. H., & Berkowitz, R. L. (1990). Delayed childbearing and the outcome of pregnancy. *The New England Journal of Medicine, 322*, 659–664.

Beydoun, H., Itani, M., Tamin, H., Aaraj, A., Yunis, K., Alameh, M., et al. (2004). Impact of maternal age on preterm delivery and low birthweight: A hospital-based collaborative study of nulliparous Lebanese women in Greater Beirut. *Journal of Perinatology, 24*(4), 228–235.

Blickstein, I. (2003). Motherhood at or beyond the edge of reproductive age. *International Journal of Fertility & Womens Medicine, 48*(1), 17–24.

Blondel, B., Kogan, M., Alexander, G. R., Dattani, N., Kramer, M. S., & Macfarlane, A. (2002). The impact of the increasing number of multiple births on the rates of preterm birth and low birthweight: An international study. *American Journal of Public Health, 92*(8), 1323–1330.

Bowman, M., & Saunders, D. M. (1995). Are the risks of delayed parenting overstated? *Human Reproduction, 10*(5), 1035–1036.

Brown, E. R. (1993). Long-term sequelae of preterm birth. In A. R. Fuchs, F. Fuchs & P. G. Stubblefield (Eds.), *Preterm birth: Causes, prevention, and management* (2nd ed., pp. 477–492). New York: McGraw-Hill.

Brunt, J. H., & Shields, L. E. (2000). Epidemiology in community health nursing: Principles and applications for primary health care. In M. J. Stewart (Ed.), *Community nursing: Promoting Canadians' health* (2nd ed., pp. 564–583). Toronto, Ontario, Canada: W. B. Saunders.

Butterfield, P. G. (2002). Upstream reflections on environmental health: An abbreviated history and framework for action. *Advances in Nursing Science, 25*(1), 32–49.

Chen, J., & Millar, W. J. (2000). Are recent cohorts healthier than their predecessors? *Health Reports, 11*(4), 9–23.

Cleary-Goldman, J., Malone, F., Vidaver, J., Ball, R. H., Nyberg, D. A., Comstock, C. H., et al. (2005). Impact of maternal age on obstetric outcome. *Obstetrics and Gynecology, 105*(5), 983–990.

Cnattinguis, S., Forman, M. R., Berendes, H. W., Graubard, B. I., & Isotalo, L. (1993). Effect of age, parity, and smoking on pregnancy outcome: A population-based study. *American Journal of Obstetrics and Gynecology, 168*, 16–21.

Cnattinguis, S., Forman, M. R., Berendes, H. W., & Isotalo, L. (1992). Delayed childbearing and risk of adverse perinatal outcome. A population-based study. *Journal of the American Medical Association, 268*, 886–890.

Cuevas, K. D., Silver, D. R., Brooten, D., Youngblut, J. M., & Bobo, C. M. (2005). The cost of prematurity: Hospital charges at birth and frequency of rehospitalizations and acute care visits over the first year of life: A comparison by gestational age and birth weight. *American Journal of Nursing, 105*(7), 56–64.

Cunningham, F. G., & Leveno, K. J. (1995). Childbearing among older women—the message is cautiously optimistic. *The New England Journal of Medicine, 333*(15), 1002–1004.

de Sanjose, S., & Roman, E. (1991). Low birthweight, preterm, and small for gestational age babies in Scotland, 1981–1984. *Journal of Epidemiology and Community Health, 45*, 207–210.

Demissie, K., Rhoads, G. G., Ananth, C. V., Alexander, G. R., Kramer, M. S., Kogan, M. D., et al. (2001). Trends in preterm birth and neonatal mortality among blacks and whites in the United States from 1989 to 1997. *American Journal of Epidemiology, 154*(4), 307–315.

Edge, V., & Laros, R. K. (1993). Pregnancy outcome in nulliparous women aged 35 or older. *American Journal of Obstetrics and Gynecology, 168,* 1881–1884.

Ekblad, U., & Vilpa, T. (1994). Pregnancy in women over forty. *Annales Chirurgiae et Gynaecologiae, 83,* 68–71.

Ekwo, E., & Moawad, A. (2000). Maternal age and preterm births in a black population. *Paediatric and Perinatal Epidemiology, 14,* 145–151.

Federal, Provincial and Territorial Advisory Committee on Population Health. (1994). *Strategies for population health: Investing in the health of Canadians.* Ottawa, Ontario, Canada: Minister of Supply and Services Canada.

Ford, D., & Nault, F. (1996). Changing fertility patterns, 1974 to 1994. *Health Report, 8,* 39–46.

Freeman-Wang, T., & Beski, S. (2002). The older obstetric patient. *Current Obstetrics and Gynaecology, 12,* 41–46.

Frisbie, W. P., Biegler, M., de Turk, P., Forbes, D., & Pullum, S. G. (1997). Racial and ethnic differences in determinants of intrauterine growth retardation and other compromised birth outcomes. *American Journal of Public Health, 87*(12), 1977–1983.

Gilbert, W. M., Nesbitt, T. S., & Danielsen, B. (1999). Childbearing beyond age 40: Pregnancy outcome in 24,032 cases. *Obstetrics and Gynecology, 93,* 9–14.

Glass, H., & Hicks, S. (2000). Healthy public policy in health system reform. In M. J. Stewart (Ed.), *Community nursing: Promoting Canadians' health* (2nd ed., pp. 157–169). Toronto, Ontario, Canada: W. B. Saunders Canada.

Goffinet, F. (2005). Primary predictors of preterm labour. *BJOG: An International Journal of Obstetrics and Gynaecology, 112*(Suppl. 1), 38–47.

Gordis, L. (2000). *Epidemiology* (2nd ed.). Philadelphia: W. B. Saunders.

Gosden, R., & Rutherford, A. (1995). Delayed childbearing. *BMJ, 311,* 1585–1586.

Hamilton, B. E., Martin, J. A., & Sutton, P. D. (2004). Births: Preliminary data for 2003. *National Vital Statistics Reports, 53*(9), 1–18.

Hansen, J. P. (1986). Older maternal age and pregnancy outcome: A review of the literature. *Obstetrical and Gynecological Surveys, 41*(11), 726–742.

Harlow, B. L., Frigoletto, F. D., Cramer, D. W., Evans, J. K., LeFevre, M. L., Bain, R. P., et al. (1996). Determinants of preterm delivery in low-risk pregnancies. *Journal of Clinical Epidemiology, 49*(4), 441–448.

Health Canada. (1996). *Towards a common understanding: Clarifying the core concepts of population health and health promotion.* Ottawa, Ontario, Canada: Author.

Health Canada. (2003). *Canadian perinatal health report 2003.* Ottawa, Ontario, Canada: Minister of Public Works and Government Services.

Heaman, M. I., Blanchard, J. F., Gupton, A. L., Moffat, M. E. K., & Currie, R. F. (2005). Risk factors for spontaneous preterm birth among Aboriginal and non-Aboriginal women in Manitoba. *Paediatric and Perinatal Epidemiology, 19*, 181–193.

Heck, K. E., Schoendorf, K. C., Ventura, S. J., & Kiely, J. L. (1997). Delayed childbearing by education level in the United States, 1969–1994. *Maternal and Child Health Journal, 1*(2), 81–88.

Jacobsson, B., Ladfors, L., & Milsom, I. (2004). Advanced maternal age and adverse perinatal outcome. *Obstetrics and Gynecology, 104*(4), 727–733.

Jolly, M., Sebire, N., Harris, J., Robinson, S., & Regan, L. (2000). The risks associated with pregnancy in women aged 35 years or older. *Human Reproduction, 15*(11), 2433–2437.

Joseph, K. S., Allen, A. C., Dodds, L., Turner, L. A., Scott, H., & Liston, R. (2005). The perinatal effects of delayed childbearing. *Obstetrics and Gynecology, 105*(6), 1410–1418.

Joseph, K. S., Demissie, K., & Kramer, M. S. (2002). Obstetric intervention, stillbirth, and preterm birth. *Seminars in Perinatology, 26*(4), 250–259.

Joseph, K. S., & Kramer, M. S. (1996). Recent trends in Canadian infant mortality rates: Effect of changes in registration of live newborns weighing less than 500g. *Canadian Medical Association Journal, 155*(8), 1047–1052.

Joseph, K. S., Kramer, M. S., Marcoux, S., Ohlsson, A., Wen, S. W., Allen, A., et al. (1998). Determinants of preterm birth rates in Canada from 1981 through 1983 and from 1992 through 1994. *The New England Journal of Medicine, 339*(20), 1434–1439.

Kessler, I., Lancet, M., Borenstein, R., & Steinmetz, A. (1980). The problem of the older primipara. *Obstetrics and Gynecology, 56*, 165–169.

Kirz, D. S., Dorchester, W., & Freeman, R. K. (1985). Advanced maternal age: The mature gravida. *American Journal of Obstetrics and Gynecology, 152*, 7–12.

Klebanoff, M. A. (1998). Conceptualizing categories of preterm birth. *Prenatal and Neonatal Medicine, 3*, 13–15.

Klebanoff, M. A., & Shiono, P. H. (1995). Top down, bottom up and inside out: Reflections on preterm birth. *Paediatric and Perinatal Epidemiology, 9*(2), 125–129.

Knoches, A. M. L., & Doyle, L. W. (1993). Long-term outcome of infants born preterm. *Bailliere's Clinical Obstetrics and Gynaecology, 7*(3), 633–651.

Kolas, T., Nakling, J., & Salvesen, K. A. (2000). Smoking during pregnancy increases the risk of preterm births among parous women. *Acta Obstetricia et Gynecologica Scandinavica, 79*(8), 644–648.

Kramer, M. S. (1987). Determinants of low birth weight: Methodological assessment and meta-analysis. *Bulletin of the World Health Organization, 65*(5), 663–737.

Kramer, M. S., McLean, F. H., Eason, E. L., & Usher, R. H. (1992). Maternal nutrition and spontaneous preterm birth. *American Journal of Epidemiology, 136*, 574–583.

Kramer, M. S., Platt, R., Yang, H., Joseph, K. S., Wen, S. W., Morin, L., et al. (1998). Secular trends in preterm birth: A hospital-based cohort study. *Journal of the American Medical Association, 280*(21), 1849–1854.

Kristensen, J., Langhoff-Roos, J., & Kristensen, F. B. (1995). Idiopathic preterm deliveries in Denmark. *Obstetrics and Gynecology, 85*, 549–552.

Lang, J. M., Lieberman, E., & Cohen, A. (1996). A comparison of risk factors for preterm labor and term small-for-gestational-age birth. *Epidemiology, 7*, 369–376.

Lansac, J. (1995). Delayed parenting: Is delayed childbearing a good thing? *Human Reproduction, 10*(5), 1033–1035.

Lewit, E. M., Baker, L. S., Corman, H., & Shiono, P. H. (1995). The direct cost of low birth weight. *The Future of Children, 5*(1), 35–42.

Luke, B., & Martin, J. A. (2004). The rise in multiple births in the United States: Who, what, when, where, and why. *Clinical Obstetrics & Gynecology, 47*(1), 118–133.

Mackenbach, J. P. (1995). Public health epidemiology. *Journal of Epidemiology and Community Health, 49*, 333–334.

Malloy, M. H. (1999). Risk of previous very low birth weight and very preterm infants among women delivering a very low birth weight and very preterm infant. *Journal of Perinatology, 19*(2), 97–102.

Mansfield, P. K., & McCool, W. (1989). Toward a better understanding of the "advanced maternal age" factor. *Health Care for Women International, 10*, 395–415.

Martin, J. A., Hamilton, B. E., Sutton, P. D., Ventura, S. J., Menacker, F., & Munson, M. L. (2003). Births: Final data for 2002. *National Vital Statistics Reports, 52*(10), 1–114.

McCormick, M. C. (1985). The contribution of low birth weight to infant mortality and childhood morbidity. *The New England Journal of Medicine, 312*, 82–90.

Meis, P. J., Michielutte, R., Peters, T. J., Wells, H. B., Sands, E., Coles, E. C., et al. (1995). Factors associated with preterm birth in Cardiff, Wales II: Indicated and spontaneous preterm birth. *American Journal of Obstetrics and Gynecology, 173*, 597–602.

Mercer, B. M., Goldenberg, R. L., Das, A., Moawad, A. H., Iams, J. D., Meis, P. J., et al. (1996). The preterm prediction study: A clinical risk assessment system. *American Journal of Obstetrics and Gynecology, 174*(6), 1885–1893.

Miletic, T., Aberle, N., Mikulandra, F., Karelovic, D., Zakanj, Z., Banovic, I., et al. (2002). Perinatal outcome of pregnancies in women aged 40 and over. *Collegium Antropologicum, 26*(1), 251–258.

Misra, D. P., O'Campo, P., & Strobino, D. (2001). Testing a sociomedical model for preterm delivery. *Paediatric and Perinatal Epidemiology, 15*, 110–122.

Mohsin, M., Wong, F., Bauman, A., & Bai, J. (2003). Maternal and neonatal factors influencing premature birth and low birth weight in Australia. *Journal of Biosocial Science, 35*(2), 161–174.

Mor, J. M., Alexander, G. R., Kogan, M. D., Kieffer, E. C., & Ichiho, H. M. (1995). Similarities and disparities in maternal risk and birth outcomes of white and Japanese-American mothers. *Paediatric and Perinatal Epidemiology, 9*, 59–73.

Moutquin, J. M. (2003). Classification and heterogeneity of preterm birth. *BJOG: An International Journal of Obstetrics & Gynaecology, 110*(Suppl. 20), 30–33.

Moutquin, J. M., & Lalonde, A. (1998). *The cost of prematurity in Canada.* Ottawa, Ontario, Canada: Society of Obstetrics and Gynaecology of Canada.

Moutquin, J. M., & Papiernik, E. (1990). Can we lower the rate of preterm birth? *Bulletin of the SOGC,* 19–20.

Mvula, M. M., & Miller, J. M. (1998). A comparative evaluation of collaborative prenatal care. *Obstetrics and Gynecology, 91*, 169–173.

Myslobodsky, M. (2001). Preterm delivery: On proxies and proximal factors. *Paediatric and Perinatal Epidemiology, 15*, 381–383.

Newburn-Cook, C. V., & Onyskiw, J. E. (2005). Is older maternal age a risk factor for preterm birth and fetal growth restriction? A systematic review. *Health Care for Women International, 26*(9), 852–875.

Newburn-Cook, C. V., White, D., Svenson, L. W., Demianczuk, N. N., Bott, N., & Edwards, J. (2002). Where and to what extent is prevention of low birth weight possible? *Western Journal of Nursing Research, 24*(8), 887–904.

Nordentoft, M., Lou, H. C., Hansen, D., Nim, J., Pryds, O., Rubin, P., et al. (1996). Intrauterine growth retardation and premature delivery: The influence of maternal smoking and psychosocial factors. *American Journal of Public Health, 86*, 347–354.

Pal, L., & Santoro, N. (2003). Age-related decline in fertility. *Endocrinology and Metabolism Clinics of North America, 32*(3), 669–688.

Paneth, N. S. (1995). The problem of low birth weight. *The Future of Children, 5*(1), 19–34.

Petrou, S., Mehta, Z., Hockley, C., Cook-Mozaffari, P., Henderson, J., & Goldacre, M. (2003). The impact of preterm birth on hospital inpatient admissions and costs during the first 5 years of life. *Pediatrics, 112*(6 Pt. 1), 1290–1297.

Petrou, S., Sach, T., & Davidson, L. (2001). The long-term costs of preterm birth and low birth weight: Results of a systematic review. *Child: Care, Health and Development, 27*(2), 97–115.

Pickett, K. E., Abrams, B., & Selvin, S. (2000). Defining preterm delivery—the epidemiology of clinical presentation. *Paediatric and Perinatal Epidemiology, 14*, 305–308.

Prysak, M., Lorenz, R. P., & Kisly, A. (1995). Pregnancy outcome in nulliparous women 35 years and older. *Obstetrics and Gynecology, 85*, 65–70.

Reproductive Health Report Working Group. (2004). *Alberta reproductive health: Pregnancies and births 2004*. Edmonton, Alberta, Canada: Alberta Health and Wellness.

Robinson, J. N., Regan, J. A., & Norwitz, E. R. (2001). The epidemiology of preterm labor. *Seminars in Perinatology, 25*(4), 204–214.

Salihu, H. M., Shumpert, M. N., Slay, M., Kirby, R. S., & Alexander, G. R. (2003). Childbearing beyond maternal age 50 and fetal outcomes in the United States. *Obstetrics & Gynecology, 102*(5 Pt. 1), 1006–1014.

Savitz, D. A., Blackmore, C. A., & Thorp, J. M. (1991). Epidemiologic characteristics of preterm delivery: Etiologic heterogeneity. *American Journal of Obstetrics and Gynecology, 164*(2), 467–471.

Savitz, D. A., Dole, N., Herring, A. H., Kaczor, D., Murphy, J., Siega-Riz, A. M., et al. (2005). Should spontaneous and medically indicated preterm births be separated for studying aetiology? *Paediatric and Perinatal Epidemiology, 19*, 97–105.

Scholz, H. S., Hass, J., & Petru, E. (1999). Do primiparas aged 40 years or older carry an increased obstetric risk? *Preventive Medicine, 29*, 263–266.

Shiono, P. H., & Klebanoff, M. A. (1986). Ethnic differences in preterm and very preterm delivery. *American Journal of Public Health, 76*, 1317–1321.

Shults, R. A., Arndt, V., Olshan, A. F., Martin, C. F., & Royce, R. A. (1999). Effects of short interpregnancy intervals on small-for-gestational age and preterm births. *Epidemiology, 10*, 250–254.

Spellacy, W. N., Miller, S. J., & Winegar, A. (1986). Pregnancy after 40 years of age. *Obstetrics and Gynecology, 68*, 452–454.

St. John, E. B., Nelson, K. G., Cliver, S. P., Bishnoi, R. R., & Goldenberg, R. L. (2000). Cost of neonatal care according to gestational age at birth and survival status. *American Journal of Obstetrics & Gynecology, 182*(1 Pt. 1), 170–175.

Statistics Canada. (2003). *Marriages, 2000—shelf tables.* Ottawa, Ontario, Canada: Author.

Statistics Canada. (2004a). *Table 282-0004—labour force survey estimates (LFS), by educational attainment, sex and age group, annual (percent change year-year).* Ottawa, Ontario, Canada: Author.

Statistics Canada. (2004b). *Table Number 1024508—live births, by age and parity of mother, Canada.* Ottawa, Ontario, Canada: Author.

Statistics Canada. (2005). *Births 2002 data tables* (Catalogue number 84F0210XIE). Ottawa, Ontario, Canada: Author.

Stoelhorst, G. M., Rijken, M., Martens, S. E., van Zwieten, P. H., Feenstra, J., Zwinderman, A. H., et al. (2003). Developmental outcome at 18 and 24 months of age in very preterm children: A cohort study from 1996 to 1997. *Early Human Development, 72*(2), 83–95.

Tommiska, V., Tuominen, R., & Fellman, V. (2003). Economic costs of care in extremely low birthweight infants during the first 2 years of life. *Pediatric Critical Care Medicine, 4*(2), 157–163.

Tough, S. C., Newburn-Cook, C. V., Johnston, D. W., Svenson, L. W., Rose, S., & Belik, J. (2002). Delayed childbearing and its impact on population rate changes in lower birth weight, multiple birth, and preterm delivery. *Pediatrics, 109*(3), 399–403.

Tough, S. C., Svenson, L. W., Johnston, D. W., & Schopflocher, D. (2001). Characteristics of preterm delivery and low birthweight among 113,994 infants in Alberta: 1994–1996. *Canadian Journal of Public Health, 92*(4), 276–280.

Valanis, B. (1999). *Epidemiology in health care.* Stamford, CT: Appleton & Lange.

Ventura, S. J., Martin, J. A., Curtin, S. C., & Mathews, T. J. (1999). Births: Final data for 1997. *National Vital Statistics Reports, 47*(18), 1–94.

Verkerk, P. H., Zaadstra, B. M., Reerink, J. D., Herngreen, W. P., & Verloove-Vanhorick, S. P. (1994). Social class, ethnicity and other risk factors for small for gestational age and preterm delivery in the Netherlands. *European Journal of Obstetrics & Gynecology, 53*, 129–134.

Virji, S. K., & Cottington, E. (1991). Risk factors associated with preterm deliveries among racial groups in a national sample of married mothers. *American Journal of Perinatology, 8*(5), 347–353.

Visscher, W. A., Feder, M., Burns, A. M., Brady, T. M., & Bray, R. M. (2003). The impact of smoking and other substance use by urban women on the birthweight of their infants. *Substance Use & Misuse, 38*(8), 1063–1093.

Wen, S. W., Goldenberg, R. L., Cutter, G. R., Hoffman, H. J., & Cliver, S. P. (1990). Intrauterine growth retardation and preterm delivery: Prenatal risk factors in an indigent population. *American Journal of Obstetrics and Gynecology, 162*, 213–218.

Wen, S. W., Goldenberg, R. L., Cutter, G. R., Hoffman, H. J., Cliver, S. P., Davis, R. O., et al. (1990). Smoking, maternal age, fetal growth, and gestational age at delivery. *American Journal of Obstetrics and Gynecology, 162*, 53–58.

White, D. E. (2004). *Direct and indirect determinants of low birth weight in a large Canadian urban health region.* Unpublished doctoral dissertation, University of Alberta, Edmonton, Canada.

World Health Organization. (2002). *The world health report 2002: Reducing risks, promoting healthy life.* Geneva, Switzerland: Author.

Ziadeh, S., & Yahaya, A. (2001). Pregnancy outcome at age 40 and older. *Archives of Gynecology & Obstetrics, 265*(1), 30–33.

Maintaining Catheter Patency Using Recombinant Tissue Plasminogen Activator

Colleen M. Astle

Introduction

Chronic renal failure is an insidious, progressive deterioration of renal function. The most common causes include diabetes mellitus, hypertension, glomerulonephritis, polycystic kidney disease, interstitial nephritis, obstructive disorders, vascular disease, and AIDS-related disorders (Central Organ Replacement Register, 1998; Lancaster, 1991). Chronic renal failure is described as insidious because it is usually not diagnosed until there is an approximately 75% loss of function and the patient's vaguely described symptoms become more pronounced. Even in the face of deteriorating numbers, the glomeruli adapt with hyperfiltration to maintain a normal homeostatic environment (Andreoli, Bennett, Carpenter, & Plum, 1997). When function has decreased to between 5 and 10%, the diagnosis of end-stage renal disease is made.

As of 1998, more than 210,000 people in the United States with end-stage renal failure were receiving treatment, the annual growth trend of the disease being 7.8%. In Canada, as of December 31, 1998, the number of patients alive on renal replacement therapy was 21,992, including 9,114 with a functioning transplant and 12,808 patients in various treatment modalities. The majority of patients were on hemodialysis (73%), and the balance was on peritoneal dialysis (27%). In 1998, there were 4025 new patients receiving treatment, representing a rate of 132.5 patients per million population. From 1981 to 1998 the annual growth rate of the disease was 6% (Central Organ Replacement Register, 1998). With the increase in life expectancy in the aging population, the United States reported a 150% increase in renal failure in people older than 60 years of age between 1984 and 1993. Thirty-six percent of those people were diabetics (Kinzner, 1998). These numbers reflect a growing trend in chronicity that will burden the healthcare system in both Canada and the United States in coming years.

The patients with end-stage renal failure require ongoing medical intervention to sustain life. The treatment options available include peritoneal dialysis, hemodialysis, or transplantation. Peritoneal dialysis involves the peritoneum as the dialyzing membrane. A sterile, physiologically prepared solution is introduced into the peritoneal cavity, and by the principles of osmosis and diffusion, fluid is removed and the blood is cleansed of its toxic impurities. The patient is required to do four or five exchanges each day. In contrast to peritoneal dialysis, hemodialysis involves passing the patient's blood through an artificial kidney where diffusion and ultrafiltration remove fluid and the waste products of metabolism, normally excreted by the kidneys. This procedure averages four hours three times per week. Both peritoneal dialysis and hemodialysis require the use of a patent, functional access, a means with which to dialyze the patient.

The three types of vascular access used for hemodialysis include the arteriovenous (AV) fistula, the synthetic arteriovenous graft, and the central venous catheter. Since 1966, the AV fistula has been, and continues to be, the preferred form of hemodialysis access (Berkoben & Schwab, 1995; Ezzahiri, Lemson, Kitslaar, Leunissen, & Toridor, 1999; Kapoian & Sherman, 1997; Laski, Pressley, Sabatini, & Wesson, 1997; Mysliwiec, 1997; Tisher, 1999). Primary AV fistulae are typically created by an end-to-side vein–artery anastomosis of the cephalic vein and radial artery or the brachial artery and the cephalic vein in the nondominant arm. They take two to six months to mature. When mature, they have long-term patency rates and are rarely associated with infectious complications. The fistulas can serve as a permanent hemodialysis access for 20 years. Not all people, however, are suitable for the creation of a fistula. Veins that have previously been used for infusion of medication, intravenous therapy, phlebotomy, or laboratory blood sampling are precluded from developing into a successful access. Also, because of an aging and diabetic population there is a lack of suitable blood vessels for creation of fistula access (Kapoian & Sherman, 1997; Konner, 1999; Polaschegg & Levin, 2000).

If the dialysis patient is unable to support a native fistula, an AV graft using synthetic materials such as polytetrafluoroethylene (PTFE) may be created. PTFE grafts are placed in the forearm, upper arm, or upper thigh, in either a straight (distal radial artery to basilic vein) or loop (brachial artery to basilic vein) configuration. Maturation requires three to four weeks. PTFE is a durable material and will withstand multiple thrombectomies and revisions, but it does have a finite functional life and will wear out with repeated needle puncture. The complications associated with grafts include infection, thrombosis, steal syndrome, formation of an aneurysm, and reaction to the graft material (Obialo, Robinson, & Braithwaite, 1998).

Central venous catheters are routinely used in the medical management of many types of patients (Farrell, Walshe, Gellens, & Martin, 1997). They provide access for the delivery of fluids, medications, blood products, chemotherapy, and parenteral nutrition. They are also useful for frequent blood sampling, hemodynamic monitoring, or hemodialysis. Central venous catheters are inserted into deep veins, such as the subclavian, jugular, or femoral veins, and are advanced into the vena cava (Brunier, 1996). They may be placed percutaneously or by using a cutdown technique. Maturation time is not required; rather they may be used immediately after placement. Associated complications include infection, thrombosis, permanent central vein stenosis, and lower blood flow rates than other accesses (Johnson, 1998).

Central venous catheter occlusion is a common complication, which can result in loss of function, delays in treatment, high costs, patient discomfort, and patient and nurse frustration. Additionally, intraluminal clotted blood and fibrin increase the risk of catheter-related sepsis (Wickham, Purl, & Welker, 1992). Thus far, various concentrations of heparin have been used to maintain the patency of the catheters. In the past, when clotting occurred in the presence of heparin as the instillation, streptokinase and then urokinase were used to lyse the clot. Presently, 2 mg/2 ml of recombinant tissue plasminogen activator (rTPA) is being used. After a specified period of time the catheter is checked for patency, and if successful dialysis is resumed. The advantage of using rTPA is that it is frequently successful in the lysis of intraluminal dialysis catheter clots. The disadvantage is the cost of the medication. For each 2-mg syringe of rTPA the cost is $54 for the Northern Alberta Renal Failure Program. The following questions then arise: What concentration of rTPA would be effective in the prevention of a thrombus in a hemodialysis catheter? What should the dwell time be for this concentration of solution?

Catheter-Related Thrombosis

The use of a central venous catheter for either temporary or chronic hemodialysis has become an acceptable bridge to internal, permanent vascular accesses (Brunier, 1996; Choudhry, Ahmed, Giris, & Kronfli, 1999; Farrell, et al., 1997; Ouwendyk & Helferty, 1996; Richard, 1986). It is easily inserted at the bedside by an experienced physician thereby reducing the need for expensive and often unavailable operating room time. It can provide long-term access in children, the elderly, the morbidly obese, or in diabetics whose vessels are not suitable for the creation of an internal fistula or graft. It is necessary for patients requiring emergency dialysis or patients who are described as access failures, having used up the vessels required to create a permanent access. Central venous catheters serve as a backup for the fistulas and grafts that require ligation due to high output failure states caused by their development and use. Further, these catheters are inserted as a temporary access while awaiting the development of the permanent access. The survival rates of these catheters are reported to be 75% at one year and 50% at two years, thereby allowing them to become alternative forms of long-term accesses (Parker, 1998). Berkoben and Schwab (1995) reported a survival rate of 47–74% at one year and 41–43% at two years. Despite the consensus that the construction of the primary AV fistulas represents the best choice for permanent vascular access, the trend since 1980 has been a continual increase in the use of these access devices. Kapoian and Sherman (1997) reported a 5% use of central venous catheters in 1980, which increased to 30% in 1993.

Catheter-related thrombosis is the most common cause of catheter dysfunction (Barendregt, Tordoir, & Leunissen, 1999; Buturovic, Ponikvar, Boh, Klinkmann, & Ivanovich, 1998; Johnson, 1998; Mysliwiec, 1997; Northsea, 1994; Parker, 1998; Twardowski, 1998b). It can result in an impaired ability to withdraw fluid from or infuse fluids through the catheter. The literature reports an incidence of thrombosis from 55 to 85% (Daeihagh, Jordan, Chen, & Rocco, 2000; Kohler & Kirkman, 1998). This broad range reflects the lack of a standardized method for evaluating and diagnosing this complication. Further, the term "catheter-related thrombosis" does not appear to be well defined. It may refer to the thrombotic occlusion of the lumen of the catheter, the formation of a fibrin sheath around the catheter, the formation of thrombus at the site of catheter insertion into the vessel, or a true thrombosis within the central vein (Wickham, et al., 1992).

Catheter clotting may result from either external or internal mechanical obstruction. Kinks in the external tubing or the catheter itself can reduce or totally obstruct flow through the lumen. Internal causes of catheter occlusion include internal malposition, catheter pinch-off syndrome caused by threading the subclavian catheter under the clavicle during insertion, drug precipitate, fibrin buildup, and blood clots (Kohler & Kirkman, 1998; Muhm, et al., 1997). Clot occlusion also occurs as a result of a retrograde flow of blood into the catheter tip during fluctuations in central venous pressure, such as when a patient coughs.

There are several sites at which thrombi are likely to form: the lumen of the catheter, the site at which the catheter enters the vein, the catheter tip, and the external surface of the catheter. The types of thrombotic occlusions include intraluminal thrombus, mural thrombus, fibrin sheath (also known as fibrin sleeve), and fibrin tail (also known as fibrin flap). A fibrin sheath can form along the external surface of the catheter and resembles a sock over the catheter (Kohler & Kirkman, 1998; Northsea, 1996). It may occur soon after insertion and extends from the insertion site to the catheter tip. This may develop within 48 hours after placement. Fibrin tail forms when fibrin adheres to the end of the catheter. Often it acts as a one-way valve, permitting infusion but not withdrawal of fluid from the catheter. Mural thrombus, which forms when the fibrin from a vessel wall injury binds to the fibrin covering the catheter surface, may lead to the formation of a venous thrombus (Wickham, et al., 1992).

Thrombus formation may be related to a number of factors. Insertion of the catheter may cause endothelial injury of the vessel wall, triggering the release of thromboplastic substances that cause platelets to aggregate at the site. Endothelial injury may also cause formation of small or large thrombi that attach to the vessel wall. Another factor may be the large-bore catheters commonly used for dialysis, which alter the blood flow in the vein and activate the release of the thromboplastic substances and platelets, thereby producing fibrin formation (Northsea, 1996; Wickham, et al., 1992).

The patients at greatest risk for the development of catheter-related thrombi are those who experience venous thrombus, enhanced blood coagulability, or trauma to the vessel wall. Venous stasis can occur when dehydration, hypotension, immobility, heart failure, or intrapulmonary–mediastinal diseases are present. Coagulability can be altered by conditions such as malignancy, sepsis, chronic renal failure, or the administration of chemotherapy (Schenk, Rosenkranz, Wolfl, Horl, & Traindl, 2000).

The vast majority of thrombi related to central venous catheters develop without symptoms. Warning signs are insidious. As the thrombus begins to form, the catheter appears problematic, causing monitoring alarms. The blood flow appears sluggish (Berkoben & Schwab, 1995; Daeihagh, et al., 2000; Northsea, 1994; Twardowski, 1998b). In some instances, it is possible to infuse fluid into the catheter, but the withdrawal is impaired. The diagnosis of catheter-related thrombosis may be based solely on symptoms or can be confirmed with the aid of imaging techniques. When the central venous catheter becomes occluded, the goal is to restore patency in a cost-effective manner with minimal risk to the patient. Catheter salvage is preferred over catheter replacement in an effort to limit the interruption to therapy, reduce the risk of trauma to the patient, reduce the risk of complications, and decrease the costs.

One factor that has been considered in the literature concerning catheter-related thrombosis is the type of catheter used (Berkoben & Schwab, 1995; Muhm, et al., 1997; Schenk, et al., 2000). In the study by Leblanc et al. (1998), blood flow and recirculation rates were reviewed in 33 well-functioning internal jugular vein catheters. The catheters described were able to maintain adequate blood flow rates between 200 and 275 ml/min without major increments or decrements in arterial and venous pressures. The study concluded that the blood flow rates were achieved because of the type of catheters chosen. Little information was provided about the characteristics of the sample population, including age, health, comorbid conditions, or diagnosis. The concern is whether the catheter used in this study could be used for a patient whose coagulability had been altered by conditions such as sepsis or malignancy.

Muhm and colleagues (1997) reviewed the use of large-bore, Dacron-cuffed catheters using the supraclavicular approach in 175 patients during an 18-month period. Five types of large-bore catheters were reviewed. There was no clinically significant incidence of central vein thrombosis or stenosis. Intraluminal fibrinolysis occurred in three cases. The supraclavicular approach has proven to be preferable to the subclavian approach and is now an accepted practice in many dialysis units.

The lock solutions used in the central venous catheters have been extensively reviewed in the literature (Buturovic, et al., 1998; Leblanc, et al., 1998; Twardowski, 1998a). The purpose of the lock solutions is to fill the length of the catheter and prevent thrombosis. Heparin appears to be the standard lock solution in most hemodialysis catheters (Barendregt, et al., 1999). Heparin prevents the clotting of blood by inhibiting factors involved in the conversion of prothrombin to thrombin. Buturovic et al. (1998) compared heparin with citrate or polygeline locks and found no difference regarding catheter patency and clot volume between groups.

Schnek and colleagues (2000) were responsible for a prospective, randomized crossover study comparing heparin and rTPA as an instillation in 12 dialysis patients over a four-month period. Blood flow rates, arterial pressure, and venous pressure were monitored at each dialysis session. The study revealed that rTPA is superior as a lock for the central venous catheters as measured by reduced blood flow problems and clotting.

Intradialytic urokinase has been extensively used in many dialysis units to lyse catheter thrombosis. Urokinase, a thrombolytic agent derived from human kidney cells, is a protein enzyme that acts on the endogenous fibrinolytic system, converting plasminogen to plasmin.

Plasmin degrades fibrin clots, fibrinogen, and other plasma properties. Northsea (1996) used urokinase to restore patency in 95 of 102 permanent or double lumen catheters. Twardowski (1998a) suggested that warfarin be used in conjunction with urokinase. Although urokinase proved to be effective in restoring catheter patency, fibrin tended to reoccur without the use of warfarin. Ouwendyk and Helferty (1996) suggested the use of baby aspirin or one-half of a 325-mg tablet of aspirin daily after central venous catheter insertion and the use of aspirin and warfarin together to prevent catheter clotting.

Since the early 1990s, rTPA has been used to restore catheter patency and lyse thrombus. As a genetically engineered enzyme, rTPA is involved in the breakdown of blood clots. It has been used successfully in the treatment of myocardial infarction, dissolving the clot and restoring the blood supply to the heart muscle. Davis, Vermeulen, Banton, Schwartz, and Williams (2000) used rTPA starting at 0.5 mg and escalating the dose to 1 and 2 mg sequentially until 50 central venous catheters were cleared and patency was restored. In 3.4% of the catheters, rTPA was unable to clear the occlusion. In a study by Daeihagh and colleagues (2000), rTPA was used to restore the patency in 49 of 56 catheters. Two milligrams was infused into each port of the catheters. The dwell time ranged between two and 96 hours. The literature supports the use of rTPA for the lysis of intraluminal thrombus, but further research needs to be done with the use of rTPA in 0.5 mg concentrations. The standard concentration used in most studies is 2 mg/2 ml. A decreased concentration of rTPA results in the added benefit of reduced costs.

Purpose of the Study

The purpose of the proposed study is to test the following hypothesis: 0.5 mg of recombinant tissue plasminogen activator (rTPA) is as effective as 2.0 mg of rTPA in the prevention of thrombosis in central venous catheters in two samples of 15 long-term, maintenance, hemodialysis patients over a two-month period. At the end of two months each group will cross over to the alternate group for study. A prospective, randomized, double-blind crossover study will therefore be performed.

Definition of Terms

Central venous catheter thrombosis is the presence of a thrombus located within the lumen of the central venous catheter that is responsible for a reduction in blood flow and fluids during aspiration and instillation of the catheter. This is evidenced by blood flow less than 200 ml/min, arterial pressure less than 2250 mmHg, and venous pressure greater than 1250 mmHg.

Recombinant tissue plasminogen activator (rTPA) is a recombinant drug used as a lock solution in concentrations of 0.5 mg and 2.0 mg in the central venous catheters of two groups of 15 hemodialysis patients during a two-month period. The selection of 0.5 mg for comparison was made because the literature suggests that this is the least amount of the drug evaluated during previous studies (Davis, et al., 2000). Two milligrams of rTPA is a standard concentration presently used in dialysis units.

Methodology

Research Design

A prospective Level III experimental design is the framework upon which this proposed study will be built. Two groups will be compared and three variables of interest will be studied. Three physiological measures and specific laboratory values concerned with clotting will be monitored during the study. The two randomized, double-blinded groups will be used to compare 0.5 mg and 2.0 mg of rTPA as a lock solution in the central venous catheters of hemodialysis patients. The formation of thrombus, as determined by catheter function, is the dependent variable, and the use of rTPA and its effect on clotting constitute the independent variable. Each sample group will consist of 15 randomly selected patients with end-stage renal failure. The physiological measures that determine catheter performance, indicating clotting, are arterial pressure, venous pressure, and blood flow because, as the thrombus forms, the catheter appears problematic and causes monitoring alarms (Berkoben & Schwab, 1995; Daeihagh, et al., 2000; Northsea, 1996; Twardowski, 1998b). The laboratory tests used to determine anticoagulation, such as hematocrit, platelet count, prothrombin time, activated partial thromboplastin time, and fibrinogen, will also be examined. Interval data will be collected from the previously mentioned tests and measures for use in the data analysis.

Sample and Setting

The representative sample to be chosen for the study will include persons with end-stage renal disease who are treated with hemodialysis and are followed by the Northern Alberta Renal Failure Program in northern Alberta, Canada. The actual field setting will be the in-center hemodialysis unit located in a large urban hospital. The patients, including both men and women, will be from various backgrounds, ethnic groups, and ages and will have various diseases. An attempt to control for extraneous variables will be possible through randomization of this convenience sample. All patients will have progressed to end-stage renal failure, thereby necessitating treatment for survival. All members of the sample will have a central venous catheter (CVC) as their dialyzing access. The catheters will be inserted using the same method of insertion by one of four experienced nephrologists. The catheters will be soft, Dacron-cuffed, dual-lumen catheters used for long-term maintenance hemodialysis. The sample patients will be approached about consent for the study within three weeks of starting treatment when it is recognized that the patients are receiving optimum treatment with maximum blood flow rates. Table F-1 includes the demographic and relevant information required for initiation in the study.

TABLE F-1
Patient Demographics and Relevant Central Venous Catheter Information:
Group A/Group B

Patient No.	Sex/Age	Causes of Renal Failure	Duration of Dialysis (days)	Dialysis Membrane	Dialysis Regimen	Duration of CVC (days)	CVC Site
1							
2							
3							
4							
5							
6							
7							
8							
9							
10							
11							
12							
13							
14							
15							

The convenience sample population will be randomized by the hospital's pharmacist using a statistical program responsible for generating a set of random numbers to determine the two groups within the study (Exhibit F-1). The patients to be excluded from the study are those who are not of legal age for consent, those with a current infective process, those with bleeding disorders that may affect patient welfare, and those with cancer in whom coagulability is altered by the nature of the disease (Schenk, et al., 2000). Children will not be included in the study because they are not representative of a hemodialysis population that is usually composed of adults. Rather, children are often redirected to the less invasive treatment and more tolerable modality of peritoneal dialysis.

The sample size will be calculated using a confidence interval of 95%, a power of 0.8, and calculated variability of 18 and difference between the means of the groups (10). The calculated variability is the standard deviation of the means of two hemodialysis samples comparing blood pump speed known as the effect size. A two-tailed test will be used because the two representative samples are hypothesized to be equal. The following formula was used in the calculations for size of the groups:

$$\frac{(Z\alpha + z\beta)}{d} = \frac{(1.96 + 0.8)}{10} \times 18 = 25$$

Za = confidence interval
zb = power
d = effect

The sample size will be 25 with an additional five for dropout (Senn, 1993). The total sample will consist of 30 hemodialysis patients, with 15 per group.

Methods

Approximately three weeks from the time of insertion of the central venous catheters, when maximum blood pump speeds are achieved, individual patients will be approached and asked to participate in the proposed study. An informed and witnessed consent will be obtained. The researcher conducting the study will fill out a demographic information sheet. Prior to the initiation of each dialysis treatment thereafter, as per unit protocol, the locking solution will be aspirated from the central venous catheter. Dialysis will commence and the patient will be monitored at least hourly for vital signs, blood flow rates, and arterial and venous pressures. This data will aid in the determination of catheter function. Blood flow rates below 200 ml/min, arterial pressures less than 2250 mmHg, and venous pressures of greater than 1250 mmHg reflect the presence of a thrombus. The blood flow rate or pump speed is a measure of how fast the pump is able to rotate based on catheter performance. Arterial pressure reflects the ease of removing the blood from the patient through the access for dialysis. The blood that is being withdrawn from the patient creates a negative or minus reading. Venous pressure is a measure of the ease of returning the patient's blood after it has gone through the artificial kidney. This pressure is interpreted as a plus value because it reflects a positive force. Systemic heparin will be administered according to individual patient clotting times to prevent clotting of the extracorporeal system and to allow patients to be monitored for bleeding. Measuring hematocrit, platelet count, prothrombin time (PT), activated thromboplastin time (APTT), and fibrinogen each month will enable patients to be monitored for anticoagulation. The same dialysis machines and bloodlines will be used for each treatment. At the completion of dialysis, the patient's blood will be returned to the patient and the catheter will be flushed with 10 ml of normal saline to remove residual red blood cells. The hospital's pharmacy department will prepare rTPA, which will be instilled into the lumen of the central venous catheter. The rTPA will dwell in the catheter until the patient returns for his or her thrice-weekly treatment. Refer to Exhibit F-2 for the unit protocol concerning catheter instillation.

Data collection will include recording interval values for blood flow rates, arterial pressure, venous pressure per patient to monitor catheter performance and thrombosis, and anticoagulation to monitor for potential clotting. The incidence of complications such as bleeding, sepsis, and clotting will be recorded and rated according to the frequency of the event. The study is divided into two stages for each of the two groups. Each stage will include the data collected for one month. At the end of two months the groups will cross over into the alternate group. Though the literature indicates that thrombus may form from catheter insertion by disruption of the integrity of vessel walls or from the material in the catheters, the incidence of thrombosis may occur at any time within the first month after insertion. A span of two to four months is optimal to determine the effects of rTPA on clotting as determined by the literature (Daeihagh, et al., 2000; Schenk, et al., 2000).

Data Analysis

The statistical analysis will use repeated-measures ANOVA to analyze and compare the data. This specific statistical test is used to compare the means of two groups using three or more variables when repeated measures are taken on each subject (Norman & Streiner, 1999). The three variables of interest are treatment, sequence of time, and period of time. The treatment variable will compare the means of the two concentrations of rTPA. The sequence of time variable will compare the measurements recorded in four separate one-month intervals. The period of time effect will include data on the specific patients within their randomized groups in one period of time, such as the first month versus the second month (Table F-2). The repeated-measures ANOVA will also be used to compare treatment, period, and sequence for hematocrit, platelet count, PT, APTT, and fibrinogen. Refer to Table F-3 for comparison of the two concentrations of rTPA. The statistical analysis of ANOVA comparing the three variables is shown in Table F-4.

Reliability and Validity

Control has been described as the key concept in experimental designs. Randomization is one method for controlling all possible extraneous variables in a Level III design (Brink & Wood, 1998). In this proposed study, the sample described will be a convenience sample selected because the patients are in end-stage renal failure, have central venous catheters, and are receiving long-term, maintenance hemodialysis. The patients will be of different ages, races, and genders, and they will have different diseases. They may not be representative of all hemodialysis patients because of the method of selection. The results, therefore, cannot be generalized to all

TABLE F-2
p Value from the Analysis of Variance of Central Venous Catheter Flow and Pressure Performance

	Treatment	Time Period	Sequence
Blood flow (ml/min)			
Venous pressure (mmHg)			
Arterial pressure (mmHg)			

TABLE F-3
Anticoagulation for Dialysis, Mean Values for Hematocrit (Hct), Platelet Count (Plt C), PT, APTT, and Fibrinogen Comparing Two Concentrations of TPA: Groups A/B (1-30 patients)

Pt no.	Hct (%) Heparin	Hct (%) rTPA 0.5	Plt C rTPA 2.0	Plt C rTPA 0.5	PT rTPA 2.0	PT rTPA 0.5	APTT rTPA 2.0	APTT rTPA 0.5	Fibrinogen rTPA 2.0	rTPA 2.0	TPA 0.5
1											
2											
3											
4											
5											
6											
7											
8											
9											
10											
11											
12											
13											
14											
15											

TABLE F-4
p Value from the Analysis of Variance of Hematocrit and Coagulation Parameters

	Treatment	Period	Sequence
Hematocrit (%)			
Platelet count			
PT			
APTT			
Fibrinogen (mg/dl)			

hemodialysis patients. After these patients are selected they will be randomized as described previously. Randomization, a control for internal validity, helps to eliminate bias by spreading variability equally across the groups.

Similar to the control achieved by randomization, incorporating a double-blind, crossover method into the study will enhance control. The use of the double-blind method eliminates bias. Neither the patient nor the researcher will be able to positively identify which patient will receive either concentration of the drug. The use of the crossover method will allow the patient to serve as his or her own control, thereby accounting for variability among the subjects and increasing equivalence between groups.

The parametric test of ANOVA will also increase control for the experimental design. This proposed study will use the repeated-measures ANOVA, which will adjust for differences between two groups and for correlation between the means (Brink & Wood, 1998). Further, because the study will be a double-blind crossover experiment, the patients will serve as their own controls for the comparison between the two concentrations of drugs to be used.

Control of experimental conditions will be enhanced by keeping procedures and equipment constant. Though four different nephrologists will perform the procedure for line insertion, the technique and actual procedure used will be the same. The type of catheter used for long-term maintenance hemodialysis will be the same: a Dacron, dual-lumen catheter. The nursing staff in the dialysis unit will be responsible for consistently performing the instillation procedure for locking the catheters. This procedure was developed and taught to all nursing staff by one clinical nurse educator, approved by the policy and procedure committee within the hemodialysis program, and is reviewed on a yearly basis. The machines and bloodlines used for the dialysis procedure will be the same. This equipment will be calibrated for accuracy as per the manufacturer's specifications and verified by an external pressure meter and by a qualified biomedical technician. The degree of error as specified by the manufacturer of the dialysis machine will allow a 10% variation in the blood pump speed and a 3% variation in the pressure readings. This will permit the measures for blood flow rates, arterial pressure, and venous pressure to be reliably tested and retested. Validity concerning anticoagulation will be addressed through specific laboratory tests that are well utilized in the health sciences field for the determination of clotting. The quality improvement program utilized within the clinical laboratory setting regularly verifies the accuracy of results. The specificity, sensitivity, and positive predictive value of the coulter hematology analyzer responsible for generating the results of the hematologic tests are reported to be 97%, 89%, and 93.5%, respectively (level III technician, University of Alberta Hospitals, personal communication, November 24, 2000). The data to be observed and recorded, measuring the function of the catheters, will be documented by one interrater observer with hemodialysis experience, enhancing the reliability of data collection.

The concern for carryover effect of the different concentrations of rTPA within the catheter will be addressed by aspirating the catheter and then flushing it with 10 ml of normal saline prior to the initiation of dialysis. A clotting time can be performed to ensure no residual rTPA was left in the catheter. The catheter will then be instilled with the new solution at the end of the treatment. A two-day span of time between treatments will also eliminate any carryover of the medication.

A pilot study is an ideal way to address some of the concerns identified in this experimental design. It could be used to identify problems in the design, refine the data collection and analysis, establish the reliability and validity of the instruments used, establish the competence of the investigator, and strengthen the case for the study being proposed. It has been calculated that a sample of 30 patients will be necessary for this study. A pilot study would require three patients or 10% of the sample population (Brink & Wood, 1998). Though the pilot study would increase efforts related to time, energy, and expenses, the knowledge gained could prove invaluable in many aspects of the finished product.

Ethical Considerations

Prior to the initiation of the study, the Health Research Ethics Board will be approached with a request for ethical review of the proposed study. Upon introduction to the study, the participants will be informed of the purpose of the study, procedures involved, risks, benefits, voluntary participation, compensation, and confidentiality. It will be stressed that the patient is under no obligation to participate and may withdraw from the study at any time, and that withdrawal from the study will not influence care given. An information sheet will be provided outlining the previously mentioned information (see Exhibit F-3). A consent-to-participate form will be signed by the participants prior to the initiation of the study and will be obtained and witnessed by a hemodialysis professional who is not involved in the study.

The risk associated with an instillation of rTPA is bleeding. Paulson, Reisoether, Aasen, and Fauchald (1993) reported that rTPA dissolves clot formation efficiently and safely, citing an 11% incidence of minor bleeding with its use. A small pilot study by Atkinson, Bagnall, and Gomperts (1990) and a prospective double-blind study by Haire, Atkinson, Stephens, and Kotulak (1994) stated there was no incidence of bleeding while using rTPA. Though the literature appears to suggest there is minimal risk associated with the use of this drug, the patient must be made aware of the potential for bleeding.

Significance of the Study

One of the limitations of this proposed study is the concern about lack of external validity or generalizability of results related to the type of sample selected. The sample will be a convenience sample, not a true representation of all hemodialysis patients with end-stage renal failure. To ensure generalizability, this type of study could be undertaken in other renal units during a multicenter trial.

The issue of cost was not addressed in this proposed study. It is well recognized that rTPA is an expensive medication, hence it is selectively used. A cost comparison concerning catheter replacement, physician time, nursing time, and radiological verification versus the use of rTPA would prove informative and may demonstrate support for more widespread use of this drug.

The insertion and removal of central venous catheters in the hemodialysis population are the responsibility of the nephrologist. The care of these catheters is the responsibility of the dialysis nurse. A high incidence of thrombosis is a well-documented complication associated with this type of vascular access. Caring for these catheters requires technical skill, problem-solving abilities, and an understanding of anatomy and catheter performance. Even for nurses armed with experience and skill, the care of central venous catheters can be a trying experience. It is understandable, therefore, that there is a search for a drug, skill, or technique that will improve catheter performance and decrease nurse frustration and patient anxiety. The use of rTPA has proven to be effective in the dissolution of clots within the catheters. The one deterrent to its widespread use is cost. If it can be demonstrated that a decreased concentration of rTPA, such as 0.5 mg, is as effective as the standard 2.0 mg, then more of it could be used, thereby improving nursing care and practice for patients in end-stage renal failure.

References

Andreoli, T., Bennett, J. C., Carpenter, C. C., & Plum, F. (1997). *Cecil essentials of medicine* (4th ed.). Toronto: W. B. Saunders.

Atkinson, J. B., Bagnall, H. A., & Gomperts, E. (1990). Investigational use of tissue plasminogen activator for occluded central venous catheters. *Journal of Parenteral Enteral Nutrition, 14,* 310–311.

Barendregt, J. N., Tordoir, J. H., & Leunissen, K. M. (1999). Antithrombotic measures for indwelling intravenous hemodialysis catheters—Columbus' egg yet to be found. *Nephrology Dialysis & Transplantation, 14,* 1834–1835.

Berkoben, M., & Schwab, S. (1995). Maintenance of permanent hemodialysis vascular access patency. *American Nephrology Nurses' Association, 22*(1), 17–23.

Brink, P. J., & Wood, M. J. (1998). *Advanced design in nursing research* (2nd ed.). Thousand Oaks, CA: Sage.

Brunier, G. (1996). Care of the hemodialysis patient with a new permanent vascular access: Review of the assessment and teaching. *American Nephrology Nurses' Association, 23*(6), 547–556.

Buturovic, J., Ponikvar, R., Boh, M., Klinkmann, J., & Ivanovich, P. (1998). Filling hemodialysis catheters in the interdialytic period: Heparin versus citrate versus polygeline: A prospective randomized study. *Artificial Organs, 22*(11), 945–947.

Central Organ Replacement Register. (1998). *Canadian organ replacement register, 1997 annual report.* Don Mills, Ontario, Canada: Hospital Medical Records Institute.

Choudhry, D., Ahmed, Z., Giris, H., & Kronfli, S. (1999). Percutaneous cuffed catheter insertion by nephrologists. *American Journal of Nephrology, 19,* 51–54.

Daeihagh, P., Jordan, J., Chen, G. J., & Rocco, M. (2000). Efficacy of tissue plasminogen activator administration on patency of hemodialysis access catheters. *American Journal of Kidney Diseases, 36*(1), 75–79.

Davis, S., Vermeulen, L., Banton, J., Schwartz, B., & Williams, E. (2000). Activity and dosage of alteplase dilution for clearing occlusions of venous-access devices. *American Journal of Health-System Pharmacy, 57*(11), 1039–1045.

Ezzahiri, R., Lemson, S., Kitslaar, P., Leunissen, K., & Toridor, K. (1999). Hemodialysis vascular access and fistula surveillance methods in the Netherlands. *Nephrology Dialysis & Transplantation, 14,* 2110–2115.

Farrell, J., Walshe, J., Gellens, M., & Martin, K. (1997). Complications associated with insertion of jugular venous catheters for hemodialysis: The value of post procedural radiograph. *American Journal of Kidney Diseases, 30*(5), 690–692.

Haire, W. D., Atkinson, J. B., Stephens, L. C., & Kotulak, G. D. (1994). Urokinase versus recombinant tissue plasminogen activator in thrombosed central venous catheter: A double-blind, randomized trial. *Thrombosis and Haemostasis, 72*, 543–547.

Johnson, M. (1998). Catheter access for hemodialysis. *Seminars in Dialysis, 11*(6), 326–330.

Kapoian, T., & Sherman, R. A. (1997). A brief history of vascular access for hemodialysis: An unfinished story. *Seminars in Nephrology, 17*(3), 239–243.

Kinzner, C. (1998). Warfarin sodium (Coumadin) anticoagulant therapy for vascular access patency. *American Nephrology Nurses' Association, 25*(2), 195–203.

Kohler, T., & Kirkman, T. (1998). Central venous catheter failure is induced by injury and can be prevented by stabilizing the catheter tip. *The Society of Vascular Surgery, 28*(1), 59–65.

Konner, K. (1999). A primer on the av fistula—achilles' heel, but also the cinderella of hemodialysis. *Nephrology Dialysis & Transplantation, 14*, 2094–2098.

Lancaster, L. E. (Ed.). (1991). *Core curriculum for nephrology nursing.* Pitman, NJ: Anthony J. Jannetti.

Laski, M. E., Pressley, T. A., Sabatini, S., & Wesson, D. E. (1997). National Kidney Foundation: Dialysis outcomes quality initiative (DOQI): Clinical practice guidelines. *American Journal of Kidney Diseases, 30*(4), S138–S237.

Leblanc, M., Bosc, J., Vaussenant, F., Maurice, F., Moragues, H., & Canaud, B. (1998). Effective blood flow and recirculation rates in internal jugular vein twin catheters. Measured by ultrasound velocity dilution. *American Journal of Kidney Diseases, 31*(1), 87–92.

Muhm, M., Sunder-Plassmann, G., Aspner, R., Kritzinger, M., Heismayr, M., & Druml, W. (1997). Supraclavicular approach to the subclavian/innominate vein for large-bore central venous catheters. *American Journal of Kidney Diseases, 30*(6), 802–808.

Mysliwiec, M. (1997). Vascular access thrombosis—what are the possibilities of intervention? *Nephrology Dialysis & Transplantation, 12*, 876–878.

Norman, G. R., & Streiner, D. L. (1999). *PDQ statistics* (2nd ed.). Lewiston, NY: B. C. Decker.

Northsea, C. (1996). Continuous quality improvement: Improving catheter patency using urokinase. *American Nephrology Nurses' Association, 23*(6), 567–571.

Obialo, C. I., Robinson, T., & Braithwaite, M. (1998). Hemodialysis vascular access: Variable thrombis-free survival in three subpopulations of black patients. *American Journal of Kidney Diseases, 31*(2), 250–256.

Ouwendyk, M., & Helferty, M. (1996). Central venous catheter management: How to prevent complications. *American Nephrology Nurses' Association, 23*(6), 572–577.

Parker, J. (Ed.). (1998). *Contemporary nephrology nursing.* Pitman, NJ: Anthony J. Jannetti.

Paulson, D., Reisoether, A., Aasen, M., & Fauchald, P. (1993). Use of tissue plasminogen activator for reopening of clotted dialysis catheters. *Nephron, 64*, 468–470.

Polaschegg, H., & Levin, N. (2000). Challenges for chronic dialysis in the new millennium. *Seminars in Nephrology, 20*(1), 60–70.

Richard, C. J. (1986). *Comprehensive nephrology nursing.* Toronto, Ontario, Canada: Little, Brown.

Schenk, P., Rosenkranz, A., Wolfl, G., Horl, W., & Traindl, O. (2000). Recombinant tissue plasminogen activator is a useful alternative to heparin in priming Quinton Permcath. *American Journal of Kidney Diseases, 35*(1), 130–136.

Senn, S. (1993). *Crossover trials in clinical research.* Chichester, England: Wiley.

Tisher, C. C. (Ed.). (1999). Clinical practice guidelines of the Canadian Society of Nephrology for treatment of patients with chronic renal failure. *Journal of the American Society of Nephrology, 10*(13), S287–S321.

Twardowski, Z. J. (1998a). High-dose intradialytic urokinase to restore the patency of permanent central vein hemodialysis catheters. *American Journal of Kidney Diseases, 31*(5), 841–847.

Twardowski, Z. J. (1998b). The clotted central vein catheter for hemodialysis. *Nephrology Dialysis and Transplantation, 13*, 2203–2206.

Wickham, R., Purl, S., & Welker, D. (1992). Long-term central venous catheters: Issues for care. *Seminars in Oncology Nursing, 8*(2), 133–147.

EXHIBIT F-1
Example of a Computerized Method for Randomizing Numbers

To generate a set of random numbers, enter the selections (integer values only):

How many sets of numbers do you want to generate?	Value—2
How many numbers per set?	Value—15
What is the number range?	Value 1–30
Do you wish each number in the set to remain unique?	Yes
Do you wish to sort your outputted numbers?	Yes
How do you wish to view your outputted numbers?	Place markers within

Randomized results:

Group A: p1 = 3, p2 = 5, p3 = 10, p4 = 12, p5 = 13, p6 = 14, p7 = 16, p8 = 17, p9 = 18, p10 = 20, p11 = 21, p12 = 22, p13 = 25, p14 = 26, p15 = 29

Group B: p1 = 1, p2 = 2, p3 = 4, p4 = 6, p5 = 7, p6 = 8, p7 = 9, p8 = 11, p9 = 15, p10 = 19, p11 = 23, p12 = 24, p13 = 27, p14 = 28, p15 = 30

EXHIBIT F-2
Procedure for Instillation of rTPA in a Central Venous Catheter

Issue date: _____

Level: Departmental

Supplies:

- Hemodialysis tray
- Tray with compartment
- 2 kelly forceps
- 3 towels and 1 fenestrated towel
- 1 package povidone-iodine (Betadine) solution
- 1 transfer forceps
- Mask
- 2 catheter caps
- Two 18-gauge needles
- 1 in Dermiclear (bridging) tape
- rTPA (prepared by pharmacy)
- 3 normal saline vials
- Sterile gloves
- Four 3-ml syringes
- Two 10-ml syringes
- Label
- 4 × 4 gauze

Procedures:

1. Mask for patient and nurse.

2. Wash hands.

3. Remove bridging tape.

4. Open hemodialysis tray.

5. Use transfer forceps on outer wrap of hemodialysis tray to pick up towels, Betadine solution, and kelly forceps. Place beside the tray.

6. Using intravenous saline from dialyzer setup, run some saline into a compartment of the tray. OR Twist open two normal saline vials and pour into a compartment of the tray.

7. Add four 3-ml syringes, two 10-ml syringes, two 18-gauge needles, and two catheter caps onto sterile field.

8. Place prepared rTPA syringes near tray.

9. Glove.

10. Pour Betadine solution into the second compartment of the tray.

11. Soak two 4 × 4 gauze with Betadine solution.

12. Prepare two 10-ml syringes with normal saline by drawing up from saline compartment.

13. While holding a catheter with a 4 × 4 gauze, position towels above and below catheter area.

14. Wrap the catheter with a Betadine-soaked 4 × 4 gauze for four minutes.

15. With catheter clamps closed, remove and discard caps.

16. While holding the wrapped catheter, lay the fenestrated towel underneath the Betadine-wrapped catheter.

17. Remove Betadine-soaked 4 × 4 gauze on catheter and attach a 3-ml syringe to each catheter extension.

18. Withdraw 3 ml from each unclamped extension of the catheter.

19. Clamp both extensions.

20. Discard the withdrawn blood onto a 4 × 4 gauze to check for clots.

21. Attach a saline-filled 10-ml syringe to each extension.

22. Unclamp and flush each extension alternately with 10 ml normal saline and clamp while instilling to remove all traces of blood.

23. Wrapping a sterile 4 × 4 gauze around the rTPA-filled syringe, instill in one continuous motion.

24. Attach new caps to leur lock connectors on clamped catheter connections.

25. Apply bridging tapes on both catheter connections.

26. Attach a label over bridging tape indicating the presence of rTPA.

27. Wrap a 4 × 4 gauze around catheter extensions and secure with tape.

EXHIBIT F-3
Tissue Plasminogen Activator Research Study Patient Information Sheet

Project title: Maintaining Catheter Patency Using Recombinant Tissue Plasminogen Activator

Principal investigator: Colleen M. Astle, RN MN Candidate

Coinvestigators: Dr. R. Ulan, Nephrologist and Associate Professor, University of Alberta

Purpose of the study: Hemodialysis is a treatment that is available to you when your kidneys have stopped working. It will replace some of the functions normally carried out by your own kidneys, such as cleaning waste products and excess fluids from your blood. To perform this procedure it is necessary to gain access to your blood. This is possible with the use of a catheter. The catheter is kept open and working by using a drug called tissue plasminogen activator. The reason for doing the study is to compare two different amounts of this drug to see which is more effective in keeping the catheter open for use.

Study procedures: Central venous catheters are a common access used for dialysis. You will have a catheter in place when this study is started. If you agree to take part in the study, an unknown concentration of the study drug will be put into the catheter to keep it open. At the end of two months you will move to the second group to use the other concentration of the drug. Neither you nor your study investigator will know which drug concentration is being used in either stage of the study.

Risks: There is a small risk of bleeding associated with the use of this medication, and one of the drugs may be less effective in preventing the catheter from clotting. You will be kept informed if any problems develop with the catheter.

Benefits: You personally may not benefit from this study at this time; however, the information gained in doing the study may help improve the care of these catheters in the future.

Voluntary participation: Taking part in the study is voluntary. Deciding not to take part will not affect the care you receive. If you decide to stop after the study has begun, your care will not be affected.

Compensation: There will be no financial cost to you for taking part in the study. You will not be charged for using the drug in your catheter or for any of the procedures. By signing the consent form you are not releasing the investigator, institution, or sponsor from their legal and professional responsibilities.

Confidentiality: The information collected for this study will be kept private. Your name will not be used. Your chart will be used to collect information for the study. If you have any questions about the study, please do not hesitate to call the program director. If you have any concerns about any aspect of this study, you may contact the Capital Health Authority patient care representative. This office has no affiliation with the study or its investigators.

Standardized Telephone Triage Practice: Impact of Protocol Implementation on Reported Job Stress and Satisfaction by Nurses in a Pediatric Oncology Outpatient Setting

By Karina Black

Introduction

Offering nursing services and advice via the telephone is a new and growing practice, yet nurses in the pediatric oncology setting lack evidence-based protocols or guidelines to support the practice. Pediatric oncology is not a low-stress work environment. Adding the anxiety and stress of dealing with complex patient issues over the telephone without guidelines to support the practice can greatly add to nurses' stress and impact job satisfaction. Ultimately, staff retention can be jeopardized.

The outpatient nurses of the Northern Alberta Children's Cancer Program (NACCP) are one such group of nurses. Nurses in the outpatient department of the NACCP can often find themselves dealing with complex and sometimes critical patient issues over the phone with children's parents. Although these nurse coordinators are experienced pediatric oncology nurses, a tool that guides their decision making is nonexistent. Uncertainty about the most appropriate advice and direction to give parents, as well as concerns regarding the accountability and potential liability, contribute to dissatisfaction and stress related to their job. Also, nurses who fill in for these nurses during times of vacation or illness have expressed feelings of great anxiety at having to deal with patient issues over the telephone and the potential for error.

Research Question and Purpose

Workplace stress contributes to organizational inefficiency, high staff turnover and burnout, absenteeism, decreased quality and quantity of care, increased costs in health care, and decreased staff morale and job satisfaction (AbuAlRub, 2004; Antai-Otong, 2001). The potential impact of high job stress and low job satisfaction at the NACCP raises the question, What is the effect of implementing telephone triage protocols on the reported job stress and satisfaction level of nurses performing telephone triage activities in a pediatric oncology outpatient setting?

Literature Review

A review of the existing literature was conducted to explore the issues of job stress, job satisfaction, and telephone triage more closely. The electronic databases CINAHL and PubMed were searched using the keywords job stress, nursing job stress, and job satisfaction, as well as telephone triage, telephone triage in pediatrics, and telephone triage in pediatric oncology. A review of selected key literature is presented here.

Stress Levels and Job Satisfaction in Nursing

Conceptual and Operational Definitions

The Merriam-Webster Online Dictionary (2004a) defines stress as "a physical, chemical, or emotional factor that causes bodily or mental tension and may be a factor in disease causation." In nursing, however, this definition is inadequate to describe stress experienced in the workplace. Nurses often have a "do everything for everyone all of the time, perfectly attitude" (Antai-Otong, 2001, p. 32). Mounting workloads, higher client acuity, inadequate staffing, job security uncertainties, and lack of control over their practice clash with this attitude and often comprise the daily stress of nurses (Antai-Otong). For the purpose of this question, however, the operational definition of the stress level for nurses in the pediatric oncology setting will be defined by the reported level of job satisfaction specifically related to the level of perceived control over work conditions, professional relationships, liability risk, and confidence in their abilities in advising patients or parents as reported by the nurses.

Review of the Literature

The nursing profession attracts motivated individuals who work in demanding environments. The ability to provide high-quality care often conflicts with the stress of diminished resources, and increased responsibilities affect job satisfaction, which in turn impacts the incidence of staff burnout (Kalliath & Morris, 2002). There are numerous references in the literature to the impact of job satisfaction and stress on staff retention and burnout. Kalliath and Morris conducted a study using surveys completed by nurses in a Midwestern US general hospital to assess the impact of job satisfaction levels on burnout among nurses. They identified six specific items that impacted job satisfaction and potentially led to burnout: work overload, lack of control, insufficient reward, unfairness, breakdown of community, and value conflict. Job satisfaction was found to be a significant predictor of burnout in nurses in this study. Based on the study outcome, Kalliath and Morris suggested that finding approaches and solutions to some of the problems nurses experience that impact job satisfaction would be of benefit.

In the pediatric setting in particular, Ernst, Franco, Messmer, and Gonzalez (2004) noted the contribution of control over work conditions, job stress, group cohesion, and recognition to overall job satisfaction, as well as the importance of considering job satisfaction in the retention of nurses. They conducted an exploratory study and surveyed a convenience sample of registered nurses at a Southeastern US children's hospital, including nurses in an outpatient clinic and after-hours telephone triage staff. After factor analysis, they found that having physicians respect their knowledge and judgments, as well as confidence in their own abilities or patient care decisions, were factors that contributed to the nurses' confidence, thereby decreasing the level of job stress. They also found a high correlation between control over nursing practice and job satisfaction.

Implications for the Pediatric Oncology Outpatient Setting

Although the literature review related to nursing stress levels was limited, the importance of addressing factors that contribute to nurses' stress was apparent. As stated earlier, pediatric oncology is not a stress-free work environment, and dealing with patient issues over the phone without specific guidelines has the potential to impact job satisfaction and stress levels and ultimately has the potential to compromise staff retention. Instituting changes to address some of the factors contributing to the stress level of the nurses working in this area is beneficial, and implementing a standardized telephone triage program and related protocols is a logical solution.

Telephone Triage

Conceptual and Operational Definitions

The word "triage" originates from the French root trier, which means to sort, to screen, or to classify (Blythin, 1988; Hartman, 2003; McMullen, 1998; Merriam-Webster Online Dictionary, 2004b). Historically, the process of triaging was initiated and practiced during times of war for sorting and classifying wounded soldiers for treatment. Today, triage is a skill that is still used in medicine and is frequently associated with treatment in emergency departments and in response to mass casualty situations. Triage is defined in the literature as the process of assessing, sorting, classifying, or prioritizing the medical needs of people while appropriately allocating available resources and services (DeVore, 1999; McMullen, 1998; VanDinter, 2000; Yurt, 1992).

Telephone triage is "one of the most rapidly growing clinical practice areas" (Rutenberg, 2000b, p. 76). Family practice physicians, pediatricians, obstetric–gynecology practices, and other specialty clinical practices are also incorporating telephone triage as part of the services available to their patients, either during regular office hours or as an after-hours service (Baker, Schubert, Kirwan, Lenkauskas, & Spaeth, 1999; DeVore, 1999; Lee, et al., 2003; Leibowitz, Day, & Dunt, 2003; McMullen, 1998; Melzer & Poole, 1999; Phelan, 1998; Richards, et al., 2002). In one study, managers who favored medical offices utilizing daytime telephone advice services stated the approach provides "better continuity of care, increased likelihood of knowing the patient, provides access to the patient's medical information . . . and facilitates giving advice that is consistent with the practice of the callers' clinician" (Valanis, et al., 2003, p. 222), all of which would be applicable to the pediatric oncology outpatient setting.

Telephone triage is described as the process of screening and collecting a caller's symptoms over the telephone to evaluate the urgency of a health problem and to determine the most appropriate advice and treatment based on the described symptoms (Briggs, 2002; Coleman, 1997; O'Connell, Johnson, Stallmeyer, & Cokington, 2001; Wilkinson, Przestrzelski, Duff, & Hite, 2000). For the purpose of this study question, the operational definition of telephone triage is the same as previously stated: the process of screening and collecting a caller's symptoms over the telephone to determine the urgency of the health problem and the most appropriate advice and treatment direction. The main difference in the pediatric oncology setting, however, is that the caller is typically the parent and not the patient.

Review of the Literature

Why Develop a Standardized Telephone Triage Program?

Assessing a patient only through a telephone conversation is different from a face-to-face assessment. The nurse is restricted to using just one sense during the patient assessment—hearing—and must make accurate decisions with limited sensory input (DeVore, 1999; McMullen, 1998; Rutenberg, 2000b; Wheeler, 2000; Wilkinson, et al., 2000). The problem is that we all have different skills and could give different advice after listening to the same information (Dale, Williams, & Crouch, 1995). As Briggs (2002) further states, advice based on what the nurse thinks is appropriate may actually be harmful. All nurses are not equal in education or knowledge base, assessment skills, or communication skills and may miss something in the assessment. Using organized, approved protocols helps to ensure a systematic, thorough assessment establishing consistency and a standard of care.

Benefits

As stated earlier, there is considerable consensus in the literature regarding the potential benefits of a standardized telephone triage process and protocols. Systematic patient assessment is critical when providing services by phone to ensure safe and effective patient care to decrease the likelihood of a problem going unnoticed (Rutenberg, 2000a). Developed protocols in a practice area outline the information required by the nurse to provide meaningful, safe advice (Wilkinson, et al., 2000). Protocols use an algorithm to elicit responses to assessment questions and therefore appropriately manage specific health concerns (Levy, et al., 1979; Mayo, Chang, & Omery, 2002; McMullen, 1998). Protocols facilitate standardization and organization and promote consistency in telephone triage practice (Larson-Dahn, 2001; Levy, et al.; McMullen).

Development of Protocols

In the development of protocols, McMullen (1998) suggests that the protocols need to be realistic, "symptom-based, offer relevant subjective and objective data associated with the problem, give possible differential diagnoses, and outline appropriate management strategies" (p. 253). Protocols need to be developed collaboratively between the nursing and medical staff through a careful review of the literature on the topics of concern in that setting (Cady, 1999; VanDinter, 2000). After protocols have been developed based on current standards of practice, they must be updated and reviewed regularly (i.e., annually or every two years) to ensure accuracy and continued compliance with standards of care (McMullen).

Liability Issues

A standardized telephone triage program may also have liability concerns. "When a nurse–client relationship is established with a caller, the nurse is professionally and legally accountable for the advice given" (Canadian Nurses Protective Society [CNPS], 1997, p. 1). Liability occurs when poor telephone procedures, lack of thorough assessment, and inadequate documentation occur. Having a standardized telephone triage process with clearly defined protocols and documentation requirements can be the best protection from liability for the nurse and employer (DeVore, 1999; Gobis, 1997; VanDinter, 2000). In addition, proper orientation, continuing education for nurses, and ongoing quality improvement should also be incorporated into the program (Cady, 1999; Zimmermann, 1999).

No matter what the area of practice, the purpose of documentation is "to clearly and accurately record and communicate to other healthcare providers information exchanged during encounters and defend the nurse if litigation occurs" (Larson-Dahn, 2001, p. 145). CNPS (1996) affirms that "since every nurse is legally accountable for care rendered, proper and thorough documentation may prove to be your best defense if a lawsuit ensues" (p. 2). Established and standardized tools for documentation of telephone triage encounters are not readily available in the literature, possibly due in part to the newness of this area (Larson-Dahn). Regardless of the format of the tool, the checklists and questions would remind the nurse of what questions to ask and ensure complete documentation (Wheeler, 2000). Documentation tools and forms must be developed according to institutional policies. CNPS (1997) does recommend that the documentation include the date and time of the call; name, phone number, and address of the caller; information received; advice or information given, including referral and follow-up; and the name and designation of the nurse. They also recommend that the record be retained for future reference.

Using Telephone Protocols

There is mention in the literature of the need for nurses to have access to a physician for consultation when telephone triage is being performed (Greenberg, 2000; Scott & Packard, 1990). A study by Edwards (1994) that examined the decision-making process of nurses performing telephone triage duties showed that risks in this setting are heightened by the fact that decisions are often made in an environment that demands accurate and fast decisions based on minimal information. But he also noted that the risks were also heightened when executed in the absence of medical support. Nurses in the study expressed vulnerability, unease, and uncertainty with making decisions over the phone. Of note were expressions of not only professional accountability in this setting but also "personal anxiety at the responsibility they feel for outcomes over which they have limited control" (Edwards, p. 54). Having physician collaboration in development of protocols for a practice setting would address some of this issue, as would ensuring the availability of a physician for consultation and advice to the telephone triage nurse.

Two separate studies by Dale, Crouch, and Lloyd (1998) and Mayo et al. (2002) evaluated the use of protocols in telephone triage practices and came to similar conclusions. The protocols in both studies were readily available and designed to support the nurses in obtaining assessment information. The studies reported that the nurses used the protocols most of the time (65%). Although the protocols were designed to guide decision making, they were not meant to replace the nurses' clinical judgment.

As noted in the aforementioned studies by Dale et al. (1998) and Mayo et al. (2002), the telephone triage protocols are not meant to replace the nurse's clinical judgment. The nursing process is a practical framework that has been ingrained into every nurse at the outset of nursing training. It is therefore a familiar process, requiring only some situational flexibility. The nursing process involves assessment, diagnosis, plan formation, intervention, and evaluation. Although the approach may be different with telephone triage, the process is not (Coleman, 1997; Mayo, et al.; Rutenberg, 2000a). As Rutenberg (2000b) articulates, although protocols serve to remind the busy nurse of all elements that must be considered, the accountability for putting it all together and making the best decision for each individual patient rests with the nurse. Inflexible protocols that limit nursing judgment should be avoided. This point is echoed by Simonsen-Anderson (2002), who states that mindlessly following protocols will not decrease nurses' liability. Although the nurse relies on protocol and standardized policies to assess the caller's condition, the nurse must also use professional judgment given the caller's situation and override the protocol if the situation warrants it.

Gaps in the Literature

In summary, we know that developing a reference manual or protocols and documentation record for telephone triage supports continuous quality improvement, provides a standardized approach, and supports nurses' legal responsibility. From a practical perspective, protocols and algorithms aimed at addressing the most frequent and serious symptoms or health concerns would be developed by nurses and physicians. The context for each protocol would be based on current standards of practice and institutional policies and procedures and would provide standardized, approved direction for the telephone triage nurse dealing with frequent patient issues. The documentation tool would cue inquiries about key information and provide a permanent record of the call information.

There are gaps in the literature, however. First, there are few established protocols or documentation tools readily available in the literature. This is a relatively new area of practice for nursing, and telephone triage in pediatric oncology nursing is no exception.

More notable, however, is the lack of reference in the literature regarding the impact of telephone triage programs on job satisfaction. Based on the issues addressed with the use of triage programs, the implementation of the standardized protocols and documentation tools would potentially address some of the issues contributing to job stress and increase job satisfaction. The guidance provided has the potential to decrease job stress because it could increase nurses' confidence in decision making, decrease liability concerns, and increase control of this aspect of their job responsibilities. This change could increase physician respect and strengthen the professional relationship, potentially leading to an increased overall confidence in one's nursing practice. The implementation of these standardized protocols and documentation tools would potentially address the issues that contribute to job stress, increase job satisfaction in the short term, and positively impact staff retention in the long term (Figure G-1).

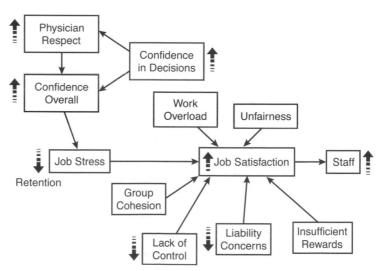

FIGURE G-1   Concept Map of Impacts of Standardized Telephone Triage Programs on Job Satisfaction and Staff Retention

The effect of implementing such programs in the high-stress environment of pediatric oncology in also unknown. It would be beneficial to know whether a standardized telephone triage program would have a positive impact on job satisfaction. The best way to answer this question is by initiating a research project on this topic.

Statement of Purpose of the Study

The purpose of this study is to examine the effect of implementing a standardized telephone triage program on the self-reported stress and job satisfaction levels of nurses who triage patient issues over the telephone at the Northern Alberta Children's Cancer Program. The study hypotheses are as follows:

H_0: The implementation of a standardized telephone triage program will have no effect on outpatient nurses' job satisfaction.

H_1: The implementation of a standardized telephone triage program will have an effect on outpatient nurses' job satisfaction.

Definition of Terms

Telephone triage is the process of screening and collecting a caller's symptoms over the telephone to determine the urgency of the health problem and the most appropriate advice and treatment direction (Briggs, 2002; Coleman, 1997; O'Connell, et al., 2001; Wilkinson, et al., 2000).

Protocols are algorithms used to elicit responses to assessment questions and therefore appropriately manage specific health concerns (Levy, et al., 1979; Mayo, et al., 2002; McMullen, 1998).

Stress level as defined for nurses is composed of the daily stress of mounting workloads, higher client acuity, inadequate staffing, job security uncertainties, and lack of control over their practice (Antai-Otong, 2001).

Job satisfaction is the nurse's rating of his or her perceived workload, job stress, control over work conditions, rewards, group cohesion, and autonomy (Ernst, et al., 2004; Kalliath & Morris, 2004) as measured for this study by the Work Quality Index.

Methodology

Design

The proposed research project is designed to assess whether implementing such a standardized telephone triage program in the Northern Alberta Children's Cancer Program (NACCP) would impact job satisfaction.

A quasi-experimental pretest–posttest design will be used to address this study question. A pretest–posttest design was chosen because all subjects will be from the same department—the outpatient department of the NACCP. Due to the constraint of a small sample in this clinical setting, the design is a quasi-experimental pilot study. Although there will be manipulation of the independent variable, there will be no control group or random assignment, a requirement of a true experimental design (Brink & Wood, 2001). Although not as rigidly designed as a true experiment design, a quasi-experimental design does introduce some research control when full experimental rigor is not possible (Polit, Beck, & Hungler, 2001).

A multicenter design would allow for a larger sample size and the potential for a true experimental design. However, there are vast differences between clinical programs, site-specific policies and procedures, and current level of telephone triage program development throughout pediatric oncology. These differences in programs make a multicenter study design unmanageable in this master's level research project.

Study Variables

The variables for this study are as follows:

Independent variable: Standardized telephone triage program, including protocols and documentation tool

Dependent variable: Self-reported job satisfaction level (as measured by the Work Quality Index)

Study Setting and Sample

Setting

This as a single-site study to be conducted at the Stollery Children's Hospital within the outpatient department of the Northern Alberta Children's Cancer Program (NACCP). The NACCP provides oncology-specific nursing care to children within a 1,139,600 km^2 area (Capital Health, 2010) stretching from Red Deer north in Alberta and including children from parts of the Northwest Territories, Yukon, Nunavut, British Columbia, and Saskatchewan. In addition to active treatment, the NACCP also includes long-term follow-up, neuro-oncology, blood and stem cell transplant preparation and follow-up, and palliative care services.

A priority of the NACCP is to ensure that nursing care is accessible, efficient, and effective. Thus, telephone contact as a care delivery method to this patient population becomes a necessity. The researcher, as an employee of the outpatient department of the NACCP, is actively involved in telephone triage and has access to the setting and potential study participants and stakeholders. Because the target population is outpatient pediatric oncology nurses performing telephone triage services, this is an ideal setting for this study. Support for this study will be sought from the administration of the NACCP (see Exhibit G-1). When support is obtained, a list of registered nurses currently employed in the NACCP (n = 5 exclusive of researcher) will be obtained for the program administration study records.

Eligibility Criteria

Inclusion Criteria

1. Registered nurse employed in the outpatient department of the NACCP.

2. Full-time or part-time status. Nurses who are employed on a full- or part-time basis in the NACCP are providing telephone triage services to pediatric oncology patients or parents on a routine basis.

3. Minimum of two years experience in the outpatient department of the NACCP.

Exclusion Criteria

1. Casual or relief staff or inpatient nurses. These nurses are rarely asked to provide telephone triage services because these duties are performed by only senior outpatient staff members.

2. Inability to read and write English. The questionnaire or telephone triage protocols will not be translated into any other language.

Regulatory Criteria

1. A letter of approval from the program director and program manager for conducting the study among the outpatient nursing staff of the NACCP must be obtained prior to conducting this study.

2. Ethics approval for Panel B of the Health Research Ethics Board at the University of Alberta must be obtained prior to conducting this study.

3. A signed informed consent must be obtained from study participants prior to inclusion in the study (see Exhibit G-2).

Sample Size

The required sample size was estimated using Cohen's (1988) power analysis. To achieve a moderate effect size of 050, an alpha of 0.05, and a power of 0.80, 88 participants would be required to ensure adequate power to the study. However, due to the constraints of the setting population (n = 5), this sample size was unattainable. Therefore, a sample was selected for a pilot study group only.

Sampling Plan and Recruitment

Because a specific target setting is being used, study participants will be selected using a convenience sampling plan. As such, every potential subject meeting the eligibility criteria will be eligible to participate (Brink & Wood, 2001).

Recruitment will begin when administrative approval and ethical approval have been obtained. Posters inviting outpatient nurses to participate will be placed in the clinic and day ward of the NACCP (see Exhibit G-3). A formal information letter will be supplied to interested participants explaining the intended study and asking for possible participation. The researcher will obtain informed consent from the participants at the time they agree to volunteer.

Data Collection

Manipulation of the independent variable, that is, introduction of a standardized telephone triage program, will allow for measurement of the dependent variable. The data to be collected are the measure of the level of job satisfaction by the participants prior to and after the standardized telephone triage program is initiated. Data collected will encompass the responses to a self-report job satisfaction questionnaire.

Instrument

The Work Quality Index (WQI) is a 38-item, seven-point Likert scale questionnaire (see Exhibit G-4). The WQI measures nurses' satisfaction with their work; their work environment; and the job properties of benefits, role enactment, work worth, professional relationships, and autonomy (Whitley & Putzier, 1994). The WQI was selected for this study because it was developed to specifically measure the job satisfaction of nurses.

The items on the WQI were distilled down to the most robust measure of 38 items related to job satisfaction, divided into six subscales. Whitley and Putzier (1994) reported that the validity of the final 38 items in the WQI were demonstrated with factor analysis through their research and that of other previous researchers.

The reliability of the WQI was determined by calculating the Cronbach's alpha for the total scale and the six subscales. The Cronbach's alpha for the complete scale was 0.94 and ranged from 0.72 to 0.87 for the different subscales (Whitley & Putzier, 1994).

Timing of Data Collection

After administrative approval, ethics approval, and informed consent have been obtained, the participants will be provided with a study package. Each study package will include a letter of support from NACCP administration (not yet obtained), a copy of the signed consent form, a study information letter, a copy of the WQI questionnaire, (Exhibits G-2, G-3, and G-4) and an addressed and stamped return envelope. Participants will be given two weeks to return the questionnaire.

After pretest questionnaires have been received from all study participants, the standardized telephone triage program will be implemented. Participants will be provided with an orientation to the telephone triage program via a group in-service. A posttest questionnaire package will be distributed to the study participants four months after the initiation of the telephone triage program. The posttest package will contain a blank copy of the WQI and an addressed and stamped return envelope. Participants will again be given two weeks to return the questionnaire.

The timing of the pretest and posttest will be designed to occur outside of summer vacation hour periods (July and August) to ensure study participants receive as close to a full four-month exposure to the telephone triage program as possible. In addition, this reduces the impact on aspects of work satisfaction due to altered workloads because of the presence of casual or relief staff in the setting.

Threats to Study Validity

Threats to internal validity include lack of control over history and selection bias. The constraints of a single-site, small sample study do not allow the researcher to address these issues with randomization or control groups. Maturation is addressed by ensuring that the sample excludes relief staff who are inexperienced with telephone triage in general and who would naturally gain confidence and comfort with the practice during the study time period, even without the standardized program. Excluding relief staff will also reduce the threat of experimental mortality because regular staff would be expected to remain in the setting for the time period of the study. Threats from changes in instrumentation are addressed by using the identical questionnaire for the pretest and posttest, thereby measuring the same data each time.

External validity is strengthened through the choice of the study instrument itself. The WQI is constructed in a format that does not reveal each subscale to the study participant (Whitley & Putzier, 1994). The subjects are not cued to the anticipated effects of the independent variable, which would change their response on the posttest or their response to the independent variable itself.

Data Analysis

Data will be entered into the statistical software package SPSS Version 12.0. Data will be entered by the researcher. Descriptive statistics (mean, median, mode) will be used to summarize the nurses' perceived job satisfaction. Descriptive statistics provide a way for the data to be analyzed for general trends, to be summarized and organized, as well as to be presented in table and graph form (Ness-Evans, 1998).

A nonparametric test will be used to determine the differences, if present, between the pretest and posttest data. The WQI provides ordinal data (Likert scale) for the six subscales as well as the total index. Due to the small sample size, a normal distribution of the population or sample data cannot be assumed, so a nonparametric test is required (Pett, 1997).

As indicated by the requirements identified by Pett (1997), the Wilcoxon Signed Ranks Test will be used because this study provides paired ordinal data from a small sample. A one-tailed z-test will then be used to test the null hypothesis (no difference in reported job satisfaction between the pretest and posttest). A one-tailed test is utilized because the study hypothesis is directional, looking for increased job satisfaction in the posttest data.

Ethical Issues

This proposal will be submitted for ethical review by Panel B of the Health Research Ethics Board (HREB) at the University of Alberta. The main ethical considerations within this proposal are data storage, confidentiality and anonymity, and informed consent. The researcher will ask the program director and program manager of the NACCP to provide a letter of support to the HREB for conducting this study.

Data Storage

All data collected will be stored in a locked filing cabinet when not in use. Computerized data, such as floppy disks or compact discs, will also be locked in a filing cabinet when not in use.

Confidentiality and Anonymity

To maintain confidentiality, no personal identifying information will be included on any questionnaires or reports. Computerized data will not contain names or personal identifying information. The researcher, who will be the only person responsible for the analysis and safekeeping of any demographic data, will maintain confidentiality of the subjects. All efforts will be made to provide anonymity where possible. For the questionnaire, each participant will be randomly assigned a study identification number, and the coding will not be known to the researcher.

Informed Consent

Participant consent must be obtained according to the guidelines as outlined by the HREB of the University of Alberta. The researcher will be responsible for obtaining informed consent. All interested participants will be provided with a full explanation of the study. All participants will receive an information sheet explaining the study (see Exhibit G-3), a letter of support from the program management, and an informed consent form (see Exhibit G-2). Participants will be asked to give informed consent by signing the form after the study information has been provided and the researcher is assured that the participants understand the implication of their participation in this study. The participant will then be supplied with a copy of the signed consent form. If a potential participant chooses not to sign the informed consent form, he or she will not be recruited to this study.

Risks and Benefits

Minimal research exists exploring the effects of a standardized telephone triage program on stress and job satisfaction in a pediatric oncology setting. Therefore, specific immediate risks and benefits of participating in the proposed study have not been identified. The participants will be informed that involvement, or lack thereof, will not affect their employment. The proposed study may provide evidence that utilizing a standardized telephone triage program is beneficial for improving job satisfaction in the pediatric oncology setting, providing an indirect, long-term benefit for the participants.

Dissemination Strategies

The researcher will contact the program director, program manager, and the outpatient nurses of the NACCP to provide information on the outcome of this study. Publications from this study will be targeted at a pediatric oncology audience but also toward a broader, multidisciplinary pediatric and nursing audience. Potential examples of targeted journals are *Journal of Pediatric Oncology Nursing, Oncology Nursing Forum, Pediatrics*, and *Journal of Nursing Scholarship*. In addition, research abstract presentation at pertinent conferences will also be sought, such as at the Association of Pediatric Oncology Nurses Annual Conference, the Alberta Pediatric Nurses Interest Group, and the Canadian Association of Nurses in Oncology Conference.

Study Limitations

The available population of study participants is a small number (n = 5), and given that everyone in the setting may not consent to participate, this number could be smaller yet. The data from this study would be used as pilot study data only. Although we cannot expect definitive causal inferences from this study design, the researcher can often achieve some knowledge using this design, and it often suggests hypotheses worth further testing (Cook & Campbell, 1979).

Future Directions

The purpose of this study is to provide baseline pilot data for studying the affect of instituting standardized telephone triage programs on job stress and satisfaction of nurses in the pediatric oncology setting. This baseline data may be used in supporting the development of a permanent standardized telephone triage program at the NACCP. This study may be used to compare the results to experiences in other centers that are developing telephone triage programs. The results may also lead the researcher to further studies at the NACCP to assess further benefits of telephone triage (i.e., cost-benefit data, quality improvement and assurance) or to multicenter studies of the effect of telephone triage program implementation with a larger sample, using a stronger research design and methodology.

References

AbuAlRub, R. F. (2004). Job stress, job performance, and social support among hospital nurses. *Journal of Nursing Scholarship, 36*(1), 73–78.

Antai-Otong, D. (2001). Creative stress-management techniques for self-renewal. *Dermatology Nursing, 13*(1), 31–32, 35–39.

Baker, R., Schubert, C., Kirwan, K., Lenkauskas, S., & Spaeth, J. (1999). After-hours telephone triage and advice in private and nonprivate pediatric populations. *Archives of Pediatrics and Adolescent Medicine, 153*, 292–296.

Blythin, P. (1988). Triage documentation. *Nursing, 3*(32), 32–34.

Briggs, J. (2002). *Telephone triage protocols for nurses* (2nd ed.). Philadelphia: Lippincott-Raven.

Brink, P. J., & Wood, M. J. (2001). *Basic steps in planning nursing research: From question to proposal.* Sudbury, MA: Jones and Bartlett.

Cady, R. (1999). Telephone triage: Avoiding the pitfalls. *The American Journal of Maternal/Child Nursing, 24*(4), 209.

Canadian Nurses Protective Society. (1996). Quality documentation: Your best defence. *infoLAW, 1*(1), 1–2.

Canadian Nurses Protective Society. (1997). Telephone advice. *infoLAW, 6*(1), 1–2.

Capital Health. (2010). *Cancer: Northern Alberta children's cancer program.* Retrieved January 11, 2010, from http://www.albertahealthservices.ca/facilities.asp?pid=saf&rid=1046087

Cohen, J. (1988). *Statistical power analysis for the behavioral sciences* (2nd ed.). Hillsdale, NJ: Lawrence Erlbaum.

Coleman, A. (1997). Where do I stand? Legal implications of telephone triage. *Journal of Clinical Nursing, 6*(3), 227–231.

Cook, T. D., & Campbell, D. T. (1979). *Quasi-experimentation: Designs and analysis for field settings.* Chicago: Rand McNally College.

Dale, J., Crouch, R., & Lloyd, D. (1998). Primary care: Nurse-led telephone triage and advice out-of-hours. *Nursing Standard, 12*(47), 41–45.

Dale, J., Williams, S., & Crouch, R. (1995). Development of telephone advice in A&E: Establishing the views of staff. *Nursing Standard, 9*(21), 28–31.

DeVore, N. (1999). Telephone triage: A challenge for practicing midwives. *Journal of Nurse-Midwifery, 44*(5), 471–479.

Edwards, B. (1998). Seeing is believing—picture building: A key component of telephone triage. *Journal of Clinical Nursing, 7*, 51–57.

Ernst, M. E., Franco, M., Messmer, P. R., & Gonzalez, J. L. (2004). Nurses' job satisfaction, stress, and recognition in a pediatric setting. *Pediatric Nursing, 30*(3), 219–227.

Gobis, L. (1997). Legally speaking: Reducing the risks of phone triage. *RN, 60*(4), 61–63.

Greenberg, M. (2000). Telephone nursing: Evidence of client and organizational benefits. *Nursing Economics, 18*(3), 117–123.

Hartman, R. (2003). Tripartite triage concerns: Issues for law and ethics. *Critical Care Medicine, 31*(S5), S358–S361.

Kalliath, T., & Morris, R. (2002). Job satisfaction among nurses. *Journal of Nursing Administration, 32*(12), 648–654.

Larson-Dahn, M. (2001). Tel-eNurse practice: Quality of care and patient outcomes. *Journal of Nursing Administration, 31*(3), 145–152.

Lee, T., Barraff, L., Wall, S., Guzy, J., Johnson, D., & Woo, H. (2003). Parental compliance with after-hours telephone triage advice: Nurse advice service versus on-call pediatricians. *Clinical Pediatrics, 42*, 613–619.

Leibowitz, R., Day, S., & Dunt, D. (2003). A systematic review of the effect of different models of after-hours primary medical care services on clinical outcome, medical workload, and patient and GP satisfaction. *Family Practice, 20*(3), 311–317.

Levy, J., Rosekrans, J., Lamb, G., Friedman, M., Kaplan, D., & Strasser, P. (1979). Development and field testing of protocols for the management of pediatric telephone calls: Protocols for pediatric telephone calls. *Pediatrics, 64*(5), 558–563.

Mayo, A., Chang, B., & Omery, A. (2002). Use of protocols and guidelines by telephone nurses. *Clinical Nursing Research, 11*(2), 204–219.

McMullen, P. (1998). Telephone triage in women's health care. *Lippincott's Primary Care Practice, 2*(3), 251–255.

Melzer, S., & Poole, S. (1999). Computerized pediatric telephone triage and advice programs at children's hospitals: Operating and financial characteristics. *Archives of Pediatrics and Adolescent Medicine, 153*, 858–863.

Merriam-Webster Online Dictionary. (2004a). *Stress*. Retrieved October 18, 2004, from http://www.m-w.com/cgi-bin/dictionary?book=Dictionary&va=stress

Merriam-Webster Online Dictionary. (2004b). *Triage*. Retrieved October 6, 2004, from http://www.m-w.com/cgi-bin/dictionary?book=Dictionary&va=triage

Ness-Evans, A. (1998). *Using basic statistics in the social sciences* (3rd ed.). Scarborough, Ontario, Canada: Prentice-Hall Canada.

O'Connell, J., Johnson, D., Stallmeyer, J., & Cokington, D. (2001). A satisfaction and return-on-investment study of a nurse triage service. *The American Journal of Managed Care, 7*, 159–169.

Pett, M. A. (1997). *Nonparametric statistics for health care research: Statistics for small samples and unusual distributions.* Thousand Oaks, CA: Sage.

Phelan, J. (1998). Ambulatory obstetrical care: Strategies to reduce telephone liability. *Clinical Obstetrics and Gynecology, 41*(3), 640–646.

Polit, D. F., Beck, C. T., & Hungler, P. B. (2001). *Essentials of nursing research: Methods, appraisal and utilization* (5th ed.). Philadelphia: Lippincott Williams & Wilkins.

Richards, D., Meakins, J., Tawfik, J., Godfrey, L., Dutton, E., Richardson, G., et al. (2002). Nurse telephone triage for same-day appointments in general practice: Multiple interrupted time series trial of effect on workload and costs. *BMJ, 325*, 1214–1219.

Rutenberg, C. (2000a). Telephone triage. *American Journal of Nursing, 100*(3), 77–78, 80–81.

Rutenberg, C. (2000b). What do we really KNOW about telephone triage? *Journal of Emergency Nursing, 26*(1), 76–78.

Scott, M., & Packard, K. (1990). *Telephone assessment with protocols for nursing practice.* Philadelphia: W. B. Saunders.

Simonsen-Anderson, S. (2002, June). Safe and sound: Telephone triage and home care recommendations save lives—and money. *Nursing Management*, 41–43.

Valanis, B., Tanner, C., Moscato, S., Shapiro, S., Izumi, S., David, M., et al. (2003). Making it work: Organization and processes of telephone nursing advice services. *Journal of Nursing Administration, 33*(4), 216–233.

VanDinter, M. (2000). Telephone triage: The rules are changing. *The American Journal of Maternal/Child Nursing, 25*(4), 187–191.

Wheeler, S. (2000). Telephone triage: Saved by the form. *Nursing2000, 30*(11), 54–55.

Whitley, M. P., & Putzier, D. J. (1994). Measuring nurses' satisfaction with the quality of their work and work environment. *Journal of Nursing Care Quality, 8*(3), 42–51.

Wilkinson, C., Przestrzelski, D., Duff, I., & Hite, K. (2000). Competency-based telephone triage curriculum. *Lippincott's Case Management, 5*(4), 141–147.

Yurt, R. (1992). Triage, initial assessment, and early treatment of the pediatric trauma patient. *Pediatric Emergency Medicine, 39*(5), 1083–1091.

Zimmermann, P. G. (1999). Telephone triage. *Journal of Emergency Nursing, 25*(4), 33.

EXHIBIT G-1
Letter to Administration of the Northern Alberta Children's Cancer Program

December 8, 2004

Program Manager
Northern Alberta Children's Cancer Program
WMC 4D4.25
8440 – 112 Street
Edmonton, AB T6G 2B7

(780) 407-6541

RE: Standardized telephone triage practices in outpatient pediatric oncology

Dear Debbie;

I am writing to seek your support for a study that I would like to conduct within the outpatient department of the Northern Alberta Children's Cancer Program (NACCP) at the Stollery Children's Hospital. The topic of my research proposal is telephone triage and the potential impact on nurses' job satisfaction and staff retention secondary to the resulting stress and anxiety associated with this practice. Telephone triage is an area of practice necessary within the NACCP given the geographic distribution of the patient population and the nature of the care required. Pediatric oncology is not a stress-free environment, and strategies to address areas affecting job satisfaction are an important area for research. I have chosen outpatient oncology nurses because of the significant proportion of time these nurses spend performing telephone triage-related activities.

My specific purpose is to explore whether implementing standardized telephone triage protocols in outpatient pediatric oncology has an impact on the nurses' job satisfaction within the NACCP. This study would involve the implementation of a standardized telephone triage program with protocols and documentation tools previously approved by the administration of the NACCP. A questionnaire package will be distributed to the full- and part-time outpatient nurses who agree to participate in the study. The package will contain an information letter as part of the informed consent, a letter of support from the NACCP administration, and two copies of the questionnaire. The participants will complete one copy of the questionnaire prior to implementation of the telephone triage program and one copy four months after implementation. The results of this study may or may not be included in a presentation or a journal publication. Confidentiality will be maintained in either case. I would also be very interested in presenting the results to you or the nursing staff at the completion of the study.

I am seeking your permission to advertise for recruitment in the 4E2 clinic and day ward. This study is not designed or intended to impact your resources. If you believe there are possible impacts on your resources, however, please do not hesitate to contact me. Funding has been approved and secured for this study. My anticipated start date is _____. I will not proceed until I have received ethical approval. I will also provide you with a copy of the letter of ethics approval for your files.

I appreciate your time and attention to my project. I look forward to hearing from you. Please do not hesitate to contact me if you would like further information.

Sincerely,

Karina Black, BScN, MN candidate

EXHIBIT G-2
Consent Form

Title: Standardized Telephone Triage Practices in Outpatient Pediatric Oncology
Principal Investigator: Karina Black, BScN, MN candidate, University of Alberta, (780) 407-8779
Coinvestigator: To be selected

Questions:

Do you understand that you have been asked to be in a research study?	Yes	No
Have you read and received a copy of the attached information sheet?	Yes	No
Do you understand the benefits and risks involved in taking part in this research study?	Yes	No
Have you had the opportunity to ask questions and discuss the study?	Yes	No
Do you understand that you are free to refuse to participate or withdraw from the study at any time? You do not have to give a reason, and it will not affect your employment.	Yes	No
Has the issue of confidentiality been explained to you?	Yes	No
Do you understand who will have access to your information?	Yes	No

This study was explained to me by: _____

I agree to take part in this study.

_____   _____   _____
Signature of research participant   Printed name   Date

Witness (if available)

_____   _____   _____
Signature of witness   Printed name   Date

I believe that the person signing this form understands what is involved in the study and voluntarily agrees to participate.

_____   _____
Signature of witness   Date

EXHIBIT G-3
Information for Study Participants

Title: Standardized Telephone Triage Practices in Outpatient Pediatric Oncology

Principal investigator: Karina Black, BScN, MN candidate, University of Alberta, (780) 407-8779

Background and purpose of study: Offering nursing services via the telephone is a new and growing practice, yet nurses in pediatric oncology lack protocols and guidelines specific to the setting. The resulting stress and anxiety associated with this practice adds to an already stressful work setting and contributes to decreased job satisfaction. Not being happy with the work environment can put staff retention at risk.

The purpose of this study is to explore whether using a formal telephone triage program in the outpatient pediatric oncology setting has an impact on job satisfaction in the Northern Alberta Children's Cancer Program (NACCP).

Procedure: All full-time and part-time pediatric oncology nurses employed in the Outpatient Department at the Northern Alberta Children's Cancer Program will be able to take part in this study. The telephone triage program used will be approved by the director and program manager of the NACCP before the start of the study. This program will be explained in full if you agree to take part in the study. If you agree to take part in the study, you will also be asked to complete two question sheets. You will complete one question sheet before the formal telephone triage program begins and one question sheet four months after the program begins. It will take about 30 minutes to complete the entire question sheet each time. If you have trouble understanding any of the questions, the researcher will be available to answer your questions. If you agree to participate, please complete the question sheet and return it within two weeks. A return addressed, stamped envelope will be provided. At any time, you may refuse to answer any questions, or if you choose, you may withdraw from the study.

Benefits: If you take part in this study, there may be no immediate, direct benefit for you. However, by taking part in this study, the researcher hopes to learn more about the effect of telephone triage protocols on job stress and satisfaction in the pediatric oncology setting. Results of this study may lead to further research that may enhance job satisfaction and patient care within a pediatric oncology setting.

Risks: There are no direct risks to you by taking part in this study. Questions about job satisfaction and stress may upset you. This is considered to be an indirect risk, and should this happen, participants will be provided with the phone number of an employee assistance program (EAP) specialist.

What are the costs? There are no monetary costs to you associated with taking part in this study. You will not receive any payment for taking part in this study.

Confidentiality: Every attempt will be made to maintain your confidentiality during and after the study. As part of maintaining confidentiality, you will be identified by a number. All information will be held confidential, except when professional codes of ethics or legislation requires reporting.

The information you provide will be kept for at least five years after the study is done. The information will be kept in a secure area (i.e., locked filing cabinet). Your name and any other identifying information will not be attached to the information you gave. Your name will never be used in any presentation or publication of the study results.

The information gathered for this study may be looked at again in the future to help answer other study questions. If so, the ethics board will first review the study to ensure the information is used ethically.

The results of this study may be included as part of a thesis or published in a scientific journal. Your name will not be mentioned in any of these documents. No participant in this study will be identified by name in either a presentation or publication.

Freedom to withdraw: If at any time you do not wish to continue in the study, for whatever reason, you may withdraw. You do not have to give a reason for no longer continuing in the study. If you withdraw from the study, it will not impact your employment.

What are my rights as a participant? Taking part in this study is completely voluntary. If at any time there is a question you do not wish to answer, please do not feel any pressure to do so. You may choose to take part or you may leave the study at any time. Regardless of your choice, this will not impact your employment. In no way does this waive your legal rights nor release the investigators, sponsors, or involved institutions from their legal and professional responsibilities.

You will be told of any new information learned during the course of this study. You also have the right to learn about the results of this study. If you are interested in learning more about when and how to get the results of this study, you may contact Karina Black at (780) 407-8779. You will receive a signed copy of the consent.

Whom do I call if I have questions or problems? I understand that Karina Black, at (780) 407-8779, will answer any questions I have about the research project. If at any time during the course of this study I feel that I have been inadequately informed of the risks or benefits or that I have been encouraged to continue in this study beyond my wish to do so, I can contact _____ (thesis supervisor) at 492-XXXX.

_____   _____
Signature of research participant   Signature of witness (if available)

_____   _____
Printed Name   Printed Name

_____   _____
Date   Date

_____
Signature of investigator or designee

_____
Date

EXHIBIT G-4
Work Quality Index

This questionnaire inquires about your level of satisfaction with 38 job-correlated factors. Please indicate how satisfied you are in your present job by circling the appropriate number.

		Not Satisfied	Satisfied
1.	The work associated with your position allows you to make contributions to:		
	.01 The hospital	1 2 3 4 5 6 7	
	.02 The profession	1 2 3 4 5 6 7	
	.03 Your own sense of achievement	1 2 3 4 5 6 7	
2.	You receive adequate praise for work well done from:		
	.01 Your peers	1 2 3 4 5 6 7	
	.02 Hospital physicians	1 2 3 4 5 6 7	
	.03 Nursing administration	1 2 3 4 5 6 7	
3.	The work associated with your position provides you with:		
	.01 The opportunity to use a full range of nursing skills	1 2 3 4 5 6 7	
	.02 A variety of clinical challenges	1 2 3 4 5 6 7	
	.03 The opportunity to be of service to others	1 2 3 4 5 6 7	
4.	The nursing practice environment:		
	.01 Allows you to make autonomous nursing care decisions	1 2 3 4 5 6 7	
	.02 Allows you to be fully accountable for those decisions	1 2 3 4 5 6 7	
	.03 Encourages you to make adjustments in your nursing practice to suit patient needs	1 2 3 4 5 6 7	
	.04 Provides a stimulating intellectual environment	1 2 3 4 5 6 7	
	.05 Provides time to engage in research if you want to	1 2 3 4 5 6 7	
	.06 Promotes a high level of clinical competence on your unit	1 2 3 4 5 6 7	
	.07 Allows opportunity to receive adequate respect from nurses on other units	1 2 3 4 5 6 7	
5.	The hospital organizational structure:		
	.01 Allows you to have a voice in policy making for nursing services	1 2 3 4 5 6 7	
	.02 Allows you to have a voice in overall hospital policy making	1 2 3 4 5 6 7	
	.03 Facilitates patient care	1 2 3 4 5 6 7	

6. You receive:

 .01 Enough time to complete patient physical care tasks 1 2 3 4 5 6 7

 .02 Enough time to complete indirect patient care tasks 1 2 3 4 5 6 7

 .03 Support for your work from nurses on other shifts 1 2 3 4 5 6 7

 .04 Support from your peers for your nursing decisions 1 2 3 4 5 6 7

 .05 Support from physicians for your nursing decisions 1 2 3 4 5 6 7

7. Good working relationships exist between you and:

 .01 Your supervisor 1 2 3 4 5 6 7

 .02 Your peers 1 2 3 4 5 6 7

 .03 Physicians 1 2 3 4 5 6 7

8. Nursing service:

 .01 Gives clear direction about advancement 1 2 3 4 5 6 7

 .02 Provides adequate opportunities for advancement 1 2 3 4 5 6 7

 .03 Decides advancements for nurses fairly 1 2 3 4 5 6 7

9. Your job offers:

 .01 Opportunity for professional growth 1 2 3 4 5 6 7

 .02 Satisfactory salary 1 2 3 4 5 6 7

 .03 Adequate funding for healthcare premiums 1 2 3 4 5 6 7

 .04 Adequate additional financial benefits other than salary 1 2 3 4 5 6 7

 .05 A satisfactory work hour pattern (8 hour, 10 hour, and so forth) 1 2 3 4 5 6 7

 .06 Adequate vacation 1 2 3 4 5 6 7

 .07 Adequate sick leave 1 2 3 4 5 6 7

 .08 Adequate in-service opportunities 1 2 3 4 5 6 7

INDEX

Page numbers followed by *t* or *n* indicate tables or notes, respectively.